THE FLOWERING OF A WARATAH

The Australian Association of Neurologists acknowledges that the publication of this book has been made possible by a generous unencumbered Educational Grant from Schering Pty Ltd.

THE FLOWERING OF A WARATAH

A History of Australian Neurology and of the Australian Association of Neurologists

M J Eadie

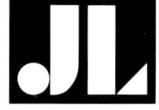

British Library Cataloguing in Publication Data

The flowering of a Waratah: the history of Australian neurology and of the Australian Association of Neurologists

1. Australian Association of Neurologists – History
2. Neurology – Australia – History
I. Eadie, Mervyn J.

616.8'00994

ISBN: 0 86196 606 6

Published by

John Libbey & Company Pty Ltd, Level 10, 15–17 Young Street, Sydney NSW 2000, Australia
Telephone: +61 (2) 9251 4099; Fax: +61 (2) 9251 4428; e-mail: jlsydney@mpx.com.au

John Libbey & Company Ltd, PO Box 276, Eastleigh, SO50 5YS, U.K.
Telephone: +44 (0)23 8065 0208: Fax +44 (0)23 8065 0259

© 2000 John Libbey & Company Pty Ltd. All rights reserved.
Unauthorized duplication contravenes applicable laws.

Printed in Malaysia by Kum-Vivar Printing Sdn Bhd, 48000 Rawang, Selangor Darul Ehsan

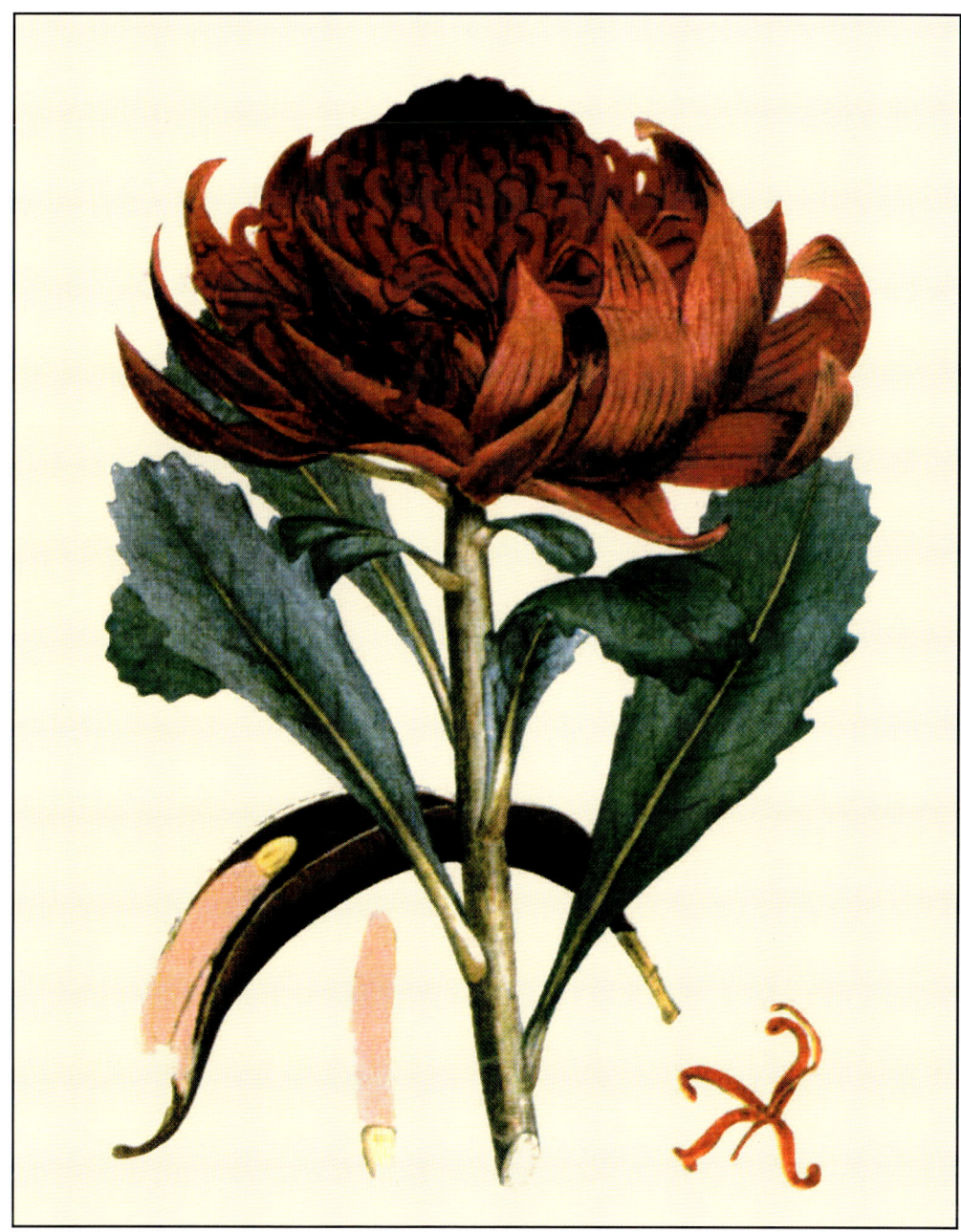

Frontispiece
The insigne of the Australian Association of Neurologists, the Waratah. The original of this illustration was prepared by James Sowerby, and appeared in *A Specimen of the Botany of New Holland*, which was written by James Edward Smith and was published in London in 1793. The illustration was based on coloured drawings and dried specimens sent to London by John White, the first Surgeon-General to the Colony at Sydney Cove.

Contents

	Foreword	ix
	Introduction	xi
Chapter 1:	Australian Neurology in the Pre-neurologist Era	1
Chapter 2:	A W Campbell: Australia's First Neurologist	43
Chapter 3:	The Founding Generation of Australian Neurologists	55
Chapter 4:	The Foundation of the Australian Association of Neurologists	77
Chapter 5:	The Decades of Growth – Australian Neurology	87
Chapter 6:	The Decades of Growth – the Australian Association of Neurologists	131
Chapter 7:	Why and How?	157
	References	161

Appendices:

I	Minutes of the Inaugural Meeting of the Australian Association of Neurologists	181
II	Programmes of the Early Scientific Meetings of the Australian Association of Neurologists	183
III	The Original Constitution of the Australian Association of Neurologists	189
IV	Amendments to the Constitution Made in 1961	197
V	Memberships of the Council of the Australian Association of Neurologists	199

VI	Dates and Venues of the Annual Scientific Meetings of the Australian Association of Neurologists	205
VII	Contents of the Journals published by the Australian Association of Neurologists (1963–1994)	207
VIII	E Graeme Robertson Memorial Lecturers and Lecture Titles	241
	Index	243

List of Illustrations:

Frontispiece The insigne of the Australian Association of Neurologists

Plate 1	G E Rennie	37
Plate 2	A W Campbell	44
Plate 3	L B Cox	58
Plate 4	E Graeme Robertson	61
Plate 5	E L Susman	65
Plate 6	Sir Kenneth Noad	67
Plate 7	G Moss	70
Plate 8	Sir Sydney Sunderland	71
Plate 9	J A Game	74
Plate 10	J Billings	75
Plate 11	Signatures on the original Constitution of the Australian Association of Neurologists	82
Plate 12	G M Selby	126
Plate 13	J W Lance	136
Plate 14	J G McLeod	136
Plate 15	B S Gilligan	136
Plate 16	J King	136
Plate 17	J P Rice	137
Plate 18	J G L Morris	137
Plate 19	R Burns	137
Plate 20	W M Carroll	137
Plate 21	Front cover of Volume 1 of the *Proceedings of the Australian Association of Neurologists*	145

Foreword

The history of a group, an organisation or an association and even a nation confers both a sense of identity and of direction with which to meet and overcome future challenges. In May 1999 at the 90th meeting of the Council of the Australian Association of Neurologists it was determined that an important part of the celebrations to mark the first 50 years of the Association should be a compilation of its history, and that of neurology in Australia. It was also resolved to ask Professor Mervyn Eadie to undertake this task, a request that he accepted with gracious celerity. *The Flowering of a Waratah – A History of Australian Neurology and of the Australian Association of Neurologists* is the agreeable consequence. It comes at an important time in the history of our Association. Not only is original material still accessible, as are most of those members of the Association responsible for its nurture during its first decade and a half and for the seeding of neurologists around Australia, but the practice of neurology is changing fundamentally. Advances in imaging technology and molecular biology are expanding the therapeutic horizons rapidly to levels which would have been almost incomprehensible to the originators of our Association 50 years ago, and yet economic and litigious imperatives and a trend to dependence on so-called evidence-based clinical pathways threaten to constrain the present-day practice of neurology.

The Flowering of a Waratah is as much a testament to the author's own contribution to Australian neurology as it is a history of neurology in Australia. Mervyn Eadie's modest description of his first appointment to the position of 'junior' to John Sutherland, Senior Visiting Neurologist at the Brisbane General Hospital, and his subsequent academic position at the University of Queensland personifies his humble, self-effacing character that has endeared him to so many students and contemporaries. Graduating with honours from the University of Queensland in 1955 he became a member of the Australian Association of Neurologists in 1961 and since then has contributed significantly to Australian neurology at every level he has engaged. Aided by Professor John Morris from Westmead Hospital and Alice Boyce (from the Australian Association of Neurologists' Secretariat), Mervyn Eadie has combined his natural percipience, ironic humour and immense experience gained over 40 years in active practice in neurology and neuropharmacology with his love of history to produce a wonderful account of the development of neurology in Australia. In doing so he has imbued it with that same crisp exciting readability which is born of an intimate and reverent knowledge of the topic and that mirrors the works of historians such as Sir Arthur Bryant.

Commencing with European settlement in Australia and the medical practitioners of that time, *The Flowering of a Waratah* traces the development of our specialty in Australia from its dependence on medical advances in Britain, Europe and North America to the present day where the high standards of clinical neurology and research are acknowledged internationally. The history not only expands on some of the personalities who have contributed to the present high international standing enjoyed by Australian neurology and some of the reasons for this reputation, including the Australian Association of Neurologists itself, but it also contains the records of membership and financial accounts and of papers presented to early scientific meetings of the Association. Important decisions and considerations of Council meetings, among which are the intriguing and recurring proposition of an independent College of Neurologists and the adoption of the Waratah insigne, are laced with personal and communicated insights into the reasoning of a particular decision or course of action.

The Flowering of a Waratah is a superbly detailed account of the history of neurology in Australia which will enrich the professional lives of future generations of Australian neurologists with a sense of 'being', as they and the Australian Association of Neurologists continue to flourish.

W M Carroll
President
Australian Association of Neurologists

December 1999

Introduction

The advent of the year 2000 marks a noteworthy occasion in the course of human history, at least to those with a mathematical cast of mind. The year also happens to coincide with the 50th anniversary of the founding of the Australian Association of Neurologists. To commemorate the latter event, that Association determined to have its own story recorded and set down in relation to the history of the overall development of neurology in Australia.

The Shorter Oxford Dictionary (1973) defined neurology as 'the scientific study or knowledge of the anatomy, function and disease of the nerves and nervous system'. However, the everyday contemporary medical use of the word 'neurology' seems largely to confine it to the scientific study, management and knowledge of *disease* of the central and peripheral nervous systems. In what follows, the word will be taken in this latter more limited sense, though work in the basic neurosciences which has obvious bearings on such clinical neurology will also be touched on.

Systematic European settlement of the Australian continent commenced in 1788. Prior to that, instances of what European medicine would interpret as neurological disease and nervous system injury must have occurred in Australian aboriginal society. However, there is no surviving record that the aboriginal inhabitants of the land engaged in any scientific study or practice, or indeed possessed any scientific knowledge, of what could be regarded as neurology. Over the period of a little more than two centuries during which Europeans have lived in Australia, the available records suggest that the development of neurology in the country can be regarded as having fallen into three overlapping stages.

The first of the three stages spanned a potential maximum of some 150 years, extending almost to the eve of the 1939–1945 World War. During that first stage, with a single most notable exception, what scientific study there was of nervous system disease was carried out by medical practitioners who did not practise exclusively, or often even predominantly, in neurology. Such practitioners became interested in, or found themselves by circumstances involved in, neurological problems, and were able to contribute to knowledge concerning these problems before reverting to their more usual fields of professional endeavour. The solitary exception to this pattern might have been passed over swiftly, almost as an aberration, except for the fact that the man who comprised that exception made a number of significant scientific contributions to neurological knowledge during his long period of clinical neurological practice in Australia. As well, before that time, whilst working overseas, he had established for himself a formidable and enduring international reputation in the neuroscience of his day. Therefore Walter Campbell, coming near the end of the first (i.e. the pre-neurologist) stage of Australian neurology, warrants separate consideration as a phenomenon in his own right.

In the second comparatively short stage of the development of Australian neurology, beginning just before the Second World War, a generation of full-time practising clinical neurologists began to appear. In 1950 they founded a professional association (the Australian Association of Neurologists), and by their endeavours established the specialty of clinical neurology in the country.

The third stage of the development of Australian neurology began about 1960. It saw neurology grow in numerical strength and maturity and achieve academic acceptance in the Australian university system. Over the same period medicine internationally became increasingly aware of the general calibre of Australian neurology, as distinct from the achievements of one or two exceptional talents among its practitioners, which had been the case in the earlier stages.

The founding generation of neurologists constituted the Australian Association of Neurologists in such a way that its members have been involved in various ways in nearly all the events in neurological medicine in the country since the inception of the Association. Thus the history of the Association largely coincides, not only temporally but in substance, with the second and third phases of the evolution of Australian neurology. Nonetheless, the Association has had a significant additional role in its own right. At the same time, since advances in neurological knowledge are not the exclusive prerogative of neurologists, discoveries about nervous system disease have continued to be made in Australia, as in earlier times, by those who were neither by training nor by mode of practice, neurologists.

The account which follows is largely arranged chronologically, in terms of the three phases of development mentioned above, though with further subdivision.

By the time of writing of this book, all but one member of the founding generation of Australian neurologists had died. Some members of the succeeding generation are also dead, or else have come to the end of their days in neurological practice. The professional lives of these men and their achievements can be seen more or less as a whole and appreciated in the context of their times and circumstances, as far as the latter are likely to become known. Admittedly, the passage of additional time before an account of their activities was produced might have allowed more mature and more ultimately valid assessment of their roles in the history of Australian neurology. However, it is when one turns to the lives and activities of those still playing an active part in Australian neurology that it becomes more difficult, and potentially more invidious, to try to form definitive judgements. In

Introduction

some ways it would have been easier not to attempt to deal with them at all, but this would have resulted in substantial gaps in the account of the past three decades. The more recent record would then have been left so unbalanced that the whole account might have been better terminated when the founding generation left the scene. On the whole, it has seemed preferable to try to deal with the achievements of living persons to the time of writing, but to set these achievements only in a contemporary and not in a more definitive perspective, and not to deal with such people from the viewpoint of their personal qualities.

The difficulties referred to immediately above prompt one to mention another limitation of this book – that it is written, as it were, from within the Australian neurological community and by one who has had immediate personal knowledge of some of the events and people described. He has numbered as close and often long-standing friends about some of whom he must write. There is thus danger that objectivity may have unwittingly been sacrificed at times to the influences of sentiment and emotion. However, to attempt to totally ablate the personal element would almost certainly have removed some sense of immediacy from parts of the text, and resulted in the suppression of some details of significance. The reader will no doubt be conscious of such considerations, and recognise that the book has been written very much from the perspective of one who is grateful to have lived out his professional life amid some of the matters recounted, and amongst some of the men involved in them.

The writer is very grateful to the Council of the Australian Association of Neurologists for inviting him to undertake the book, and for making the Association's records available to him. Mrs Alice Boyce, in the Association's office in Sydney, has been unfailingly helpful in finding documents and seeking out information. Her help has been invaluable, and her willingness to provide that help greatly appreciated. Professional colleagues have been generous in answering queries and in offering and giving assistance, and I would like to acknowledge particularly John Morris in this regard, and those who provided him with the photographs of various Australian neurologists included in the book. I am also indebted to Dr Humphrey Cramond, Honorary Curator of the Library of the Queensland Branch of the Australian Medical Association for access to that Library's collection of early Australian medical journals, and to Brenda Heagney, Librarian to the History of Medicine Library of the Royal Australasian College of Physicians in Sydney for the supply of information and photographs. For the errors in the book, and for its infelicities, I must accept blame. In compensation for exposing myself to the odium of being responsible for such shortcomings, I have had the pleasure of an awareness of finding within myself a growing empathy with the past events and life of Australian neurology.

MJ Eadie
Brisbane

December 1999

Chapter 1

Australian Neurology in the Pre-neurologist Era

If the first phase of the development of Australian neurology is taken to have terminated with the advent of the founding generation of Australian professional clinical neurologists in the 1930s and 1940s, the question arises as to when the first phase began?

Prior to the time of the first European settlement in 1788, the pattern of Australian aboriginal society was far from uniform throughout the extent of the continent. The aboriginals comprised nomadic tribal hunting peoples who lacked knowledge of agriculture and who had been isolated from the influence of the remainder of the world's population over the course of many centuries. They had no single language in common. Apart from drawings, they kept no lasting records since they lacked knowledge of writing (Abbie, 1969), and history transmitted by word of mouth is vulnerable both to loss and to inaccuracy. The aboriginal understanding of medicine, such as it was, differed considerably from the European one by the time aboriginal society came into contact with European civilisation. Basically, the aboriginals interpreted disease and death in terms of witchcraft (Abbie, 1969), a stage in the development of human culture that belonged to the past in more advanced societies elsewhere. Therefore it is hardly surprising that there remains little record of what would now be considered as neurological illness in aboriginal society, though Hogg (1902) in writing of the Tasmanian aboriginals, who had become extinct by 1876, remarked that:

> 'madness and convulsions were known by the aboriginals, and were believed by them to be due to an evil spirit.'

Abbie (1969) considered that, apart from infectious diseases, Australian aboriginals suffered from the same patterns of illness that afflicted the remainder of mankind, though the shorter life-span of the aboriginals gave the impression that degenerative disease was less common among them. As an example of persisting aboriginal medial concepts after more than a century of potential exposure to European culture, Elkin (1935) mentioned that in Australia it was quite common to see a native with a string bound tightly round his head for the purpose of relieving headaches.

As a result of the lack of surviving aboriginal records prior to 1788, knowledge of what is now regarded as neurology can be taken as not having begun on Australian soil earlier than the advent of European settlement. Sydney was the site of that original settlement, and Gandevia and Cobley (1974) described occurring there a probable neurological death in 1791, three years after the founding of the colony.

> '*Case 5*. Probably either Robert Hogg or Peter Hubbert, a convict attending on Mr White [the Principal Surgeon], in passing from his house to the kitchen, without any covering upon his head, received a stroke from a ray of the sun, which at the time deprived him of speech and motion, and in less than twenty-and-four hours, of his life. The thermometer on that day [4 November 1791] stood at twelve o'clock at $94^{3}/_{4}$ ...'

Neither the ambient temperature, nor the duration of exposure to the sun, appears sufficient for the role attributed to it. The account of the event seems more suggestive of a cerebral haemorrhage or, possibly, a massive cerebral infarction.

Epilepsy, lues and 'locked jaw' were neurological illnesses also mentioned in at least one return of the assigned causes of death in Sydney prior to 1800 (Watson, 1911). In the more northern convict settlement of Brisbane (founded in 1823), the Brisbane Hospital records indicated that there were two admissions for paralysis in 1828, and one instance of paralysis and one of hemiplegia in 1831 (Jackson, 1924), whilst there were five cases of epilepsy amongst a total of 170 admissions for the two-year period 1840–1842 (Tyrer, 1993).

Of course, the presence of instances of disease which would now be classed as neurological does not itself constitute evidence either for the existence of the discipline of neurology or for its practice on Australian soil, in that there is nothing to indicate that such cases were the subject of any particular scientific management, study or knowledge. In fact, they had occurred before the notion of 'neurology' as a medical discipline had itself taken shape elsewhere in the world. It was also at a time when the spectrum of diseases of the nervous system, i.e. what was to become the content of neurology, was substantially different from what it has now become, and was also rather more extensive than at present.

In 1778, the first edition of Samuel-Auguste Tissot's classic *Traite des nerves et de leurs maladies* appeared. His account was based on a mixed classificational basis involving both anatomy and concepts of pathogenesis. The book included, as well as chapters on epilepsy and migraine, a consideration of various disorders of 'moral' causation, which today would be considered as the territory of psychiatry. In 1789, one year after the first European settlement of Australia, Cullen brought out his *First Lines of the Practice of Physick* which was to play a major part in the education of several future generations of English-speaking medical students. Cullen's classification of nervous system diseases, for which he coined the collective term 'neuroses', was based on clinical phenomenology rather than on pathology or aetiology. Within his rubric of neuroses were included entities such as palpitations, dyspnoea, asthma, whooping cough, pyrosis, colic, diarrhoea, diabetes, mania, melancholia and other insanities, as well as disorders which would now be taken as neurological. It was almost as if nervous system disease to Cullen comprised the whole range of convulsive disorders discussed by Thomas Willis in his *Pathology of the Brain and Nervous Stock*, dating from 1684, though considerably extended to take in almost every conceivable disorder in which visceral motor overactivity occurred in the absence of macroscopic pathology; added to this in Cullen's text were many of the neurological disorders considered in Willis' *De Anima Brutorum* (1683), and as well much of the content of present-day psychiatry. To today's thinking, someone whose practice or interests embraced all of Cullen's neuroses would almost certainly be considered a general practitioner or perhaps a general physician, but certainly not a neurologist.

What is generally considered the first neurology textbook of modern times, Romberg's *Manual of the Nervous Diseases of Man* (1853), used a similar symptomatic approach to classification to that employed by Cullen, and considered a similar array of what would now be regarded a non-neurological disorders. This was so even though Abercrombie (1828) had earlier provided a reasonable and logically satisfactory account of many neurological disorders classified on a basis of pathology. In contrast to Romberg's text, by 1871 Hammond in his monograph employed a classification schema largely based on pathology to discuss nervous system disease, and it is comparatively easy to relate his categories to the content of present-day neurology. Similarly, Gowers in his great two-volume *Manual of Diseases of the Nervous System* (1886 and 1888) used a classificational approach similar to that in use today, based mainly on a mixture of aetiology and pathology. The disorders discussed in Gowers' text are reasonably similar to those to be found in a modern day textbook of neurology. The psychiatry, and the visceral functional disorders included by the earlier authors, were no longer present. Somewhere between 1850 and 1870 the issue of what disorders were to be regarded as neurological and what were not, seems to have been settled, probably largely by informal agreement. Thus the canon of neurology became determined for future generations, about the time when the present-day specialty of neurology emerged.

In Britain and in Europe it was over the years around 1860 that neurology as a recognisable medical specialty first began to appear. The National Hospital for Nervous Diseases in Queen Square, London, was founded in 1860 (Holmes, 1954; Anonymous, 1960). J-M Charcot was appointed to the world's first Chair in Neurology in Paris in 1882, at the Salpêtrière, where he had commenced the teaching of neurology in 1862 (Guillain, 1959). It was to be another six or seven decades before clinical neurology came to be generally recognised as a medical discipline in Australia. Nonetheless, in the interval contributions to neurological knowledge had been made on Australian soil, but they were made by those who were not acknowledged neurologists, and who indeed usually practised mainly in other areas of medicine. Many of these contributions were essentially opportunistic in nature, and arose when neurological illness manifested itself in ways which were peculiar to Australian conditions. However, a few contributions were deliberate attempts to grapple with neurological problems which were global in their impact. Relative to the situation in the Northern hemisphere, the delay in the emergence of neurology in Australia was probably largely a consequence of the comparatively short existence of European culture in the country, and of geographical and the resulting economic factors. At a time when communications were relatively slow and difficult, Australia was a long distance from the large European centres where neurology had first gained its status. More importantly, distances within Australia were such that the wide scatter of a relatively small number of inhabitants meant that a considerable time had to pass for sufficient population growth to allow the critical mass of patients capable of supporting the activities of even one neurologist to accumulate in any given locality.

The present chapter attempts to deal with the neurological work that went on, and the neurological discoveries of some significance which were made by non-neurologists from 1880 onwards, up to the eve of the Second World War. It also touches on the few men in the Australia of those times who, at least for a period in their professional lives, had a major interest in neurological disease.

During the years prior to World War II, communication between Australia and Europe or North America was relatively protracted and sometimes rather uncertain. Although Australian medicine in those times clearly kept aware of overseas knowledge and trends, its own research tended to be published in its own local medical journals. This was probably partly because of publication delays if papers were submitted to overseas journals and because of the potential uncertainties of maintaining communication with journal editors. The pre-war *Medical Journal of Australia*, which first appeared in 1914, and its predecessors, the Melbourne-based *Australian Medical Journal*, which appeared between 1856 and 1895, and reappeared between 1910 and 1914, seemingly being replaced in the interval by the *Intercolonial Quarterly Journal of Medicine and Surgery* (1894–1896) and the *Intercolonial Medical Journal of Australasia* (1896–1909), and the Sydney-based *Australasian Medical Gazette* (1881–1914), appear to have served a greater educational and local professional news dissemination role than later became the case for Australian medical publications. Perusal of the contents of the old journals gives something of the flavour of the medicine of the time, with its heavy dependence on British, and to a lesser extent Western European and American medicine. A very significant portion of the papers published on neurological topics were thorough and contemporaneous reviews of matters which should have been of considerable educational value to the Australian medical community, but which did not claim to break new ground based on original Australian achievements. Such reviews sometimes did happen to contain, almost incidentally, details of their authors' personal experiences, or of small clinical experimental studies they had carried out, or of original ideas they had developed about the topics they were considering.

Chapter 1 Australian Neurology in the Pre-neurologist Era

The latter type of review thus included the sort of material that modern-day writers would have made into the main themes of research-type papers, and in which the educational matter relating to the topic would have provided the background to the new information instead of being the dominant feature of the publication. Thus there sometimes is Australian neurological research to be found in the old writings, which seemingly were intended mainly for educational purposes. It must be acknowledged that after reading enough of the material published, at least in the inter-war period, one gains the impression that younger specialists, probably in the process of building up their practices after returning from overseas training, would attempt to enhance their reputations locally by publishing ostensibly educational material which as a side issue tended to testify to the author's clinical expertise in the area. The old literature sometimes also contained observational type research on what was perceived as new or unusual disease patterns, which were at least sometimes the outcomes of peculiar local circumstances. There were virtually no deliberate experimental studies reported until Royle and Hunter's investigations in the 1920s which will be considered in some detail later in this chapter. The old journals also included numerous case reports which fell into two classes. Firstly, there were formal accounts of individual unusual cases or of small collections of cases. These accounts sometimes also involved some discussion of the topic. However, they often merely reported the case details only and read as though they had been presented to local medical meetings and had simply been submitted simultaneously to the journal for publication. Secondly, there were also numerous brief reports of local medical meetings at which interesting cases had been described. These reports provided a précis of the case description and sometimes of the related discussion. This affords the present-day reader some idea of the level of local medical knowledge, even though no formally developed consideration of the topics was published. Such material, though interesting to read, breaks no new research ground. However, it gives some indication of the pattern of disease which was occurring locally at various times, and what the presenters judged would interest their colleagues.

On the basis of such material, one can build a picture of Australian neurological knowledge, thought and discovery in the period before neurologists appeared in clinical practice in the country.

Australian neurological knowledge and practice

In the years prior to, and soon after World War I, the authors of neurological articles and reports in the pages of the *Medical Journal of Australia* and its immediate predecessors usually did not quote references at all extensively, and if they quoted them did not set them down in much detail. It was not unusual for a substantial paper to contain no, or almost no, references. When reference to authoritative sources was considered necessary, the works most frequently cited were the contemporary editions of Osler's textbook, or Gowers' *Manual of Diseases of the Nervous System* (the first volume of which had first appeared in 1886, and the second two years later). When any original publications from the literature were cited, they were usually of British or German origin, at least until after World War I. Later, works such as Kinnier Wilson's *Modern Problems in Neurology* (1928) seem to have become influential, and in the references cited there was clear evidence of considerable familiarity with the international literature.

The range of neurological conditions discussed in the Australian journals in the latter part of the 19th century and in the earlier part of the 20th century differed from that which would be expected in today's journals, mainly in that infectious diseases of the nervous system received distinctly more emphasis, and cerebral vascular disease, notably stroke, was almost totally ignored. In the inter-war period, the types of neurological disorder reported increasingly took on a pattern similar to that of recent years, with the exception of HIV-related syndromes. The enormous therapeutic progress after World War II resulted in the virtual elimination of neurosyphilis and poliomyelitis, and a great reduction in the menace of bacterial meningitis and intracranial suppuration, all of which had received frequent mention in earlier years.

Over the 60 years prior to World War II, as judged from the contents of the local medical publications, one can trace trends in what the Australian medical community considered was of interest and importance to it.

Headache

In the Australian journals, there was very little discussion of the general topic of headache, now the bread and butter of neurological practice, until after World War I. The systematic account of headache given by McWhae in 1924 did not involve nearly as much emphasis on migraine as might have been expected, tension headache as such was not mentioned, nor was cluster headache under any of its acknowledged synonyms, and there was more attention given to ocular and nasal sinus headache than would be the case today. In 1934 an Adelaide ophthalmic surgeon, Barham Black, gave a thoroughly competent account of migraine and discussed the various contemporary theories of its pathogenesis and treatment. The account would not have seemed particularly out of date two decades later. There was also some observational research on migraine mechanisms which will be discussed later. Ergotamine was recommended, sometimes in a rather distant manner, for the treatment of attacks of the disorder, but there seemed little awareness of the possibility of migraine prophylaxis by pharmacological agents.

Trigeminal neuralgia was well recognised before the turn of the century, though at least one published description of it reads more like cluster headache (Hawkes, 1903). By 1910, Campbell was treating trigeminal neuralgia by the injection of alcohol into the main trigeminal nerve or one of its branches. Later, Clark (1937) recommended a course of action for its management which comprised the exclusion of any local source of sepsis, the use of simple analgesics in milder cases, then butylchloral hydrate with gelsemium, with the inhalation of trichlorethylene for severe paroxysms, and ultimately injection of the Gasserian ganglion. In his view, injection of the trigeminal nerve or of its peripheral branches was to be eschewed. As early as 1893, O'Hara had reported surgical curettage of the Gasserian ganglion to relieve the condition.

Epilepsy

The Australian writings on epilepsy from quite early times showed awareness of the entity of Jacksonian motor seizures. However, until much later there seemed on the whole to be little appreciation of the consequences of Hughlings Jackson's (1870) insights into the nature of epilepsy, and into the implications that Jackson's concept of localisation of function in the cerebral cortex held for the understanding of epilepsy. Springthorpe, of Melbourne, was one exception to this generalisation. In 1886 he plainly indicated his acceptance of Jackson's interpretation of epileptogenesis. In the following year he (Springthorpe, 1887) put the matter in slightly more forcible terms than Jackson probably would have chosen – the main pathological state in epilepsy was:

> '... An over-explosability of the cells in the cortical layers of the brain.'

Springthorpe seemed to take a particular interest in epilepsy, and in 1888 referred to his collection of 50 cases of the disorder.

There seemed perhaps less emphasis on the idea that epilepsy was idiopathic, or a disease in its own right, than was the case in contemporary Britain, and more ready acceptance that convulsions were an epileptic phenomenon. Angel Money (1896), in Sydney, argued that all distinctions between epilepsy, convulsions, eclampsia, epileptiform and epileptoid seizures should be subsumed into the general term 'cerebral paroxysms'. In his account of epilepsy, Youngman (1942) quite obviously accepted the local origin of epileptic seizures in the brain, but did not seem to think through the further implications of this. He was aware of the electroencephalographic changes reported to be present in different types of epileptic seizure. Later this same author (Youngman, 1945) seemed to take the position that in those with epilepsy there was an intrinsic underlying tendency to seizures which was developed to different degrees in different sufferers, and that there existed a great variety of potential seizure-provoking factors. As a result, epilepsy could appear to be a symptom with a number of possible causes, but there was always an underlying intrinsic tendency to it in those who suffered from it. Such an interpretation seems to have been the result of deduction or intuition rather than actual analysis of data.

From at least several years prior to 1873 (Smith, 1873), bromide had been the mainstay of antiepileptic therapy, particularly for major as compared with minor epilepsy (Hawkes, 1905), though the use of chloretone (chlorobutanol) was advocated by Bentley (1911, 1912). Borax had proved successful in a case where bromide therapy had failed (McAdam, 1895), but the agent did not become popular. Bentley

(1911) summarised the then contemporary situation regarding the treatment of epilepsy thus:

> 'The greatest optimist must admit that the treatment of epilepsy is in a thoroughly unsatisfactory condition.'

However, to some extent, this situation improved with time. 'Luminal' (phenobarbitone) came into use a little afterwards, and seems to have been regarded as superior to the bromides in efficacy. By 1942, Youngman was clearly familiar with the use of phenytoin ('Dilantin'), which had become available overseas only two or three years previously. By 1947 troxidone ('Tridione') was in use for the treatment of *petit mal*.

Trepanning of the skull was carried out in quite early times (Maund, 1856; Whitcomb, 1862), in the latter case successfully, at least in the short term, for epilepsy associated with depressed fractures of the skull.

Cerebral vascular disease

Stroke and other cerebral vascular disorders appeared a relatively neglected topic until after World War I, probably not because medical men were ignorant of them, but because they were already well enough recognised and there had been no diagnostic or therapeutic advances in relation to them over many years. Reeves (1861) had written on his 14 cases of corpus striatum softening encountered amongst 113 instances of brain softening, but held the view that such softening did not always have an ischaemic basis. Robertson (1881) described two instances of stroke, simply from the point of view of their phenomenology. Interestingly, as early as 1906 McDonald had adduced physiologically-based arguments against attempting to reduce the blood pressure after cerebral haemorrhage. Dawson's (1937) discussion of cerebral arteriosclerosis tended to be orientated towards its role in producing higher level cerebral disorder. By 1938, De Crespigny's account of cerebral vascular disease read much as a present-day version might, except that today syphilitic vascular disease would scarcely merit mention, there would be more emphasis on disease of the posterior circulation, and there would not be such paucity of therapeutic options.

Cerebral aneurysm and subarachnoid haemorrhage received little attention until the inter-war years, though Williams (1881) briefly described the autopsy features of a ruptured posterior inferior cerebellar artery aneurysm. Prior to the introduction of lumbar puncture, it was difficult to recognise the presence of subarachnoid blood during life, and diagnosis of cerebral aneurysm in the living had to await the advent of angiography shortly before World War II. Graeme Robertson (1936) described a case series of intracranial aneurysms, stating that no diagnosis of cerebral aneurysm had been made at the Melbourne Hospital prior to 1929, though he knew of 31 instances of ruptured cerebral aneurysms at the hospital between 1929 and his time of writing. Cleland a year later (1937) reported 19 instances of small aneurysms on the circle of Willis or its branches in 3670 autopsies in Adelaide. Only two of these aneurysms had not ruptured and caused subarachnoid haemorrhage.

Infections

Syphilis

From quite early times a good deal was written concerning syphilis of the nervous system (e.g. Jamieson, 1895–6; Morgan, 1920; Minogue, 1926), particularly general paresis of the insane, and tabes dorsalis. Stoller and Emmerson (1969) published a description of the history of general paresis of the insane in Victoria, based on their survey of mental hospital records. The first possible instance they traced dated back to 1859, more than a decade before the designation 'general paresis' came into use. They noted that this particular diagnosis had first been recorded in 1867, and was made frequently after 1872.

There was a good deal of interest in the malarial treatment of general paresis in the 1920s and 1930s (Ellery, 1926; Dawson, 1928) and a little later in its treatment by electrically-induced fever (Prior, 1937). When Cox (1949a) reviewed the treatment of neurosyphilis he indicated that penicillin was beginning to supplant the older agents (mercury, arsenic, bismuth and potassium iodide). In that same year, Susman (1949) vigorously extolled the virtues of penicillin in neurosyphilis, and stated that arsenic and bismuth had become obsolescent.

Meningitis

Bacterial, mainly meningococcal, meningitis (often called 'cerebro-spinal fever') occurred sporadically (Hood, 1902), and in epidemics in Australia (Fairley and Guest, 1915; Cleland, 1916; Calov, 1940), and tuberculous meningitis was reported at times. In the period 1938–1940 there was a small flurry of publications attesting to the efficacy of the newly available sulphonamides in treating various forms of bacterial meningitis (Anderson and English, 1938; Robinson, 1939; Hamilton, 1940a; Lowe, 1940). Soon after, Milroy and Hughes (1945) reported on the cure of pneumococcal meningitis by injected penicillin, and in the next year Turner (1946) described its effectiveness in childhood purulent meningitis.

Sawers and Thomson (1935) reviewed four previous Australian reports of torula (cryptococcal) meningitis, the first dating back to Swift and Bull (1917), when they added a fifth instance of the disorder. Soon after, De Crespigny (1944) devoted a Rennie Memorial Lecture to the topic of torula meningitis and a little afterwards Cox and Tolhurst (1946) published a monograph on the subject.

Encephalitis and myelitis

There were also outbreaks of viral encephalitis at times in Australia, but these will be discussed separately later, because of their particular interest. Aseptic meningitis did not seem to be diagnosed as such during the times under consideration, possibly because instances were categorised as non-paralytic poliomyelitis.

Poliomyelitis occurred in epidemic form in some of the years under consideration, and will be discussed below.

Rabies

Rabies has never been an appreciable problem in Australia, because of the effective quarantine practices that have been in operation. However, Crowther (1946) described a set of events which occurred in Hobart long before his time, and which raised the spectre of the dreaded disorder. Crowther's account, based on reports in the local newspapers, deserves to be read in its entirety, partly for its discursive charm. In January 1867 a boy in Hobart was bitten on the lip by a half-bred spaniel. One month later, the boy became ill with symptoms suggestive of rabies, and died within a few days. The dog, which also died soon afterwards following further wayward behaviour, had in the interval bitten two other citizens. There was consternation, and an anxious wait for the whole community, to say nothing of those bitten, until it became apparent that neither of these persons had become ill. In retrospect, Crowther thought the boy had died of tetanus, but the majority of the local medical profession at the time was convinced that he had suffered from rabies.

Tumours

Cerebral tumour was not a prominent topic in the old Australian medical literature, though there were isolated reports of interesting cases, suggesting that the condition did not go unrecognised, e.g. Robertson (1860). From quite soon after the time of the initial overseas reports of the successful surgery of cerebral tumour, beginning with Macewen in 1879, there had been reports of isolated craniotomies for tumour carried out in various parts of Australia, sometimes in rural areas. For instance, in 1892 Parry, in rural New South Wales, had operated unsuccessfully on a cerebral hydatid cyst in a nine-year-old boy. Rudall (1859) had earlier demonstrated a cerebral hydatid cyst at autopsy. Syme (1895), in Melbourne, reported the successful removal of what almost certainly was a meningioma. Harold Dew, later to be Professor of Surgery in the University of Sydney, reported an operative series of 85 cerebral tumour cases, 55 per cent of them gliomas, in 1922. In the 1930s, there was a considerable increase in the amount written about cerebral tumour in Australia, much of it from the pen of Leonard Cox (see later) and the initial generation of Australian neurosurgeons, e.g. Gilbert Phillips, Rex Money and Douglas Miller, whilst Dew (1936) returned to the topic and reviewed the biology of the meningiomas in a Bancroft Oration.

Involuntary movement disorders

Parkinsonism

Curiously little was written of Parkinson's disease during the earlier part of the period under discussion, though the disorder was recognised (Huxtable, 1892a).

Parkinsonism followed in the wake of the Australian epidemic of encephalitis lethargica (see later), but attracted no especial local interest. The treatment of Parkinson's disease comprised various agents with anticholinergic properties (Hughes, 1940). Interestingly, in 1948 the Sydney neurosurgeon W Lister Reid reported favourable results in 15 patients from an experimental procedure, the surgical excision of Brodman's cerebral cortical area 6.

Chorea

When Stawell (1915) at a medical meeting in Melbourne expressed the belief that he had provided the first description of Huntington's disease in a patient in Victoria, psychiatrists in his audience promptly announced that there were other cases to be found in Victorian mental institutions. Jones (1917) described a Tasmanian family affected with the disorder. Brothers (1964) traced the history of the disease in Tasmania and Victoria to a family of Huguenot origin which had emigrated to Tasmania from Somerset in the west country of England in 1842 (Brothers gave the date as 1848, but it was subsequently corrected by Pridmore in 1990). Brothers did not make it clear whether this was the same Tasmanian family reported earlier by Jones (1917). The first instance of the disease in the family had been recognised in 1878. It is perhaps of some interest that there was no record of Huntington's disease in the convicts shipped to Australia in earlier times.

Sydenham's chorea was known in Australia in the latter half of the 19th century (Jamieson, 1873). Its relationship to rheumatic fever was recognised (Williams, 1937). Fulton (1879) had used injections of curare in an attempt to relieve choreic movements.

Wilson's disease

There were a few reports of clinically recognised progressive lenticular degeneration (Swift, 1917; Macdonald, 1927; Minogue, 1927). Most of them lacked any indication of the presence of a similar disorder in the affected person's family. Often the clinical details appeared insufficient to sustain the diagnosis that had been made.

Demyelinating disease

Frith (1988) published a careful account of the history of multiple sclerosis in Australia. Newman had discussed the disorder of multiple sclerosis in the pages of the *Australian Medical Journal* under the old designation of insular sclerosis in 1875, but described no Australian case. The clinical diagnosis in the earlier reported Australian instances of what was then termed insular or disseminated sclerosis often appears quite uncertain from the details provided (e.g. Huxtable, 1892b; Officer, 1903), but a pathologically-confirmed instance of the disorder was described by Flashman and Latham in 1915. As early as 1886 James Jamieson, of Melbourne, had reported two instances of unusual peripheral neuritis, in the second of which he had at first thought the diagnosis was that of disseminated sclerosis. Frith with some justification pointed out that his initial diagnosis appeared a great deal more probable than the one under which the case was published. Until the mid-1920s reports such as those of Griffiths (1922) and Maudsley (1925) seemed not to reveal any appreciation that the essentials of the clinical diagnosis of the common relapsing-remitting form of the disorder depended on there being evidence of the presence of disease which had affected multiple areas of the central nervous system at different times in the sufferer's life. By 1926, matters appeared to change so that clinically probable instances came to be described (Hurley, 1926; Maudsley, 1927; Sewell, 1926; Johnston, 1927). However, the formal clinical diagnostic essentials were not acknowledged as such.

Cox et al. (1949) carried out a therapeutic trial of anticoagulation in an attempt to prevent worsening of disability in multiple sclerosis. The rationale for the treatment lay in the idea that intracranial venous thrombosis was causally related to the demyelination of the disorder. The investigators concluded that the treatment was ineffective, though by present-day standards their trial design was deficient and there was no proper statistical analysis of the results.

Pathologically proven diffuse sclerosis was reported in Australia by De Crespigny and Woollard (1929) and by Holmes à Court and Latham (1935), with a clinically diagnosed instance by Flynn and Greenaway (1935). Just prior to, and during World War II, E Weston Hurst, in Adelaide, with various co-workers, reported instances of various types of demyelinating disease, whilst Hurst himself described the new entity of acute haemorrhagic leucoencephalitis (Hurst, 1941a,b). Hurst's experimental work is discussed later in this chapter.

Tropical neurological disorders

There were Australian reports of uncommon neurological disorders not often encountered in more temperate climates, e.g. tick-bite paralysis (Cleland, 1912; Eaton, 1913), to be discussed further a little later in this book. In the earlier part of the period under consideration certain common tropical diseases tended to go unrecognised in Australia. Those at that time practising medicine in the country had often been trained in Europe or in Britain, or later in Melbourne (which produced the first Australian medical graduates). In these places tropical diseases were not likely to be seen by students. Therefore when graduates from these institutions began to practise in Australia and first came across instances of certain tropical diseases, they were not familiar with the disorders and failed to make their diagnosis. This was, in particular, the case for leprosy.

Leprosy

In Australia, leprosy appears to have first been encountered in Chinese seamen in the country's sea-ports, and in Chinese and Polynesian immigrants, but after a time it was also recognised among the aboriginals in northern Australia. Thompson (1898), in his review of the history of the disorder in Australia, stated that it had not occurred in Australian aboriginals until 1892, when an instance was noted at

Chapter 1 Australian Neurology in the Pre-neurologist Era

Maryborough, in Queensland. Possibly leprosy-affected persons from tropical countries to the north of Australia had made their way into the country other than through the ports, and in so doing had come in contact with the local aboriginals and infected some of them. Creed (1889) stated that there were no known lepers in Australia in 1856, with the exception of 13 in Victoria. By his time of writing there were still five in that State, and 10 in New South Wales, but none in South Australia or Tasmania. He could not obtain figures for Queensland. Creed also stated that only one European was to be numbered amongst the leprosy sufferers, in conformity with the statement of Shields (1889):

> 'In reference to the prevalence of leprosy in Australia, the disease is, with few exceptions, confined to the Chinese. It is known in one case only, and that in New South Wales, to infect a European. In Victoria there are five lepers (all Chinese) in the leper camp at Point Nepean.'

However, Joseph Bancroft, of fame for his discoveries in relation to filariasis, wrote in 1892 of how, when he had first taken up duty in the old Brisbane Hospital in 1868, he had failed to recognise leprosy in a patient of German origin. From his reading of the earlier Brisbane Hospital records, Bancroft mentioned that he considered that there had been an even earlier unrecognised instance of the disease in a patient of Chinese origin admitted to the Hospital as early as 1855. In contrast to these figures concerning the rarity of leprosy in persons of European origin, according to an Editorial in the *Australasian Medical Gazette* in 1892, there were eight affected white persons in New South Wales, all of whom were detained in lazarets. In earlier years, it had been widely and reassuringly accepted that leprosy in Australia was to be found only in Asian immigrants and in persons from the South Sea islands. There was consequently some consternation when the first instance of the disorder occurred in an Australian-born citizen of European descent. By 1926 there were 16 persons in the lazaret of the Coast Hospital in Sydney, and a total of 13 white lepers in New South Wales, 51 in Queensland, two in West Australia and none in the remaining three States (Molesworth, 1926). Sufferers from leprosy had to be quarantined in lazarets situated well away from the remainder of the community and kept there for the remainder of their lives unless, as occasionally appeared to happen, they apparently became cured. This situation continued until the advent of sulphone therapy after the end of World War II.

Beri beri

Instances of beri beri neuritis were also reported in Asian seamen, and in Chinese immigrants in Melbourne in 1888 and in Sydney from 1890 on (Graham, 1893; Paton, 1894). As was the case for leprosy, the cause of the polyneuritic disorder was not recognised for a time.

Miscellaneous neurological disorders

In the latter part of the 19th century and the early decades of the 20th century the case reports which appeared in the pages of the *Medical Journal of Australia* and its precursors the *Australian Medical Journal*, the *Australasian Medical Gazette* and the *Intercolonial Medical Journal* included instances of many neurological conditions which would even today be regarded as uncommon and of interest to the general medical community. Further, the clinical details of the descriptions as published suggest that the diagnoses made usually would withstand the scrutiny of modern knowledge. There were, for instance, reports of myasthenia gravis (Hogg, 1906), polyneuritis, which often probably was due to the Guillain-Barré syndrome, which was not well recognised until after the end of World War I (Crago, 1890; Thomson, 1898; Mills, 1919), Duchenne muscular dystrophy (Smith, 1871; Jamieson, 1894), myotonia congenita (Fleetwood, 1889; Campbell, 1919), epiloia (Lind, 1924), paramyoclonus multiplex (possibly simply a severe Janz syndrome – Verco, 1912), Leber's optic atrophy (Pockley, 1915; Hogg, 1915, 1928; Morlet, 1921), carotido-cavernous fistula (Gibson, 1896, 1905), Friedreich's ataxia (Stawell, 1895; Spark, 1897; Litchfield *et al.*, 1917), Marie's cerebellar ataxia (largely equivalent to what was later called olivo-ponto-cerebellar atrophy – Morris, 1908), amyotrophic lateral sclerosis (Howson, 1918; Murphy, 1924), geniculate zoster (Findlay, 1933), post-herpetic neuralgia (Marten, 1897), subacute combined degeneration (Evans, 1925), diabetic pseudo-tabes (Bostock, 1926), diptheritic paralysis (Jamieson, 1883), arsenical neuritis (Hughes, 1927), meralgia paraesthetica (Rennie, 1902) and congenital word blindness (MacLeod, 1920).

There was no record of botulism in the country until 1942, when two outbreaks occurred, both associated with the eating of canned beetroot (Gray, 1948).

As well as the reports of unusual and interesting disorders, new treatments of real value came into use at times. Thus in, 1938, Leonard Cox (1938b) was in a position to report on the effectiveness of injected neostigmine in relieving the manifestations of myasthenia gravis. At an earlier stage, ephedrine and potassium chloride had been used for the disorder. At much the same time, neostigmine was also tried, and allegedly provided benefit, in certain forms of myopathy (Taylor, 1938).

Neurological investigations

Over the period under consideration, various ancillary investigations became available to assist in the diagnosis of neurological disorders, and the recognition of certain conditions during life became possible by virtue of these investigations.

Radiology was available in Australia from quite early times. Within a few months of the announcement of Rontgen's discovery in 1895, Balls-Headley (1896) in Melbourne described the use of X-rays to demonstrate a needle buried in a girl's foot and Clendinnen (1897) reported the use of the method to display the cranial blood vessels post mortem. In the following year Hopkins (1898) gave an account of Clendinnen's use of the technique to locate a bullet within a living patient's brain.

Whilst it was not necessarily for the first time in Australia, a lumbar puncture for cerebro-spinal fluid examination was recorded as having been carried out in Victoria in 1907 (Stoller and Emmerson, 1969), more than a decade after the procedure was first described by Quinke (in 1891). Later, there was interest in the chemical composition of the cerebro-spinal fluid, notably in its protein content (Phillips, 1937) and in its Lange colloidal gold reaction (Buchanan, 1937), which was then important in the diagnosis of neurosyphilis. John Fullarton Mackeddie (1868–1944), Physician to In-Patients at the Alfred Hospital in Melbourne, who played a very influential part in the foundation of the Baker Institute (Kennedy, 1944), wrote of the technique of cisternal puncture in 1926, and of myelography (using 'lipiodol') by the cisternal and the lumbar routes in 1927, 1929 and 1931. Edye (1926) of Sydney, independently described the technique of cisternal puncture. Ventriculography, described by Dandy in 1918, was the subject of reports by Noble and by Monson, both of whom described the same patient from Sydney, in 1926. Pneumoencephalography was described by Buchanan, of Sydney, in 1929, though there are intimations that Leonard Cox, in Melbourne, had used the technique earlier. The Adelaide neurosurgeon, Leonard Lindon, in 1936 published an account of cerebral arteriography using 'Thorotrast' as contrast medium, some six years after Moniz had first described his work with the technique.

In 1939, almost a decade after Berger had described the possibility of recording the electrical activity of the human brain, the neurosurgeon Gilbert Phillips wrote of the appearance of the electroencephalogram in epileptic seizures, as did the psychiatrist N V Youngman soon afterwards (1942). However, from these two accounts it is difficult to know whether the authors were already using the technique in Australia when their papers appeared. Geoffrey Trahair (1910–1950) a psychiatrist who died young and who was the first acknowledged electroencephalographer in Australia (Phillips, 1951) made it clear that the electroencephalograph had been in use in Sydney in the hands of Phillips and A K McIntyre (Trahair, 1950), though not elsewhere in Australia, as early as 1941 or 1942 (Trahair and Garvan, 1948).

In general, there appears to have been a lag of some five to 10 years between the time when a new neurological investigational technique was reported overseas, and when the first accounts of its use in Australia appeared, though of course the method may have been employed previously in the country but its use was not recorded in an accessible source.

Investigations into topics of global relevance

Spasticity and its attempted surgical relief

The first deliberate and sustained effort in Australia to investigate a neuroscience question of international significance, and at the same time provide a therapeutic benefit for patients, was made in the Department of Anatomy of the University of Sydney in the third decade of the 20th century. The attempt derived from a finding in a serpent and, like a much earlier event which was instigated by a serpent, produced enticing prospects which culminated in disaster. The story can be pieced together from a series of papers which began to appear in the *Medical Journal of*

Australia in 1924 and 1925, and later in two obituaries published in the same journal.

In 1879 Tchiriew had discovered two types of nerve ending in snake muscle, the familiar motor end plates in which myelinated fibres from anterior horn cells terminated, and in addition a new type of ending, *terminations en grappes* (Hunter and Latham, 1925). The nature of the latter endings, and their functional significance and relation to the sympathetic nervous system, became a controversial matter, particularly as knowledge of nerve and muscle physiology accumulated, largely stimulated by Sherrington's work in Britain. In a series of papers from 1909 onwards, the Dutch histologist Boeke described evidence that skeletal muscle possessed a double innervation which comprised both myelinated and unmyelinated fibres. The unmyelinated fibres ended in the *terminations en grappes* and were sympathetic in nature. However, others disagreed with this interpretation. The members of the Department of Anatomy at Sydney University became interested in the matter and J T Wilson, who had held the Challis Chair of Anatomy at that institution for some 30 years, subsequently published a major review dealing with the question. A Sydney orthopaedic surgeon, Norman Royle (Burkitt, 1944), who had previously been a Demonstrator in Anatomy in Wilson's department became interested in the problem of spasticity and the possibilities for its treatment. Royle began to do experimental work on the matter of spasticity in the Department of Anatomy. Around 1920 a young medical student of exceptional ability and energy, John Irvine Hunter (Anonymous, 1924), born in 1898, was also working in the Department as a Prosector in Anatomy whilst in the process of completing his medical course. Hunter almost certainly became aware of Royle's work on the anatomical background to spasticity somewhere around this time. Whilst still a medical undergraduate Hunter, patently possessed of some considerable measure of genius, had already carried out a number of experimental anatomical studies. On graduation in Medicine from the University of Sydney in March 1920, he was almost immediately appointed Demonstrator in Anatomy. Shortly afterwards he became Associate Professor of Anatomy in the University.

In 1920 Wilson was appointed to the Chair of Anatomy at the University of Cambridge and resigned his post in Sydney. The University of Sydney did not replace him immediately, but arranged for Hunter to spend some time overseas, part of it in Wilson's department in Cambridge, part with Grafton Elliott Smith, a Sydney graduate of an earlier day and by then Professor of Anatomy at University College, London, and part with Ariens Kappers at Amsterdam. In these places Hunter carried out further anatomical research, including a study of the fore-brain of a kiwi which earned him a Doctorate of Medicine from Sydney. He then returned to Sydney in 1923, and at the early age of 25 became Wilson's successor in the Challis Chair of Anatomy. He brought back with him to Sydney a slide given to him by Kuchinsky in London. This slide demonstrated the dual innervation of python muscle. Hunter also brought back the information that Kuchinsky had concluded that the myelinated and unmyelinated nerves in muscle never ended on the same muscle fibre. Hunter seems to have seen a possible application for Kuchinsky's conclusion in relation to the work that Royle continued to do on the basis of spasticity in what had now become Hunter's department.

At that time there was a school of thought which considered that muscle tone involved two elements, contractile tone and plastic tone. If there was a double innervation of skeletal muscle, with two different types of terminal nerve fibre (originating from anterior horn cells and the sympathetic nervous system, respectively) supplying two separate classes of muscle fibre, it seemed reasonable to hypothesise that the anatomical background to the two types of tone might lie in this pattern of double innervation. It was already well known that division of the fibres emanating from anterior horn cells would produce paralysis, but would section of the sympathetic fibres alter tone in a clinically useful way? Hunter and Royle began to collaborate. Royle produced spasticity in experimental animals by spinal cord section and later by decerebration, and then studied the effects of previous or subsequent sympathectomy on the spasticity produced. Royle became convinced that the surgery did reduce the spasticity in his animals. Meanwhile Hunter apparently carried out some experimental studies of his own on fowls and embarked on a program of histological studies on the innervation of muscle in conjunction with Oliver Latham (whose career is discussed later).

Royle reached a stage where he felt justified in carrying out sympathectomies on two patients with spasticity. He convinced himself, and provided cinematographic evidence sufficient to satisfy others, that the disability from spasticity in these patients was reduced. The work was presented at a meeting of the New South Wales branch of the British Medical Association held in the Anatomy Department of Sydney University on 23 October 1923, and subsequently published (Hunter, 1924a; Royle, 1924a). At this meeting, a very distinguished visitor was present – Sir William Macewen, Regius Professor of Surgery in the University of Glasgow, arguably the greatest innovator in all the history of surgery, the founding father of neurosurgery and the first man ever to successfully remove a diseased whole human lung. Macewen, a shrewd old man, as judged from the precis of his comments reported after the presentation, was a little hesitant to commit himself too enthusiastically about the discoveries and seemed rather to try to skirt around the issue. However Hunter's youth and transparent genius, the obvious practical importance of Royle's surgery and its potential benefits to neurological patients, and the fact that, for the first time, Australian research had produced an outcome of international significance, had a major impact in local medical circles. The report of the meeting seemed to catch the spirit in which the research appears to have been appreciated in local medical circles (Craig, 1924, *Medical Journal of Australia*, p. 98):

> 'Dr R Gordon Craig, in thanking Dr Royle and Professor Hunter for their splendid demonstration, said that the Medical School at their University was emerging from its infant into its adult life ... Formerly they had been content to depend for their scientific information on the researches conducted in the

old world. Now they had among them men who were able to contribute to knowledge.'

A little later the results of the surgery also produced a very considerable impression on a delegation of visiting American surgeons, including William Mayo. This resulted in Hunter and Royle being invited to travel to New York in October 1924 to deliver the J B Murphy Lecture to the American College of Surgeons as a vehicle for making their findings more widely available. Before they did this they had presented further relevant material at a regional meeting of the British Medical Association at Lismore in northern New South Wales on 12 April 1924. There Royle (1924b) largely confined himself to extensive details of the surgical operations he was carrying out to divide the grey rami of the sympathetic trunk, though he mentioned that he had performed additional successful operations since the two described in his initial communication some months previously. Hunter (1924b), however, gave a very long and competent account of the relevant background literature concerning the procedure and briefly described some experimental observations of his own relating to the effect of sympathectomy on the wing posture of the fowl. In the same issue of the *Medical Journal of Australia* he also provided comments on the anatomy relevant to Royle's operative procedure (Hunter, 1924c). One cannot but wonder whether an audience which presumably comprised mainly local general practitioners might have been rather overwhelmed by the amount and depth of the scientific data provided for their edification. From the material published to this point, one might have gained the impression that Hunter's role had been largely to stimulate and facilitate Royle's work and to explain its theoretical background in anatomy and neurophysiology with great lucidity. But in the meantime Hunter had been carrying out histological research in conjunction with Oliver Latham as mentioned above (Hunter and Latham, 1925), though this work did not appear in print until after the events to be recounted below. The conclusion to Hunter and Latham's paper summarised their findings:

> '... As far as our work goes these two types of nerve terminations *en grappes* and *en plaques* do not exist in the same muscle fibres but each supply separate groups and we have found little evidence incompatible with the theory that these striped musculatures are divided into alternate groups of muscle fibres served respectively by branches from the somatic and sympathetic nervous systems ...'

Thus they considered they had established the microscopic evidence which provided the rationale for the procedure of sympathectomy in the treatment of spasticity.

After their presentation to the American College of Surgeons in New York, Hunter (not long married) and Royle travelled to Britain. There the lecture Hunter had been invited to give in London had to be cancelled because the young man had become ill. He died in University College Hospital on 10 November 1924, just before the lecture was due. At the time, it was believed he had contacted enteric fever and had died from it. However in Boston Royle also became ill and remained so for long enough to prevent his contributing to the tributes to Hunter which were paid by his senior colleagues at the University of Sydney over the ensuing weeks (*Medical Journal of Australia*, 10 Jan 1925). Royle was later able to return to work, remained productive and carried out further sympathectomies for spasticity and other disorders, e.g. retinitis pigmentosa (Royle, 1930, 1932a, b), and for what he had diagnosed as disseminated sclerosis (Royle, 1933). He also carried out some experimental neuropharmacological work, using ephedrine to reduce spinal cord oedema which he postulated was the cause of anterior horn cell injury in acute poliomyelitis (Royle, 1935), and engaged in experimental physiology studies (Royle, 1937). Sadly, Royle's career came to a premature termination, for he began to develop manifestations of post-encephalitic Parkinsonism from 1930 onwards. When this became known, there arose speculation, at least among those who were then members of Hunter's former Department in Sydney, that both Hunter and Royle had contracted encephalitis lethargica whilst in America, where the disorder was then occurring. It was thought that Hunter had died in the acute phase of the illness, whereas Royle had experienced a mild initial illness but later suffered its progressive and debilitating extrapyramidal consequences.

Thus the whole splendid endeavour to relieve spasticity ended in disaster for those involved in it. For Hunter, the disaster was immediate, though it spared him the realisation that his work was invalid and his conclusions incorrect. For Royle, the disaster was more delayed and protracted, and possibly compounded by the realisation that he had survived long enough to become aware that neither aspect of the work for which such high hopes had been held, the neuro-anatomical findings and the surgical treatment, had proved sustainable or consistently reproducible in the hands of others. As early as 1926, in the face of criticism of Hunter and Royle's work, Editorial comment in the *Medical Journal of Australia* found it desirable to mount the argument that failure of a surgical procedure to provide an expected benefit did not necessarily prove that the rationale for the procedure was invalid (Anonymous, 1926). Royle (1927), seemingly wounded by criticism of his results and of their theoretical basis, including that from the neurophysiologist E D Adrian (subsequently Lord Adrian, and a Nobel Laureate), threw down the challenge that no one else had done sympathectomies in goats, the species in which he had obtained his experimental relief of spasticity. In Melbourne, Tiegs and Coates (1928) responded by failing to show that sympathetic ramisection in goats altered limb posture, the knee jerk or the tension in the tendo achilles. Their report triggered correspondence from Royle (1928), with the support of A W Campbell (1928a), which tried to explain the discrepancies in the findings of the two groups of workers. Gradually, it became established that, although unmyelinated sympathetic nervous system fibres went to skeletal muscle, there they innervated blood vessels and not the muscle fibres. As well, the future neurosurgeon Gilbert Phillips (1931), working in the Anatomy Department of Sydney University, demonstrated that the sympathetic nervous system did not constitute the efferent limb of the reflex subserving posture.

Why Royle's operations should have appeared to relieve spasticity is unclear. It was suggested that it was the post-operative physiotherapy rather than the surgery which produced the benefit, for Royle had been a physical education teacher before he studied medicine, and was interested in the application of physiotherapy. However, Royle countered by pointing out that the benefit from the operation was present even on the first post-operative day. Some years after his original work with Hunter, Royle (1933) finally came to acknowledge the correctness of the investigation to be described below which showed that there was no sympathetic innervation of voluntary muscle. However, Royle then ascribed the relief of spasticity produced by sympathetic ramisection to the improved spinal cord circulation which the procedure produced, arguing the faster local circulation gave oxygen less time to act in the spinal cord so that neuronal function tended to be suppressed (1937). It was an explanation which seems physiologically untenable. Perhaps Royle's surgery, in avulsing the grey rami communicantes of the sympathetic trunk (for he avulsed them rather than simply divided them), disturbed the function of gamma efferent fibres or even those from alpha motor neurons. Interestingly, Royle's early account of the surgery (Royle, 1924a) mentioned muscle twitchings in the leg on the sympathectomised side after the operations, suggesting that motor nerve fibres had been affected by his procedure. The long-term outcomes of Royle's own surgery do not appear to have ever been reported in detail. Unfortunately, neither Hunter nor Royle appears to have examined his experimental animals to see what damage to neural structures the surgery had produced before making their results public. Underlying their concept seems to have been the assumption that, because there were unmyelinated nerve fibres in muscle, and unmyelinated fibres in the sympathetic nerves which went to muscle, the two sets of unmyelinated fibres were the same fibres.

Despite its imperfections and its ultimate abandonment, the work of Hunter and Royle was a courageous and imaginative attempt to deal with a very significant global medical problem. Hunter, widely admired for his personal qualities and something of a contemporary local idol because of his enormous talents and already considerable scientific achievements, was to be transformed into a figure of almost legendary stature in the memory of the Sydney School of Medicine. The fact that he and Royle were ultimately proven incorrect was largely lost sight of in the regret evoked by the awareness of the unfulfilled promise of a life of genius so prematurely and abruptly cut off. Herbert John Wilkinson (1891–1963), the foundation Professor of Anatomy in the University of Queensland (Hickey, 1963) had been a medical student in Hunter's Department during the latter's brief period in the Challis Chair of Anatomy. After his own graduation Wilkinson became a member of the academic staff of that Department. In later life, Wilkinson spoke of Hunter to his own students and conveyed almost a sense of reverence and hero worship. Yet long afterwards, one of Wilkinson's own former junior colleagues in the Queensland Department of Anatomy, Geoffrey Kenny (1988) published information which he must have received through his contacts with Wilkinson. This information yielded the insight that a third, though much lesser, calamity emanated from the Sydney work on the dual innervation of muscle, and that the victim of that latter calamity was Wilkinson himself.

After Hunter's death Wilkinson, as a young academic in the Sydney Department of Anatomy, had taken up, almost by inheritance, the question of the double innervation of skeletal muscle. After very careful and detailed investigation in Sydney and overseas he came to the definite conclusion that the sympathetic nerves which entered muscle supplied the blood vessels only, and not the muscle fibres themselves (Wilkinson, 1929). Thus he found himself in the situation that, in the pursuit of truth, he had come to erode, as it were from within, a major part of the intellectual edifice on which rested the fame of the local hero and idol John Irvine Hunter. It must have been very difficult for Wilkinson, and also for his colleagues in the Sydney Department of Anatomy, and in the University more largely. Moreover, it involved Wilkinson in an ongoing controversy with Boeke, so that it was quite a number of years before the essential correctness of the former's views became generally accepted. Wilkinson's subsequent academic career was made away from Sydney, first in Adelaide from 1930 as Elder Professor of Anatomy, and then in the University of Queensland from 1936 to 1959, where he seemed to be almost at pains to avoid mentioning to students the major role he had come to play in correcting Hunter's mistake.

Thus Sydney men in the end came to correct the earlier error of Sydney men, and the first Australian systematic research into a major neuroscience problem ultimately produced a valid and scientifically sustainable outcome, though one disappointing in terms of the earlier high expectations. However, the man who first obtained the correct answer received (and indeed seemed to expect) far less fame than the earlier investigators who drew mistaken conclusions and yet who, through the intervention of fate, became the heroes of a seeming catastrophe. Yet it was a catastrophe which had the effect of heightening Australian consciousness of, and pride in, the capacity and promise of its medical science. Interestingly, and almost as an accidental byproduct of the endeavour, according to Greenwood's (1967) interpretation Royle's operation had opened up the possibility of sympathetic trunk surgery instead of peri-arterial sympathectomy, for the relief of vasospastic disorders.

Poliomyelitis and Sister Kenny

The occurrence of poliomyelitis in epidemic form was noted in the latter part of the 19th century in the Australian medical literature, and in the first half of the 20th century there were a number of well-documented outbreaks of the disorder during the Australian summers (e.g. Ham, 1905). The disease came to be greatly feared in the community. The advent of the injected Salk vaccine in the latter 1950s, and of the oral Sabin vaccine a little later, completely transformed the situation. It is now only the members of an ageing generation in the country who can recall the anxieties which their parents experienced each summer, fearing that their children might contract the dreaded 'infantile paralysis'.

Australian neurology, and indeed Australian medicine, had little or no notable impact on knowledge of the biology or treatment of poliomyelitis. However, one Australian woman, Elizabeth Kenny, brought about a transformation in the management of the disorder, and in the quality of life of those who were, or were in immediate danger of being, handicapped by it (Macnamara, 1953).

Elizabeth Kenny was born in 1880 and lived out much of her life in country towns in south-east Queensland and northern New South Wales. As a young woman she found her way into the nursing profession through rather informal means. However, after joining the Army Nursing Service during World War I she was ultimately promoted to the level of nursing sister, and thereafter was usually referred to as Sister Kenny. In the post-war years she worked as a nurse in small country towns on the Darling Downs in Queensland. There she found her way to an original approach to treating the disability of poliomyelitis (and also that of spasticity). From an early stage in the illness she replaced the conventional initial therapeutic inactivity, or the use of immune serum in the pre-paralytic phase (Macnamara, 1929), and the subsequent immobilisation of limbs, and the splinting (Vickers, 1921; Clubbe, 1925), with massage, the application of heat, and rather intensive passive and active exercises. She found increasing support for her methods in the general community as time passed. Local people became convinced of their efficacy, and she also received support from some local medical men, though the majority of the medical profession was opposed to her methods, and these methods were condemned by a Queensland Royal Commission in the mid-1930s.

Elizabeth Kenny appears to have been a woman of some considerable strength of character and inner conviction, and her attitudes hardened in the face of medical opposition to her approach. The story of the struggle has been told, from the standpoint of one who had access to the Queensland Health Department records, by Ross Patrick (1985). With growing local community and some medical support, and State Government backing, clinics utilising Sister Kenny's approach to the management of poliomyelitis were opened in certain cities in Queensland. The State Government gave her an introduction to health authorities in the United States of America and there, after some delay, her methods were taken up on a much larger scale than in her homeland. Gradually she became a famous and revered public figure in the United States, whose President at the time, Franklin Delano Roosevelt, had been crippled by poliomyelitis earlier in his life.

By the time of her death in 1952 it seems to have become fairly generally accepted that Sister Kenny's methods were more successful than those which they had displaced. In contrast, her novel ideas of the pathogenesis of poliomyelitis, viz. that the disability in the disorder was due to viral damage to peripheral tissues, were recognised as scientifically unsustainable. Her fame may have rested on a false theoretical premise, but she had empirically, and by the strength of her personality and conviction, very significantly improved the outlook for many afflicted by a crippling neurological disorder. From an international community viewpoint, Elizabeth Kenny would probably appear the most famous figure concerned with neurological disease ever produced by Australia, though from a more scientific standpoint that assessment could scarcely be warranted.

Investigations into peculiarly Australian disorders

Childhood lead poisoning

At the third session of the Intercolonial Medical Congress of Australasia held in Sydney in 1892 one of the papers presented was entitled *'Notes on lead poisoning as observed among children in Brisbane'*. There were five authors, of whom the first named was J Lockhart Gibson. The purpose of the presentation was to report an unusual event, the fact that 10 instances of lead poisoning had been admitted to the Hospital for Sick Children in Brisbane in the first seven months of 1892. The dominant feature of the poisoning was reported to be the gradual onset of a reasonably bilaterally symmetrical paresis of the distal muscles of the limbs with the development of associated muscle wasting. The weakness usually began in the lower limbs. In half of the cases, before the development of the paralysis, there were attacks of abdominal pain usually accompanied by vomiting, and associated with convulsing in two cases. Lead was found in the urine of the two children in whom its presence was sought. Such a disorder had not previously been recognised among children in Brisbane, though the authors of the presentation confessed that they might have missed the true diagnosis on occasions in the past. Further cases continued to occur in Queensland and additional communications concerning the matter appeared in the local medical literature. It became clear that the clinical spectrum of the disorder was more extensive than the original description had suggested. In particular, an encephalopathic presentation was recognised, dominated by the manifestations of intracranial hypertension. A possible example had been reported in the June 1891 issue of the *Australasian Medical Gazette*, a case of acute ophthalmoplegia with double optic neuritis, the latter term being used for what would now be called bilateral papilloedema. The author of the report was F Antill Pockley, a Sydney ophthalmic surgeon, and the patient was a six-year-old girl brought to him in 1888 with the rapid onset of total blindness (Pockley, 1891). When living in Brisbane five weeks previously she had developed sudden abdominal pain and persistent vomiting. Two weeks later a temporary squint appeared and on the next day she had a convulsion. Further convulsions and screaming fits occurred and it was realised that the child had become blind. When examined in Sydney she had severe bilateral papilloedema, almost total loss of external eye movements, and was completely blind. Intellectually she was normal and there was no other abnormality on examination. Afterwards there was some return of eye movements and the papilloedema gave way to bilateral optic atrophy. This was perhaps the first recorded example of a type of case history which became commonplace in Brisbane over the next few years, but in this early instance the possibility of lead poisoning was not considered. Similar events in Brisbane were first reported as instances of 'localised basal meningitis' (Gibson *et al.*, 1892). By

1897 it had become clear to Turner and Gibson that the entity represented by this diagnosis was an expression of lead poisoning (Turner, 1897).

In the *Medical Journal of Australia* for 11 February 1922 the Council of the Queensland Branch of the British Medical Association endorsed a report in which the unnamed authors described in some detail the course of the Queensland outbreak of childhood lead poisoning up to that time (Anonymous, 1922). By 1908 some 262 instances of lead poisoning had been admitted to the Hospital for Sick Children in Brisbane (Turner, 1908). At this time 20 new cases a year were appearing, and affected children had been referred from various Queensland towns as well as from Brisbane. Later a series of cases was reported from Townsville in North Queensland (Breinl and Young, 1914). From 1917 to 1926 no less than 428 children with lead poisoning were admitted to the Brisbane Hospital for Sick Children, whereas over the same period there were only four such admissions to the Royal Alexandra Hospital for Children, in more populous Sydney, and three to the Melbourne Children's Hospital (Nye, 1933). Coincident with these events, there had been no outbreak of lead poisoning in Australian adults, the few instances which occurred being explained by industrial exposure, particularly that occurring at the mining town of Broken Hill. The clinical picture recognised by 1908 involved more than the abdominal symptoms and muscle atrophy which featured prominently in the initial report. There was greater emphasis on convulsions, which were termed eclampsia after the then contemporary use of that word, and on the encephalopathic pattern of presentation of the poisoning mentioned above with its headache, papilloedema, and bilateral abducens palsies, going on to blindness. At lumbar puncture, the intracranial pressure was raised (Gibson, 1912). Also, the presence of anaemia and transitory albuminuria was mentioned, with the possibility of chronic interstitial nephritis as a rare complication, though the passage of time proved the latter to be far from rare (Nye, 1933).

The interest in this relatively localised outbreak of lead poisoning did not lie so much in the matter of diagnosis, which became clear enough early on, but in why so many cases should occur in Queensland children but not in Queensland adults or in children elsewhere in Australia. Because the symptoms lessened or disappeared when the affected children were hospitalised, and might recur after they returned to their homes, it seemed likely that the lead exposure occurred somewhere in the domestic environment (Turner, 1897). Originally it was suggested that the affected children had chewed the tin foil which was used for the wrapping of various sweets, and cigarettes (Turner, 1897). However, there was never adequate evidence to sustain this hypothesis. The next possibility raised was that the children had drunk water which contained lead. At the time, the roofs of Queensland houses were often made of galvanised iron which was fixed to the underlying roof timbers with lead-headed nails. Rain water from the roof was collected into galvanised iron tanks for domestic use, and it was thought that Queensland children might have been exposed to lead from drinking this water. This might have explained why Queensland children, but not children from more southerly parts of Australia, where iron roofing was less common, developed lead poisoning. It did not explain why their parents and often their siblings escaped. At one stage the Queensland Government Analyst did report the presence of lead in the water from galvanised iron tanks, but this finding was later found to be due to analytical error. What proved to be the probable cause of the lead exposure was first suggested by Turner in 1899, but then forgotten until it was resurrected by Gibson in 1904. The proposed mechanism was as follows, in Turner's (1908) words:

> 'Nearly all the dwellings in Queensland are built of wood, and in the towns the wood is covered by paint, consisting largely of white-lead. Exposed to our hot summer sun, this paint rapidly weathers, and becomes reduced to a powdery condition. This is particularly noticeable on verandah railings. The verandahs are favourable playgrounds for young children, who clasp the railings with their moist hands, which become covered with poison. Thence it finds its way to the child's mouth, especially in children who suck their fingers or bite their nails.'

This putative mechanism was never fully established by rigorous scientific proof and the controlled studies which would satisfy present-day standards of medical evidence. Nonetheless, the Queensland medical profession was convinced that the circumstantial evidence and the gravity of the situation justified its launching a publicity campaign to educate the public, to ban the use of lead paint, particularly on the external surfaces of dwellings, and to have such paint removed, or covered over. The pages of the *Medical Journal of Australia* of 11 March and 1 April 1922 contain a deal of rather acrimonious, though courteous, correspondence between Dr S A Smith of Sydney and a number of members of the Queensland Branch of the British Medical Association in Australia. The controversy centred on the source of the lead exposure, though it spilled over into other areas. Smith had sought a higher level of scientific proof of lead ingestion than was available. Nevertheless, Queensland Government action and legislation to the desired end followed, later in 1922. Thereafter the incidence of cases of acute lead poisoning gradually diminished and after some years the illness ceased to be a local medical problem. Unfortunately, residual consequences of lead exposure in earlier life continued to account for cases of chronic kidney disease in Queensland until after the time of the Second World War.

Queensland childhood lead poisoning constituted a unique outbreak of neurotoxicity due to heavy metal exposure, which came about as a consequence of employing a European domestic practice in a tropical environment. The problem was investigated by those on the spot, and in time they came to understand its basis and produced an effective solution for it.

Pink disease of childhood

Australian medicine in its pre-neurologist days made a significant contribution to world knowledge of pink disease, another childhood disorder with neurological connotations. Unlike the situation with lead poisoning of childhood, where the novel features were the circumstance of occurrence of the phenomenon and the factors responsible for it, pink disease appeared to be a new phenomenon which was first described in Australia, though its true cause was ultimately determined by workers in other countries.

In 1914, Harry Swift, an Adelaide physician and paediatrician (Newland, 1937), described a condition which he called 'erythroedema', a name he continued to advocate (Swift, 1923) even when others preferred to call the disorder 'pink disease' or 'acrodynia'. Swift (1914) stated that in the previous two years he had seen 14 instances of a disorder in children aged between six and 15 months. The symptoms began with loss of appetite, restlessness, crying, fretting and sleeping poorly. After a few days the hands and feet became swollen and red, though they were cold and clammy to the feel. The skin of the palms of the hands became sodden and tended to desquamate. Swift noticed the resemblance between the appearance of the fingers and hands and that found in patients with peripheral neuritis. The muscles, particularly the larger ones in the limbs, became wasted and hypotonic. Movement became slow and prolonged effort could not be sustained. The prognosis in all cases proved to be favourable. Recovery after hospitalisation occurred slowly over a period of months. Diagnostically, Swift remarked on the affinities between the disorder and peripheral neuritis, but also recognised that there were certain differences. He concluded that the disorder was 'an intestinal toxaemia giving rise to an angio-neurosis', without explaining the basis of his pronouncement.

At the time of Swift's account, the disorder was thought to be a new disease, though Littlejohn (1923) noted that there had been anecdotal reports of the same condition in Australia over the three decades previous to his own time of writing. Clubbe, of Sydney, had coined the name 'pink disease' for it. After Swift's report, there were additional published descriptions of the disorder both from Australia and overseas. In 1931 a monograph by Rocaz appeared and two years later was translated into English by Wood, who had reported further Australian cases from Melbourne in 1921. Rocaz believed that the first description of the disorder had been given by a German physician, Selter, who had named it 'tropho-dermatoneurosis'. However, Rocas acknowledged the important role of the Australian physicians in making the condition known in the world literature, though the subsequent flood of publications concerning the disorder came mainly from Europe and the United States. McDonald (1933) provided a competent account of knowledge of the condition in the *Medical Journal of Australia*, and discussed the postulated aetiologies, indicating that none appeared satisfactory. Penfold *et al.* (1932), at the Baker Institute in Melbourne, had searched unsuccessfully for a bacterial cause of the disorder. Later there were suggestions that a fungus growing on cereals, a virus (whose nature was unspecified), or vitamin B1 deficiency was responsible. However, Southby (1949) reverted to favouring a viral aetiology for the disorder (Clements, 1940). A decade later Cheek (1950) and Cheek and Hicks (1950) in Adelaide found evidence of hyponatraemia in children affected by pink disease, and considered that the disorder was due to adrenal deficiency. A year after that, Williams *et al.* (1951) in Melbourne failed to confirm Cheek's findings.

In 1960 Clements published Australian hospital admission data for cases of pink disease and also Australian and British mortality data for the disorder. Both the incidence and the mortality had declined from the early 1950s onwards. For practical purposes the condition disappeared after various lines of evidence established that it was a toxic effect of mercury contained in teething powders given to children. Once the practice of using these powders ceased, and the powders themselves became unavailable, the disorder ceased to occur. Although the laboratory work which established the presence of excessive levels of mercury in affected children was carried out overseas, it is of some interest that Clements (1960) mentioned that Bancroft, of Brisbane, in 1881 had reported to the local Board of Health that he:

> 'sees many children brought to death's door from the parents dosing them with a powerful powder of mercury'

whilst Evans (1931) in discussing the differential diagnosis of pink disease, commented:

> 'Lastly, the blame may be laid at the door of the homely old-fashioned tooth in its process of eruption',

words more prophetic than was realised at the time.

Thus the Australian role in the understanding of this now extinct peripheral neuropathy of infancy was essentially that of the clinical observation of new phenomena, though it was observation on a comparatively large scale and it brought the disorder to international notice. There was also a continuing, though ultimately unsuccessful, Australian attempt to determine the disorder's cause.

Australian 'X' disease

In 1917 and again in 1918, and also in 1925, outbreaks of what appeared to be a novel viral encephalitis occurred mainly in northern and western Queensland and in western New South Wales. The disorder came to be known as 'X' disease, though it was sometimes referred to in the literature as the 'mysterious' disease. A number of reports of local outbreaks appeared in the *Medical Journal of Australia,* and it was studied in the laboratory first by Breinl in Townsville and later by Cleland and Campbell in Sydney, who after the outbreak published overviews of the events. The disorder occurred at a time when the pandemic of encephalitis lethargica had been occurring in the Northern Hemisphere (from 1915 to 1926), and this inevitably at first led to suspicion that this disorder had also appeared in Australia (Wilson, 1918). However, from the old records, and from subsequent events, it is quite clear that 'X' disease was not encephalitis lethargica, though the latter did occur in Australia, but later than in Europe and North America. There was no significant

Australian contribution to research on encephalitis lethargica as such. In contrast, the investigation of 'X' disease, which appears not to have been recognised elsewhere in the world at the time, was entirely in Australian hands throughout. More or less synchronously with 'X' disease, an influenza pandemic (the Spanish or black 'flu) was raging in Australia and elsewhere, but this does not seem to have led to difficulty in recognising the presence of an Australian outbreak of encephalitis.

Encephalitis lethargica

The first recorded instance of encephalitis lethargica in Australia (at least along its eastern seaboard, appears to have occurred in Tasmania in May 1919. It involved a soldier who had returned from service overseas in World War I (*Medical Journal of Australia* 1: 204, 1920). Shortly after, in the same year, there was a series of reports of the disease from Victoria (Downing, 1919; Hiller, 1919; Stawell, 1919, 1920; Wilkinson, 1920), and until 1923 further cases occurred in that State (Stawell, 1923). In New South Wales 35 cases were admitted to Sydney Hospital in 1922 and 1923 (Holmes à Court, 1923) and other cases were described (Smith, 1920; Mills, 1922). Revisiting the situation a little later, Collins (1928) stated that 50 instances of encephalitis lethargica had been admitted to the Royal Prince Alfred Hospital, Sydney, between 1919 and 1927, with nine deaths occurring. Latham (1934) reported that he had received for examination in his laboratory in Sydney 80 brains from persons with encephalitis lethargica. The earliest reports from Queensland came from the Ipswich area, a little way west of Brisbane, where in May 1922 some 31 cases of an acute encephalitis had been seen in the previous few months (Trumpy, 1922). Mathewson (1922) considered that some of these cases resembled clinically the instances of 'X' disease he had seen a few years earlier. However, some of the cases had clinical findings which made encephalitis lethargica more likely, and Cleland (1923) believed that this disorder accounted for the outbreak. From personal experience of patients with post-encephalitic Parkinsonism, it would appear that there were instances of encephalitis lethargica in nearby Brisbane at much the same time, and for two or three years afterwards. According to Cleland's (1923) evidence, the State of Victoria bore the brunt of the Australian outbreak of encephalitis lethargica. This outbreak did not occur synchronously with 'X' disease, and the geographical distributions of the two disorders differed. Encephalitis lethargica tended to appear mainly in the more populous areas, whereas 'X' disease occurred in north Queensland and in rural areas along the Darling River basin. Moreover, Parkinsonism tended to develop after a time in those who became ill with what was often regarded as influenza at the time when local cases of encephalitis lethargica occurred, whereas with one exception Parkinsonism did not occur as a sequel of 'X' disease. The exception was reported by Burnell (1922) in a seven-year-old girl in Broken Hill in south-western New South Wales, whom he had diagnosed as suffering from 'X' disease in 1918. Much later, serological evidence from patients with post-encephalitic Parkinsonism provided no evidence that the virus believed responsible for 'X' disease had played a part in the aetiology of Australian Parkinsonism (Eadie *et al.*, 1965).

The 'X' disease outbreaks

The first recognised case of 'X' disease was reported from Bourke, in western New South Wales, in 1917 (Litchfield, 1917). Breinl, from the Australian Institute of Tropical Medicine in Townsville in north Queensland issued a preliminary report of a local outbreak of acute encephalitis one week later (Breinl, 1917). Burnell (1917) reported 16 cases from Broken Hill and Cleland (1917) found a total of 57 (of whom 34 died) in the State of New South Wales in the 1917 outbreak. Breinl (1918) described another nine instances in Townsville, Anderson (1917) 14 at Goondiwindi in western Queensland near the New South Wales border which had occurred between February and May 1917, and there were said to be 17 childhood cases in Brisbane, in the extreme south-east corner of Queensland after the end of March, with a 65 per cent mortality (Matthewson and Latham, 1917). The outbreak of acute encephalitis lasted some four months, beginning in mid-summer, reaching a peak in February and March, with cases ceasing to appear after May 1917.

In the following summer, the set of events was repeated in western New South Wales with cases being reported again from Broken Hill by Burnell (1918). Although fewer individual reports appeared in the local medical literature, when Cleland and Campbell (1920a) described the epidemiology of the outbreaks they were aware of a total of 134 cases in New South Wales. This suggests that another 77 had occurred in that State in 1918, again in the summer months.

Further cases were described in 1925 in Townsville (Baldwin and Heydon, 1925) and in Broken Hill (Kneebone and Cleland, 1926). Thereafter, for a generation, the disease in Australia disappeared from medical notice.

The clinical features

Clinically, the disorder behaved as a viral polioclastic encephalomyelitis. Cleland and Campbell (1920a) described it as follows:

> '... The disease was abrupt in onset and severe. Children chiefly were affected (ninety-five cases) but adults did not escape (thirty-nine cases). General signs of cerebro-spinal irritation, namely, convulsions, rigidity, increased reflexes, mental obfuscation and loss of consciousness, accompanied by high fever, were the dominant features. Paralysis of voluntary muscles did not occur in more than one out of ten cases. Four and a half days was the average duration of the illness, and it was fatal in no less than 70 per cent of cases, fatality figures which were more than double those of any recorded epidemic of acute poliomyelitis (infantile paralysis).'

Breinl (1918) examined the cerebro-spinal fluid in several of his cases of 'X' disease and reported that it always appeared to be under normal pressure though it sometimes contained a mild excess of lymphocytes, or lymphocytes and leucocytes. It was always sterile on culture for the presence of bacteria.

The pathogenesis

The main initial investigations into the nature of 'X' disease were carried out by Anton Breinl, at the Australian Institute of Tropical Medicine in Townsville, and by J Burton Cleland and Walter Campbell, in Sydney.

Breinl (died 1944) was an Austrian who had commenced a career in the investigation of tropical diseases whilst based in the School of Tropical Medicine at Liverpool. He came to the Townsville Institute as Director in 1911 and over the next decade carried out a number of studies into local and nearby tropical health problems. His life story, and that of his Institute, were described in some detail by Douglas (1977). Cleland at the time was Principal Microbiologist to the Department of Public Health, New South Wales. Later he had a very distinguished and productive career as Professor of Pathology in the University of Adelaide. Campbell was a very great neuroscientist whose career is described in the next chapter.

Breinl (1918) carried out autopsies on seven of his cases of 'X' disease, and described histological appearances in their brains and spinal cords, mainly perivenous cuffing with round cells, which he interpreted as consistent with poliomyelitis. However, he recognised that the brain was involved more extensively than was usual in poliomyelitis. The pia mater might show leucocyte and round cell infiltration and the brain substance might contain pinpoint haemorrhages. Cleland and Campbell (1919) generally concurred with these findings, but added the observation that changes in anterior horn cells were distinctly less frequent than in poliomyelitis.

Breinl (1918), and also Campbell *et al.* (1918) demonstrated that the causative agent in nervous tissue and cerebrospinal fluid was transmissible to monkeys by intracerebral inoculation, and in these animals produced an encephalitic illness. On this basis, and taken in conjunction with his clinical and histological data, Breinl concluded that the illness was a clinically aberrant form of acute poliomyelitis, though he was careful to point out the unusual severity of the brain involvement. In contrast, as they accumulated further evidence, Cleland and Campbell (1919) increasingly inclined to the view that the disease was a new and discrete entity. Not only was the course of the illness different from that of poliomyelitis, with a greater mortality and less risk of residual paralysis, but histologically the damage to anterior horn cells was less severe, and the causative agent could be transmitted to species such as a sheep, a calf and a foal (Cleland and Campbell, 1920b) to which the virus of poliomyelitis could not be transmitted. Thus the existence of a new viral encephalitis peculiar to part of Australia was established.

Noting the geographical distribution of the cases in consecutive years, and the seasonal occurrence, Cleland and Campbell (1920a) took thought concerning the mode of transmission in humans. In this paper they discussed the possibility of there being an animal reservoir of the virus, and of its human dissemination by travel along the Australian railway network. However, no firm conclusion was possible.

There, despite the 1925 cases, and Macfarlane Burnet's (1934) suggestion that the louping ill virus might have been responsible for the outbreaks, the story rested for a little over a quarter of a century, which takes the matter to just beyond the temporal confine imposed on the present chapter. Also, contrary to the notion that the present chapter deals with neurology in the hands of non-neurologists, an Australian neurologist, E Graeme Robertson, was involved in the later stages of the study of the matter, though not in the principal role. Despite these considerations, the events of 1951, and later, will be pursued here, albeit briefly, as they almost certainly complete the record of Australian 'X' disease.

Murray Valley encephalitis

In 1951 an outbreak of acute encephalitis occurred in the Murray River valley in southern New South Wales and northern Victoria. Clinically and histopathologically it behaved as an acute viral encephalitis and resembled Australian 'X' disease (Anderson, 1952; Anderson *et al.*, 1952; French, 1952; Robertson, 1952; Robertson and McLorinan, 1952; McLean and Stevenson, 1954). By this time, much more sophisticated facilities for virological investigation were available in Australia, and evidence accumulated that this Murray Valley encephalitis was an arthropod-borne viral infection closely allied to Japanese B encephalitis. The latter infection is believed to be endemic in New Guinea and Northern Australia (Anderson *et al.*, 1960). It becomes epidemic when seasonal weather conditions cause wild birds carrying the virus to migrate south, which they do principally to the Murray-Darling River basin (Miles and Howes, 1953), and when the residual level of immunity in the local communities has again become low enough. Sporadic cases and small outbreaks have continued to be reported since 1951 (Burrow *et al.*, 1998). It has become widely accepted the 'X' disease and Murray Valley encephalitis are the one and same illness (Burnet, 1952a, b).

Other original work

Headache

Francis Hare, of Brisbane, in a series of three papers on the paroxysmal neuroses (1903), attempted to forge a unifying concept of a vasospastic pathogenesis for a variety of disorders which embraced epilepsy, migraine and asthma, among other conditions. The word 'neuroses' apparently was taken in Cullen's old general sense of a nervous system disorder, or of a nervous system disorder for which no pathological basis could be detected at the time. With the exception of migraine, the range of disorders Hare considered was more or less the spectrum of illness which Willis long before (1684) had considered convulsive in nature. Hare's concept of their pathogenesis really represented a return to ideas in vogue a century previously. These ideas at that earlier time had never had adequate experimental confirmation, and Hare failed to provide one except in the case of migraine. The observations he made about the effects of temporary occlusion of various scalp arteries by local pressure during migraine attacks proved very reminiscent of those later described by Wolff (1963) in his classic *Headache and Other Head Pain*. Probably, having been published in a colonial medical journal in a country far from the mainstream of medical intellectual activity, Hare's ideas and observations about the mechanism of migraine went largely unnoticed internationally. Possibly they were also to some extent submerged by Hare's other observations and conclusions which must not have appeared satisfactory even in the state of then contemporary knowledge. Yet, though Hare's observations were uncontrolled, and were not expressed in quantitative terms as would be seen desirable if not essential to modern-day research standards, they still appear valid and would demand consideration in any adequate explanation of the pathogenesis of migraine.

There were also some small-scale Australian investigations into the treatment of headache. Sippe (1938), a Brisbane physician, believed that migraine had an allergic basis. He therefore tested the efficacies of various diets which were designed to eliminate the intake of specific items of food in preventing attacks of the disorder. In 105 cases managed in this way he reported a 61.9 per cent cure rate, though he seemed aware that he had tended to select the cases in whom he used the treatment. As well, he studied no control group. Lister Reid (1940) described the success of repeated subcutaneous injections of histamine in the prevention of recurrent migraine in five subjects, again without any control observations. Kelly (1942) investigated the effectiveness of injecting local anaesthetic into tender areas in the posterior neck muscles in the relief of what he categorised as chronic traumatic and rheumatic headache in 40 patients. It would be difficult to translate the diagnoses in his subjects into modern-day headache categories.

Epilepsy

Hare (1903) chose to reject the theories of the primary neurogenic origin of epileptic seizures that had come into vogue by his time, as a result of the studies of Hughlings Jackson and Gowers. He preferred to return to the earlier vasomotor hypotheses of the origin of the disorder. The ideas he espoused were really variants of Brown-Séquard's (1860) concept of epileptogenesis, rather than an original hypothesis, and by Hare's own admission were based primarily on what he recognised was an assumption that:

> 'I shall assume provisionally that in epilepsy, as in most cases of migraine and asthma, there is an initial widespread area of vaso-constriction ...'

Hare's ideas attracted some temporary local interest in Australia, but they patently lacked the necessary evidential basis to be developed further in relation to epilepsy, and led nowhere.

George Rennie (1905a), a man apparently of a more sober cast of mind, addressed the question as to whether epilepsy could be cured. He raised the important issue of what phenomena should be embraced within the rubric of 'epilepsy'. Was it to be only those instances in which no underlying pathology could be found to explain epileptic seizures, the view taken by Delasiauve (1854) and Reynolds (1861) some half-century earlier? And what constituted a 'cure' for epilepsy? For how long needed the sufferer remain seizure free to be considered cured? These were matters which should have been raised sooner and far more often in the international literature than they had been, and Rennie's considering them in 1905 gives some indication of his intellectual qualities.

Within the mental hospital system, some work was also done on metabolic changes, specifically in relation to calcium concentrations in the blood, in epilepsy (Prior and Jones, 1916). In this connection 'epilepsy' referred to convulsive seizures as they occurred in patients who needed to be confined to such institutions. There seemed little recognition on the part of the authors that their conclusions might not be applicable to epilepsy as it was present in the general population. Lalor and Haddow (1920), again working in a mental hospital environment, argued for a toxaemic causation for idiopathic epilepsy on the basis of their measurements of the urinary excretion of urea in epileptic patients.

Various encephalitides

The Australian outbreaks of 'X' disease and encephalitis lethargica seemed to lead to a continuing interest in the topic of the encephalitides over the next decade, or rather longer. From the local varieties of encephalitis, interest first extended to the viral encephalitides in general (Duhig, 1922) and then to the various acute disseminated demyelinative encephalomyelitides, whose autoimmune basis was then unknown, e.g. those associated with varicella (Lockwood, 1931) and measles (Chinner, 1940), and a localised brain stem variety reported by De Crespigny and Hurst (1942). The neuropathologist Oliver Latham took up the subject from a diagnostic and a pathogenic standpoint on several occasions (1927, 1930, 1931). E Weston Hurst, in Adelaide at the Institute for Medical and Veterinary Science in the latter 1930s, did investigational work on the production of experimental demyelination. He achieved this in experimental animals by means of repeated sublethal exposures to cyanide, or sodium azide. Before Hurst had completed his investigations, he described them (1941a, b) in the initial Rennie Memorial Lecture given to the Royal Australasian College of Physicians. This lecture contained an admirable and critical account of demyelinating diseases in animals and humans. Incidentally, in this lecture Hurst remarked on the unexpectedly low prevalence of multiple sclerosis in South Australia, as compared with the United Kingdom and other countries, an observation confirmed by epidemiological studies carried out three decades later.

The Argyll–Robertson pupil

H J Wilkinson was mentioned previously in this chapter for his role in correcting Hunter's misinterpretation of the role of sympathetic nerve fibres in skeletal muscle. Whilst still in the Anatomy School of Sydney University, Wilkinson (1927) carried out a series of physiological and neuroanatomical studies which led him to the conclusion that the afferent pathways from the retina (for light) and the proprioceptive pathway from the extrinsic eye muscles (important for convergence) reached the oculomotor nuclei through different routes in the periaqueductal region of the midbrain. At this site, syphilitic inflammation was therefore able to involve the former pathway selectively to inactivate the pupillary response to light, whilst allowing preservation of the response to accommodation.

Cerebral vascular disease

In 1937, A A Abbie, who later became Professor of Anatomy in the University of Adelaide, published detailed studies of the arterial blood supply of the deep central regions of the human cerebral hemispheres which corrected certain errors contained in the earlier accounts of Duret and Heubner (both in 1874 – see Abbie, 1937). Abbie also showed that the lenticulo-optic artery of Duret did not exist. Abbie's work was significant from the point of view of interpreting the consequences of vascular lesions of the internal capsule and neighbouring brain areas.

Peripheral nerve pathology

Goulston (1930) published in the *Medical Journal of Australia* a long and detailed account of the damage caused to peripheral nerves in experimental animals by the effects of radiation from radium needles inserted near the nerves studied.

Myasthenia gravis

Corkill and Ennor (1937) described their investigation of blood esterase activity in two cases of neostigmine-responsive myasthenia gravis. The esterase activity was not increased. Despite this finding, the researchers were not prepared to discount the possibility that the disorder could be due to increased circulating esterase activity, or decreased acetylcholine production. Competition for post-junctional acetylcholine receptors was not raised as an additional possibility.

Tick-bite paralysis

Instances of paralysis associated with tick bites had been reported from Eastern Australia as early as 1884 (Bancroft, 1884). Of these, at least two had been fatal (Bancroft, 1884; Ferguson, 1924). Probably prompted by this knowledge, Clunies Ross, in the Veterinary Science Department of the University of Sydney, carried out an investigation which led to the recognition of the existence of a tick-derived neurotoxin as the causative agency (Editorial, 1927). Later the Sydney paediatrician Donald Hamilton (1940b) reviewed the topic and added further cases of the disorder to the literature.

Myotonia

Covernton and Draper (1947) reported a comprehensive clinical and experimental study of myotonia in animals and humans which was extracted from the former's

MD thesis (from the University of Adelaide). Some of the pharmacological observations, e.g. relating to the effects of neostigmine, adrenaline and carbaminyl chloride, were of theoretical importance.

Finger-cherry blindness

From 1894 onwards (Flecker, 1944), instances were reported of sudden bilateral blindness which affected children a few hours after eating the fruit of the finger-cherry plant *(Rhodomyrtus macrocarpa)* which grew in north Queensland. The toxicity appeared restricted to the optic nerves. The resultant blindness was permanent and was accompanied by bilateral optic atrophy. The disorder ceased to occur after 1915, when an educational campaign was mounted to alert children to the dangers of ingesting the fruit of the plant. The nature of the toxin does not appear to have been determined.

Bromide clinical pharmacology

The modern medical mind is attuned to the notion that the study of clinical pharmacology is a post-World War II development. It may therefore seem a little surprising to some that, as long ago as 1932, Sippe and Bostock, in Brisbane carried out what was in essence a clinical neuropharmacological study of the toxicity of bromides, which were at that time still in use in the treatment of epilepsy. Whilst these workers could not establish an optimal bromide concentration in blood which correlated with clinical benefit, they did obtain some evidence of a bromide threshold concentration of 200 mg per 100 ml, above which neurotoxicity was likely.

Forerunners of the Australian clinical neurologists

Leaving aside Walter Campbell, who will be dealt with in the next chapter, over the period before men began to practise exclusively in clinical neurology in Australia there were certain physicians who achieved local reputations for their interest and skill in neurological matters. These physicians included George Rennie, Sidney Sewell, Henry Maudsley and James Froude Flashman. There was also a neuropathologist Oliver Latham, who was involved in numerous neurological collaborations over the course of half a century. In those times there were also other persons who had been accorded the title of neurologist to various institutions within Australia. Some of these were primarily psychiatrists, e.g. Grey Ewan at Newcastle, John Bostock in Brisbane, Reg S Ellery in Melbourne. Some were physicians, such as H K Fry (1886–1959), who between 1920 and 1924 held the appointment of Honorary Assistant Physician in Neurology at the Adelaide Hospital (Rischbieth, 1994). When Fry resigned the position, though remaining as a Physician to the Hospital, he was not replaced. This particular neurological appointment was not mentioned in Burston's (1988) obituary of Fry. It has been difficult to trace information about any original contribution to the advancement of neurology that Fry made, locally or more globally. There was also the anatomist

John Irvine Hunter, who briefly held the title of Honorary Neurologist to the Lewisham Hospital in Sydney. None of these men was a committed neurologist in the modern sense, Rennie probably being the closest approximation.

George Edward Rennie (1861–1923)

George Rennie (Plate 1) appears to have been the first medical man in Australia to have taken a major and sustained interest in organic neurological disease, though he continued to practise as a general physician throughout his career. Details of his life have been obtained from his obituaries (Anonymous, 1923; Crago, 1923; Clayton, 1923) and the introductions to some of the lectures commemorating his memory which are given at intervals at meetings of the Royal Australasian College of Physicians.

Born in Sydney in 1861, educated at Sydney Grammar School and the University of Sydney, where he received a BA degree in 1882, Rennie went on to University College, London, to take medical qualifications (the University of Sydney at the time had no full medical course). In 1887 he became MB (London) and a Member of the Royal College of Surgeons. In the following year he was awarded a Doctorate of Medicine by the University of London.

After returning to Sydney in 1889 Rennie worked as a pathologist and physician, becoming Honorary Assistant Physician to the Royal Prince Alfred Hospital in 1894, and being appointed Honorary Physician to that institution four years later. However, in that same year he returned to London to take the Membership of the Royal College of Physicians (of which he later became a Fellow). When he returned to Sydney in 1900 he reverted to being an Honorary Assistant Physician at the Royal Prince Alfred Hospital. In 1906 he again became Honorary Physician to that hospital and was its Senior Physician from 1912 until 1921, when he retired under the age limit rules.

Throughout his consultant career Rennie's main professional interest appears to have been in clinical neurology, and he seems to have been regarded as the leading neurological opinion in the New South Wales of his time. There is a good deal of testimony concerning his abilities as a clinician and medical teacher. He seems to have been a man of integrity and honour who served his community well. For over a dozen years, as well as conducting his practice and working at his hospital, he edited the *Australasian Medical Gazette* whilst it grew from a monthly to a weekly journal, the major one in the Commonwealth of Australia until it was subsumed into the *Medical Journal of Australia* in 1914, when Rennie relinquished its editorship.

Over the years Rennie published a significant number of neurological papers. Some were essentially reports of unusual cases, e.g. exophthalmic goitre associated with myasthenia gravis – 1919) or of small case series, but several were significant reviews of important topics in the applied physiology of the nervous system. Thus he wrote, for example, on death after apparently minor head injuries (1895), the

Chapter 1 Australian Neurology in the Pre-neurologist Era

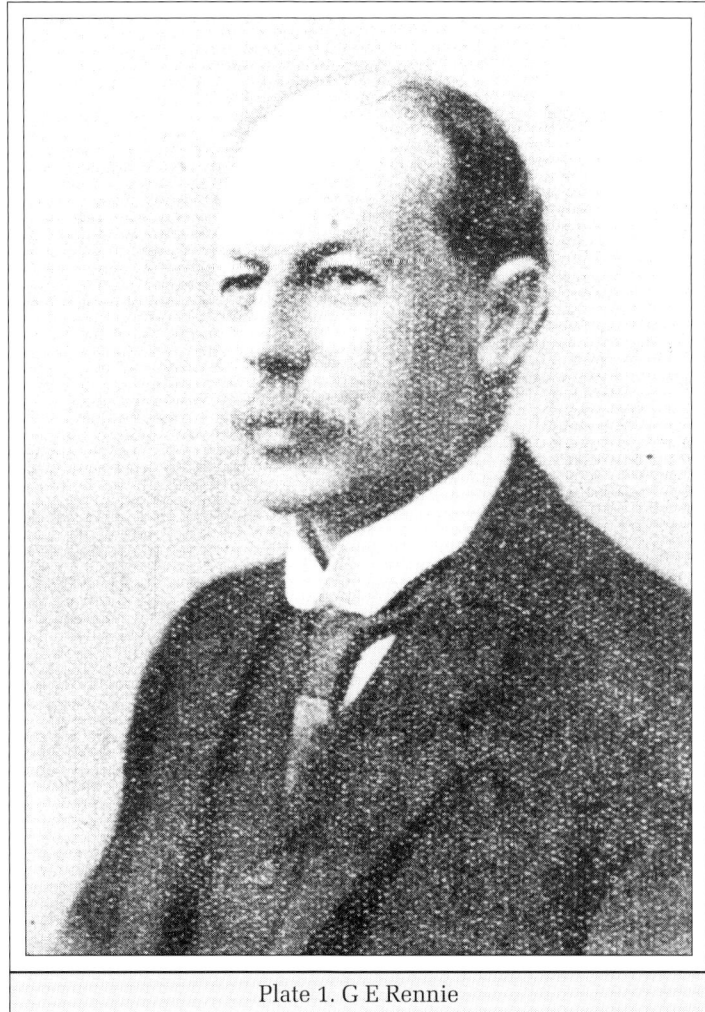

Plate 1. G E Rennie

functional anatomy of the cerebellum (1897), meralgia paraesthetica (1902), the physiology of voluntary movement (1903), the curability of epilepsy (1905a), the treatment of peripheral nerve diseases (1905b), the possibility of occupation and peripheral trauma determining the site of syphilitic cerebral pathology (1915), and the effects of spinal cord transection (1921). His discussion (Rennie, 1905b) of the possibilities of treating chronic neurological disorders revealed how limited the range of therapeutic options then was, largely comprising mercury and potassium iodide, and massage, exercise and electricity. There were also so-called 'nerve-tonics'. Curiously, he did not mention the use of bromide for epilepsy. Rennie's papers showed thorough familiarity with the then contemporary literature, and considerable ability to collate facts and to reason from them. However the papers contained no indication that Rennie had carried out any original investigative work, or that he had reasoned his way to new insights about the nervous system. There is every reason to infer from his publications that he would have been an excellent teacher of students, but great teachers are seldom remembered beyond the generations that they teach unless their teaching is perpetuated in some durable form and also continues to remain relevant.

Rennie's sustained publication record, and his practice interests, might allow one to argue that he was the first Australian neurologist. He had begun his professional activities in Australia a decade earlier than Campbell. However, throughout Rennie's career, and sometimes in the same volume of the journals in which he published his neurological writings, there appeared his papers on topics such as the open air treatment of acute pneumonia, tuberculosis, the ductless glands, deafness in children, and pernicious anaemia. This suggests that Rennie is better regarded as a physician with a strong neurological interest than as a man committed predominantly to neurology. There appears to be little evidence that his contributions to neuroscience would allow neurology to make any stronger claim for his inclusions in its ranks than this, meritorious though his life clearly was.

Sidney Sewell (1880–1949)

Sidney Sewell was born in Melbourne, educated at Caulfield Grammar School, and studied Medicine at the University of Melbourne from which he graduated MB ChB in 1906, subsequently taking that institution's MD in 1910 (White, 1949). After a period on the resident staff at the Melbourne Hospital, he spent a year with the pioneer neurosurgeon and neurophysiologist Sir Victor Horsley at University College Hospital in London and also worked at the National Hospital for Nervous Diseases at Queen Square, and with F W Mott. On his return to Melbourne he commenced practice in Collins Street, and over some months held an appointment as Honorary Neurologist to St Vincent's Hospital before becoming Outpatient Physician to the Melbourne Hospital. Early in his consultant career in Melbourne he gave postgraduate lectures in neurology and also lectured to medical students on the nervous system. He wrote on the effects of transverse lesions of the spinal cord on the bladder (Sewell, 1915). These activities led to his fairly rapidly building up a substantial neurological consultant practice. However, after the First World War, though he clearly retained his interest in neurology and was described as Neurologist to the Base Hospital in St Kilda Rd, Melbourne (Sewell, 1920), he became very concerned about the welfare of sufferers from pulmonary tuberculosis and devoted considerable energy to advancing their cause. Nevertheless, he returned to a neurological theme, the localisation of function in the cerebrum, in his Listerian Oration (Sewell, 1937). Sewell also became involved in the activities of the Association of Physicians, and was a major driving force in that body's developing into the Royal Australasian College of Physicians, of which he was to become the second President. His example was a significant factor in Graeme Robertson's taking up of neurology. Sewell was knighted four years before his death.

Chapter 1 Australian Neurology in the Pre-neurologist Era

Sewell's professional interests ranged well beyond neurology, and history would probably regard his main achievements as being in relation to the foundation of the Royal Australasian College of Physicians and the development of tuberculosis services in Victoria. Nonetheless, his own example and his endeavour to advance Graeme Robertson's career were significant factors in getting neurology underway as a specialty in Australia.

Henry Fitzgerald Maudsley (1891–1962)

Maudsley came from a distinguished medical lineage, his father being a knighted Melbourne physician who, in 1906, had published a detailed interpretation of what probably was red nuclear tremor (Maudsley, 1906), though he seemed unaware of Gordon Holmes' then recent work (1904) concerning the phenomenon. The younger Henry Maudsley was educated at Melbourne Grammar School and the University of Melbourne, graduating MB BS from the latter in 1915. He served in the Army during World War I, and took the Melbourne MD in 1920 before going to London where he passed the Membership of the Royal College of Physicians and the Diploma of Psychological Medicine. During the inter-war years he was Honorary Physician in Charge of the Neurology and Psychiatry Clinic at the Melbourne Hospital, and Honorary Neurologist to the Victorian Eye and Ear Hospital. He became a Fellow of the London College of Physicians in 1937 and a Foundation Fellow of the Australasian College of Physicians in the following year. During World War II he was consultant in Psychiatry to the Australian Army.

Although by all accounts Maudsley was competent in neurology, his main professional activity was in the field of psychiatry, and he was the chief founder of the Royal Australian and New Zealand College of Psychiatrists, of which he was elected President on two occasions. He did not publish a great deal in connection with neurology, though his name often appeared among the discussants at the neurological presentations in Melbourne which were recorded in the pages of the *Medical Journal of Australia*. He wrote in that journal on ocular signs in neurological diagnosis (1928), and on the consequences of encephalitis lethargica (1926). It seems possible that Maudsley's neurological abilities were a factor which delayed for some years the appointment of a dedicated neurologist at the Melbourne Hospital.

J Froude Flashman (1870–1917)

In Sydney around the end of the first decade of the 20th century, whilst Campbell was practising as a neurologist, and George Rennie as a physician and neurologist, a third man appears to have entered the practice of neurology, though only for a short period. The advent of World War I, and premature death in it, cut short that man's neurological career. However, the evidence of his publications, and the testimony of the unnamed writer of one of his obituaries, leave little doubt that

James Froude Flashman was a man of considerable talent and organising ability, a productive neuroscientist and a capable clinician. Had he returned from war service, who knows how Australian clinical neuroscience might have developed under his leadership, if his obvious gifts in that direction had not been seduced by circumstances into some other direction of professional life.

Flashman was born at Braidwood in New South Wales in 1870, and took, consecutively, first level degrees in Arts, Science and in Medicine from the University of Sydney, the latter degree in 1894, and then proceeded to a Doctorate in Medicine in 1897 (Anonymous, 1917). Near the end of his life he took the Membership of the Royal College of Physicians of London whilst serving in Britain with the Australian Army Medical Corps. This latter fact indicates his interest in continuing the clinical side of his career. Much of Flashman's professional life was spent in the service of the Lunacy Department of the State of New South Wales. Over much of his career his major interest lay in pathology. In 1900 he became the first director of the Pathology Laboratory of the State Lunacy Department, whose sympathies clearly lay in the biological rather than the psychodynamic approach to psychiatry. Flashman arranged for the laboratory to be sited in the Medical School of the University of Sydney and there he, and Oliver Latham, carried out various neuropathological and clinical pathological investigations into the basis of insanity. They combined to publish the first account of pathologically confirmed multiple sclerosis in Australia (Flashman and Latham, 1915). Flashman also worked on the comparative anatomy of the brain of the Australian aboriginal, though these particular studies were never completed. He instituted serological testing for syphilis – the old Wasserman reaction – in the inhabitants of the various institutions for the mentally retarded in New South Wales and published on this and various other clinical pathological topics, as well as on morphological pathological matters. Latham (1934), in his Beattie Smith Lectures, almost incidentally listed Flashman's published work (including some that is not readily accessible) and his investigational interests. For a time Flashman acted as a locum tenens for the Professor of Pathology at Sydney University, and in 1910 he entered private practice in neurology and pathology in Sydney to better provide for the future of his family. He enlisted in the Army in 1915 and, with the rank of Lieutenant-Colonel, was sent to England. There he showed great foresight and organising ability in setting up arrangements and facilities for the care of the Australian wounded from the battlefields of France. Those who wrote his obituaries (MacLaurin, 1917; Mills, 1917) concentrated heavily on this aspect of his career, perhaps in part reflecting the preoccupation at that time of men who were serving in a war. Nonetheless, it would seem that Flashman had made a very major contribution to the care of the Australian wounded, and that not enough time had elapsed for this to be officially acknowledged before death from pneumonia carried him off at Boulogne, in France, on 12 February 1917.

How much clinical neurology J Froude Flashman had practised in Australia, and what impact he had on that specialty, are not clear, partly because of the brevity of his time in its practice. Certainly he deserves some mention in the record of the development of Australian neuroscience. Reading his obituary leaves one with a sense of regret for what might have been.

Oliver Latham (1877–1974)

Despite his being a well known figure in Australian clinical neuroscience over more that half a century, details of Latham's career are now hard to obtain. The difficulty seems to arise because he outlived not only his own generation but most of the succeeding one, so that by the time he died there was no one to write his obituary whose knowledge of him spanned his whole career. In particular, his quite extensive publication record went almost completely unmentioned in the available accounts.

Latham was born in Dublin and educated there and at Harrow, where Winston Churchill was also a boy at the same time (Noad, 1975). Latham graduated in Medicine from the University of Sydney in 1903, and soon joined Flashman in the Pathology Laboratory of the State Lunacy Department, where he continued to spend his entire professional life. He seems to have been known as a learned and well liked man whose life was devoted to the morphological neuropathology that was so important in his time. During his career he published on a considerable variety of topics, often in the form of case reports to which he added detailed and beautifully illustrated neuropathological descriptions, but there were also studies on histological methodology and on clinical pathology. In the pages of the Australian medical journals of his time one can find his name associated with topics such as the Wasserman reaction in mental hospital patients, modification of the Widal test, methods for estimating glucose in urine and test meals in the insane, as well as more formal neuropathology topics as diverse as glial biology (1926), Friedreich's ataxia (Litchfield et al., 1917), the various encephalitides (Hogg and Latham, 1923; Latham 1922, 1927, 1930, 1931), encephalomyelitis (Dawson and Latham, 1931), dementia and other disturbances related to cerebral tumour (Wallace and Latham, 1914; Nowland et al., 1924), multiple sclerosis (Flashman and Latham, 1915), Australian 'X' disease (Mathewson and Latham, 1917), the general pathology of the cerebellum (Latham, 1941), cerebello-olivary atrophy (Hall et al., 1945), olivo-ponto-cerebellar atrophy (Lambie et al., 1947), cerebellar degeneration with epilepsy (Minogue and Latham, 1945), cerebellar laminar degeneration (Hagen et al., 1951), haematomyelia (Latham, 1939), the reactions of the small calibre cerebral blood vessels (Latham, 1938), acute haemorrhagic encephalomyelitis (Shallard and Latham, 1945), dementia praecox (Dawson and Latham, 1943), and Alzheimer's disease (Edwards and Latham, 1943; Himmelhoch et al., 1947). He also carried out the studies on muscle histology mentioned earlier in this chapter in collaboration with John Irvine Hunter in the Anatomy Department at the University of Sydney (Hunter and Latham, 1925). On occasions Latham also provided the pathology reports appended to various published case studies, e.g. Mathewson and Latham (1921), Blackburn and Latham (1922), Hogg and Latham (1923) and Bell and

Latham (1928). His 1934 Beattie-Smith Lectures incorporated his vast experience of diverse types of morphological neuropathology, and reveal something of his professional activities over the course of a third of a century. During his long career his publications in the pages of the *Medical Journal of Australia* covered a great deal of the recognised range of morphological neuropathology.

Latham may not have done a great deal of original experimental work in his lifetime, but that seems to have been the norm for a neuropathologist of his day. He constituted the main source of the pathological knowledge and experience which underpinned Australian clinical neurology for half a century. Clearly, it was he who, more than anyone else, carried Australian neuropathology forward from almost its earliest times to the emergence of the Australian Association of Neurologists, of which he was elected an Honorary Member in 1951, one year after the Association itself was founded.

Chapter 2

A W Campbell: Australia's First Neurologist

As mentioned in the Introduction, Alfred Walter Campbell's career and achievements in the international neurological science of his day constitute the major exception to the generalisation that, prior to the threshold of the Second World War, Australian contributions to the accumulating corpus of international neurological knowledge came from those who were not professional neurologists.

Campbell's life

Campbell's career was described in some detail in the obituaries produced by his friend and physician L R Parker and by Professor W S Dawson, both published in the *Medical Journal of Australia* of 22 January 1938. Further information appeared in a later obituary written by John Farquhar Fulton in the American Medical Association's *Archives of Neurology and Psychiatry* (1938). The fact that this eminent Yale neurophysiologist, who was Cushing's biographer, was motivated to write of Campbell as he did gives some indication of the latter's standing more that three decades after he had disappeared from the world stage. Some additional biographical material and his photograph (Plate 2) became available as the outcome of a personal communication from Mrs Veda Hope, Campbell's elder daughter.

Alfred Walter Campbell was the son of a pastoralist, David Henry Campbell, and his wife Amelia, nee Breillat. He was born on 18 January 1868 at his parents' station at Cunningham Plains, near Harden, in New South Wales. His primary education took place at Oakland School, near Mittagong, where his headmaster was the son of Robert Southey, the English poet. Campbell apparently determined on a medical career only three years after the University of Sydney had opened its Medical School and before it had produced the first graduates from its own medical course, though the University of Melbourne had already done so, a few years earlier (Young *et al.*, 1984). At the age of 18 Campbell therefore followed a rather common practice among aspiring Australian medical practitioners of the time, and entered the

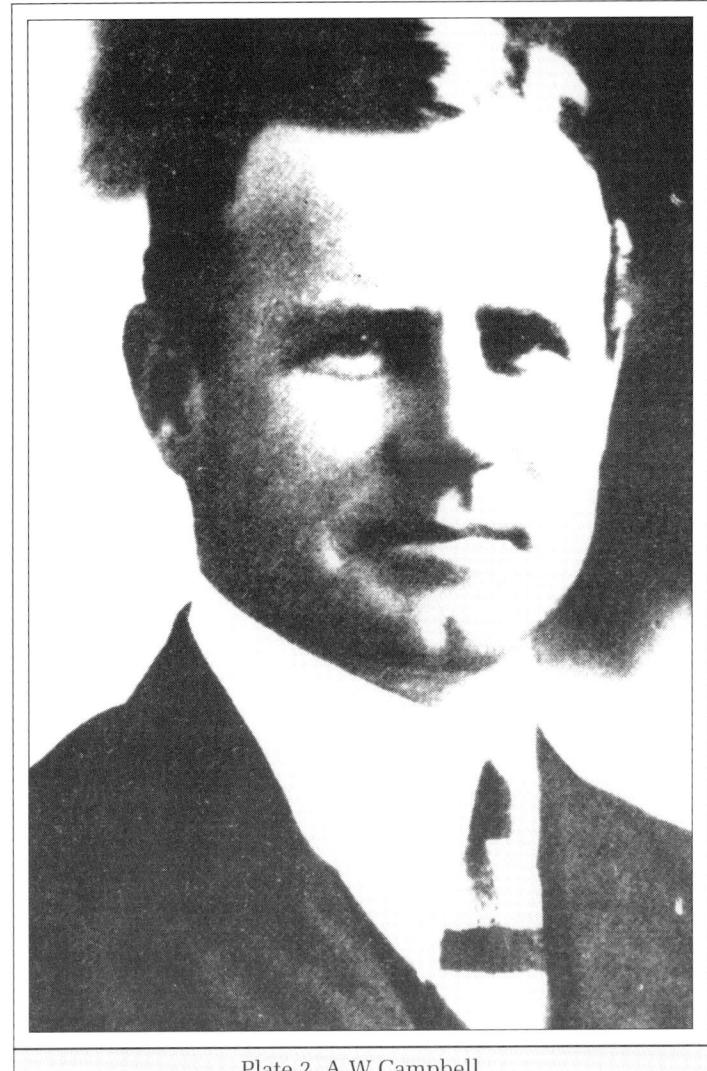

Plate 2. A W Campbell

University of Edinburgh as a medical student. Four years later, in 1889, he graduated, taking the degrees MB, ChM, with honours. During his time in Scotland, Campbell appears to have been a rather considerable sportsman. He captained both the cricket and the football teams at Edinburgh University. After graduation he worked as an assistant in several British mental hospitals. He also seems to have attended the ward practice at the National Hospital for Nervous Diseases, Queen Square, London. There he had some contact as 'a newly fledged graduate and ward follower' with John Hughlings Jackson, whose genius he recognised and to which he paid tribute long afterwards, near the end of his own life (Campbell, 1935).

Chapter 2 A W Campbell: Australia's First Neurologist

Campbell then proceeded to further his neurological studies in Europe, working for a time as assistant to Krafft-Ebing in Vienna. Afterwards he became a member of the staff of the State Asylum in Prague. He returned to England in 1892 and, at the age of 24, his thesis entitled *The Pathology of Alcoholic Insanity* was awarded the degree Doctor of Medicine of the University of Edinburgh with high commendation, and a University gold medal. Campbell was appointed Resident Medical Officer and Director of the Pathology Laboratory at the Rainhill Asylum, Liverpool and remained in that position till 1905. Over those 13 years in Liverpool he conducted the series of investigations which brought him recognition as one of the foremost neurohistologists and neuropathologists in the world. In his obituary of Campbell, Parker (1938) stated that his laboratories 'became a place of visitation and study by specialists from all parts of the world'.

In 1904 Campbell applied for the post of Inspector-General of the Insane in Victoria, but withdrew his application when he knew that there was a local contender for the post. A year later, at the age of 37, and having lived overseas for a little more than half his life, he finally returned to Australia, to reside in Sydney. There he commenced practice as a specialist in neurology and mental diseases, though he described himself as a neurologist. He occupied rooms at 183 Macquarie Street for over 30 years until he retired in 1937. During this period he was appointed Honorary Neurologist to the Royal Alexandra Hospital for Children, the Coast Hospital and the Department of Repatriation, though not to the longer established and more prestigious Sydney and Royal Prince Alfred Hospitals. There is evidence from the contents of the *Medical Journal of Australia* over some three decades that he played a significant part in the local medical affairs of the day, particularly as they related to neurology and, to a much lesser extent, psychiatry. Over a number of years he was responsible for the selection from the international literature of the Abstracts on Neurology and Psychiatry which were a regular feature of the issues of the *Medical Journal of Australia* of those times.

One year after returning to Australia, Campbell had married Jenny Mackay, a childhood friend who had been brought up on 'Wallen Been', the pastoral holding adjoining that on which Campbell had spent his youth. According to Campbell's daughter, Mrs Veda Hope, Campbell's future wife and her mother had spent a considerable amount of time overseas and presumably had seen something of Campbell in Britain. The newly married couple went to live at 'Wallendoon', Rose Bay, Sydney, and had two children, both daughters. At the age of 46, at the commencement of the 1914–1918 War, Campbell enlisted in the AIF and served with the Army in Egypt with the rank of Major before returning to Australia, where he continued in clinical practice till 1937. His health then began to fail, and he died on 4 November 1937 from cancer which, judging from Parker's obituary, probably had spread to involve his central nervous system.

Campbell's personal characteristics are probably of some importance to any attempt to understand the pattern of his life. He was described as saying relatively little, though his diction was careful and his words well-chosen. He was fluent in French,

German and Italian. Those who wrote or spoke of him on a basis of personal experience seem generally agreed that he was a rather reserved man. His daughter said that he was 'frightfully shy and reserved and loathed publicity'. Parker mentioned how Campbell once said that he could not have borne to be a teacher because:

> 'It would have taken too much out of me, the constant dread that I should leave something out, or say something which might not be true.'

Campbell's scientific career

Campbell's career in neurology fell into two reasonably clear-cut parts – the European, mainly Liverpool, years between 1889 and 1905, during which he did nearly all of the scientific work on which his international fame was based, and the Sydney years from 1905 to 1937 in which his main activity appeared to be that of a clinical neurologist.

The European years

After his early studies on *The Pathology of Alcoholic Insanity*, which gained for him a doctorate from the University of Edinburgh in 1892, Campbell worked on various neuropathological subjects. In 1894, no less than three major papers appeared under his authorship, as well as several more minor works. In the *British Medical Journal*, forming one of a pair with a paper by the London neurologist J S Risien Russell, Campbell (1894a) provided a detailed description of the tract degenerations consequent on local lesions of the human cerebellum. For this work he had studied five cases of recent thrombotic, embolic or haemorrhagic softening of the cerebellum, and had followed the resultant tract degeneration in serial sections of the brain stem and spinal cord which he had stained by the Marchi technique. The *Journal of Mental Science* published his prize-winning essay *A Contribution to the Morbid Anatomy and Pathology of the Neuro-muscular Changes in General Paresis of the Insane*. In this paper (Campbell, 1894b) he described peripheral nerve changes in 12 cases of general paresis of the insane. Campbell's third major paper for the year (Campbell, 1894c) was entitled *On Vacuolation of the Nerve Cell of the Human Cerebral Cortex*, and was published in the *Journal of Pathology and Bacteriology*. This study was based on the histological examination of the brains of 47 cases of pulmonary tuberculosis and 13 cases of acute lobar pneumonia. Vacuolation, which was present in cortical neurons in nearly all these brains, was considered by Campbell to be a toxaemic phenomenon.

> '.... with so much positive and direct evidence, is one, therefore, not justified in concluding that, in the case of the highly organised cortical nerve cell, so intrinsically dependent on a pure and untainted supply of blood for its healthy maintenance, such a harassing factor as toxaemia must not only play a most important pathogenic role, but actually induces the remarkable vacuolatory change in all these conditions.'

In that prolific year, papers also appeared on changes in the senile brain, on thrombosis of the inferior cerebellar artery and on the breaking strain of the ribs of the insane. Thereafter, Campbell continued to produce work on a range of neuropathological topics, and some non-neurological ones (e.g. acute pancreatitis, dysentery). As well, there were publications dealing with neuropathological technique (the use of formic aldehyde in the laboratory), spinal heterotopias, disseminated sclerosis, amyotrophic lateral sclerosis, the relationship between syphilis and general paresis of the insane, the anatomy and pathology of the pineal, the histology of cerebral tumours, and the effects of pernicious anaemia on the nervous system. It was a wide ranging coverage of neuropathological territory, culminating in 1897 in a learned and detailed review *On the Tracts of the Spinal Cord and Their Degeneration*, which was published in the journal *Brain*.

In 1900 Henry (subsequently Sir Henry) Head's great work on the dermatomes appeared, also in *Brain*. The title was *The Pathology of Herpes Zoster and its Bearing on Sensory Localisation,* and Head's co-author was Campbell, though the latter's role in this investigation is sometimes passed over whilst Head's is remembered. The paper comprised a lengthy (170 pages) correlation of Head's clinical observations with Campbell's 21 autopsy studies. It remains one of the chief sources of our knowledge of the distribution of the dermatomes in humans.

As judged from his publication record, from 1900 onwards, Campbell's interests appear to have been increasingly focused on the anatomy and pathology of the cerebral cortex. In 1895 Charles Scott Sherrington had been appointed as Holt Professor of Physiology in the University of Liverpool. In 1901, Sherrington's studies on the physiology of the cerebral cortex in higher apes appeared. Campbell subsequently examined the brains of Sherrington's animals. This material formed part of his own investigation of cerebral cortical architecture. Campbell set down his reasons for undertaking his study of the microscopic structure of the cerebral cortex when he wrote:

> 'Particularly do I hope that those who, like myself, have pledged their energies to the apparently hopeless task of elucidating problems connected with mental disease will derive benefit from this research for it was only after several valuable years had been spent in the cause of scientific research in a laboratory attached to an asylum for the insane that I recognised that it was necessary for some worker to begin at the beginning, and attempt to piece together our disjointed knowledge of the cortex ... .'

For his investigation of the microscopic organisation of the cerebral cortex Campbell cut three complete normal human cerebral hemispheres into approximately 50 blocks, and embedded them in celloidin. A 25-micron-thick section was cut every millimetre through each whole hemisphere. Alternate serial sections were stained for myelinated fibres by the Wolters-Kulschitzky technique and for cell-bodies, by means of thionin. The examination of each individual hemisphere occupied Campbell for six months. Three further normal complete hemispheres were cut in serial section and stained for nerve fibres only, whilst parts of another two normal hemispheres were cut in serial section and stained for both nerve cells and fibres. Campbell also cut in serial section the relevant regions of cerebral cortex from two cases of amyotrophic lateral sclerosis, three cases of tabes dorsalis, one case of internal capsule infarction, two cases of long-standing blindness and from seven patients who had amputations of an extremity at least two years previously. The cerebral hemispheres of two chimpanzee and one orang monkey, and those of a cat, a dog and a pig were also studied in detail, employing the same meticulous neuroanatomical techniques. All of this enormous collection of material was examined microscopically, an undertaking which must have involved prodigious labour and the expenditure of a vast amount of time. Hand drawings were made of the sections with the aid of a special eyepiece, because the then available photographic techniques could not adequately display each individual section in its entirety.

On the basis of his examination of this material, Campbell considered himself justified in dividing the human cerebral cortex into some 12 major areas on histological grounds. He correlated these areas with what evidence of localisation of function he could derive from knowledge of comparative anatomy, experimental physiology and the consequences of human disease. His thinking was not purely in terms of morphology at a microscopic level, but sought to correlate neurohistology with localisation of function.

Sherrington communicated the outcome of Campbell's great investigation to the Royal Society in 1903, and it was published in an abstract in the Society's Proceedings (Campbell, 1903). However, the work, *in toto*, was regarded as too extensive for publication in the *Philosophical Transactions of the Royal Society*. Instead Sherrington, who had already become influential in the councils of the Society of which he was later to become President, obtained a grant from the Society which allowed the work to appear in 1905 as a separate monograph under the insignia of the Cambridge University Press. It was titled *Histological Studies of the Localisation of Cerebral Function*, and comprised 360 pages of 11.5 inch by 9 inch dimension, with 29 whole page plates. Before the book was available in print, Campbell had resigned his post in Liverpool and returned to Australia.

The Sydney years

Some additional papers on cerebral anatomy and pathology appeared in 1905, the year of Campbell's return to Australia. These (on the homologies of the Rolandic region, on the brain of the cat compared with that of man, on cerebral sclerosis and on cortical localisation) were probably the results of work already carried out in Britain. Thereafter, as judged from the list of his 66 publications and presentations appended to his obituary which appeared in the *Medical Journal of Australia*, Campbell's research output seemed to cease for several years. However, there is good evidence that this was not the case. Despite the distractions of establishing himself in consultant practice and bringing up two young children, Campbell continued to do original investigational work during his first few years back in his homeland. The list of publications in Campbell's obituary is incomplete, at least for the period in question. It omitted papers on the labyrinth (1924a), and on the injection of alcohol into the trigeminal nerve and various of its branches for the relief of trigeminal neuralgia (1910), a technique he had learned in Paris from Ostwalt.

Much more importantly, in the *Transactions of the Ninth Australasian Medical Congress* held in Sydney in 1911 there is a description of a very considerable piece of Campbell's research which must have involved the expenditure of considerable time and effort (Campbell, 1911). It was one which went unmentioned in his obituary and which seems to have escaped notice elsewhere. The publication's title was *On the Localisation of Function in the Cerebellum*. Bolk, of Amsterdam, had made use of a principle employed by Thomas Willis in his *De Anima Brutorum* (1683) and had drawn deductions about the function of parts of the cerebellum by correlating their degrees of development in different animal species with the capacities of these species to carry out certain motor activities. On this basis Bolk had assigned responsibility for various parts of the body to particular areas of the cerebellum. Campbell had taken this type of approach further in an exhaustive anatomical and histological study of the cerebellum of the frog, lizard, albatross, turkey, platypus, native-cat, wallaby, rabbit, cat, dog, pig, gorilla, and man. It was a natural sequel to his work on the cytoarchitectonics of the cerebral cortex. As far as can be ascertained, this extensive investigation carried out by Campbell was never published except in the *Transactions* of what would have been regarded as a relatively obscure colonial medical society. For this reason the study probably escaped the international notice that had greeted Campbell's work on the cerebral cortex. None of Campbell's obituarists, including Fulton, mentioned the work on the cerebellum, yet its validity and worth are incontestable. Gordon Holmes in his 1922 Croonian Lectures on the cerebellum (Holmes, 1956) devoted considerable space to refuting Bolk's views, but seemed quite unaware that Campbell a decade earlier had arrived at and published a similar conclusion. Campbell's fellow Australian, Abbie (1941), in discussing the lack of validity of Bolk's deductions about localisation of function in the cerebellum, made no reference at all to Campbell's work on the topic. Campbell put the matter of localisation of function in the cerebellum thus:

> 'My conclusion, therefore, from an impartial consideration of all the evidence is that the surface of the cerebellum cannot be cut up into functional territories. I would subscribe to the belief that the cortex of the cerebellum subserves a function which is sensory in kind. I would regard it as a general receiving station for impressions from muscles, bones, and joints, and from the vestibulum. It is my belief that these impressions are not delivered at special stations, but are diffusely distributed in the cortex of each homolateral hemisphere. From the cortex these impressions are transferred to the intrinsic nuclei from which the efferent tracts lead to other parts of the nervous system, and thence again to the muscles, &c. So a great reflex arc is completed, the function of which is to regulate and co-ordinate movement.'

Admittedly the outcome of Campbell's extensive investigation was a negative one, but it was nonetheless important. Regrettably, Campbell appears not to have been a man to put himself forward, and on this occasion there was no Sherrington to ensure that the results of the investigation were published where they would be noticed. Thus a great study seems to have wasted its sweetness on the desert air of a former British colony remote from the centres of Northern Hemisphere medical thought.

Campbell described a case of syringomyelia in the *Australasian Medical Gazette* in 1913, and gave an account of his examination of the gorilla brain in 1916 which was published in a relatively inaccessible report. In that same year he wrote on his experience of neurosis and psychosis under the stress of war (Campbell, 1916). There was a case report of Friedreich's ataxia in the *Medical Journal of Australia* in 1917 (Litchfield *et al.*), one on probable myotonia congenita in that same journal in 1919 and one with N Dowling on nervous or hysterical fever in 1920. Campbell collaborated with J B Cleland, later Professor of Pathology in the University of Adelaide, in a series of investigations into the transmission of the poliomyelitis virus in 1918 (Campbell *et al.*, 1918), and into the aetiology and pathology of Australian 'X' disease (as mentioned in Chapter 1). They defined the pathology of that condition, and demonstrated very clearly that it was not an aberrant form of poliomyelitis (as had been suggested by Breinl in 1918) but was a novel type of encephalitis. These investigations were published in stages in the *Medical Journal of Australia* between 1918 and 1920, with a final major review paper in the *Journal of Hygiene* in 1920, and a report of the epidemic in the 1920 *Proceedings of the Royal Society of Medicine*. After this, Campbell published no further scientific work, though he contributed to the clinical neurological literature from time to time in his latter years, dealing with topics such as cerebral palsy (Campbell, 1924b), childhood epilepsy (Campbell, 1927a), nervous disease in childhood (Campbell, 1927b), ocular signs in neurological diagnosis (Campbell, 1928b), cerebrospinal syphilis (Campbell, 1930), affections of peripheral nerves (Campbell, 1931), the nervous child (Campbell, 1933a) and the treatment of migraine (Campbell, 1933b). Near the end of his life, in 1935, he produced a gracious account of the life and achievements of John Hughlings Jackson, whom he appears to have long admired (Campbell, 1935).

The significance of Campbell's neuroscience

Campbell's range of investigations over the years covered a goodly part of the territory of classical neuropathology. Much of the work was descriptive, but that does not detract from its value at a time when the corpus of available knowledge in the area was not as great as it now is. And underlying a deal of it was a concern for reconciling morphology with normal and with disordered function. It was his investigation of the dermatomes carried out in conjunction with Henry Head, and even more so his study of the cytoarchitectonics of the cerebral cortex, on which Campbell's reputation rests. His only real rival as a contributor to knowledge of the neuronal arrangements in the cerebral cortex was Korbinian Brodman, and at least some authorities preferred to accept Campbell's views of the matter.

Nearly a century after its publication, the validity of Campbell's great work on cerebral cytoarchitectonics stands unchallenged. His drawings of cerebral cortical histology still appear in textbooks of neuroanatomy. In his obituary of Campbell which appeared in the *Archives of Neurology and Psychiatry* (1938), John Farquhar Fulton, Sterling Professor of Physiology at Yale, paid a great tribute to a man who had long faded from the sight of the international scientific community by quoting the words of Lorente de Nó.

> 'The only really good cytoarchitectonic pictures are those of Campbell, who – let me put it in capital letters – HAS BEEN THE ONLY CYTOARCHITECTONIST WHO HAS DESCRIBED FACTS AND ONLY FACTS. The German cytoarchitectonist has mixed facts with theory in such a manner that nobody can tell where facts end and theories begin. I must say that there are perhaps no more than a dozen photographs out of hundreds in which the layers of the cortex have been properly and consistently labelled. On the other hand Campbell's ink drawings, besides being good, are easily reproduced.'

Von Bonin (1970) assessed the value of Campbell's work thus:

> 'Campbell's subdivisions of the primate cortex were not as fine as those of the German school, but modern architectonics has time and again decided in favour of his sober views'.

When Webb Haymaker and Francis Schiller collected the biographies of those whom they regarded as the greatest 146 neurologists and neurological scientists of the past and published them in the most recent edition of *The Founders of Neurology* (1970), there were only two Australians included. Both were contemporaries, and both were New South Welshmen. One was Grafton Elliot Smith (1871–1937), who graduated in Medicine from the University of Sydney, but spent almost all the remainder of his life in Egypt and England, studying the comparative anatomy and evolution of the nervous system. The second Australian was Alfred Walter Campbell. When one considers the magnitude of Campbell's achievements in relation to the level of knowledge, the opportunities and the career expectations of the neuroscientists of his day, it is difficult to quarrel with Haymaker and Schiller's assessment. Moreover, it was a judgement that apparently was made in ignorance of Campbell's study of the comparative anatomy of the cerebellar cortex.

It could, of course, be argued that a substantial part of Campbell's original neuroscience, and that part of it which was of the greatest importance to posterity, was not carried out in Australia, and therefore should not be considered a contribution made by Australian neurology. Clearly there is some force in that argument, and the decision about the matter is left to the reader. Nonetheless, Campbell did live out his early life in Australia, served his country in a War, and in his homeland practised as a neurologist and carried out further neuroscientific work over more than three decades, including a great study of the cerebellar cortex which, had it become known internationally, must have enhanced the reputation of Australian neuroscience.

Campbell as a clinician

In practising clinical neurology in Australia nearly a century ago, Campbell was in many ways a man before his time. He had almost no local colleagues with similar interests with whom he could discuss matters or compare professional standards, and for the most part he had to depend on medical journals for contemporary information about neuroscience. For much of Campbell's period in practice, neurology was an almost entirely clinical art with plain skull radiography and cerebrospinal fluid examination as the only relevant ancillary investigations. By the close of his career ventriculography and pneumoencephalography had become available, but Campbell must have had to attempt to achieve diagnosis by purely clinical means throughout nearly all of his life in clinical practice. As well, neurological therapeutics were distinctly limited at the time. Campbell probably had not received as extensive a clinical neurological training as might have been desirable for the situation in which he placed himself, though his neuropathological knowledge would have been extraordinarily profound even by today's standards. From what can be gleaned, Campbell's contemporaries and juniors seemed to have sensed that his clinical performance fell somewhat short of their expectations. Whether what they hoped for was realistic in the circumstances and whether the limitations were his or theirs, or largely reflected the thoughts of their seniors, are other questions. After the lapse of more than half a century, the late Sir Kenneth Noad recalled Campbell sometimes writing 'NYD' (not yet diagnosed) on the hospital records of children with obscure neurological illnesses, though Noad commented that Campbell took the histories of children with neurological illnesses in meticulous detail, though his physical examinations were perhaps more brief. Reading Campbell's clinical writings long afterwards gives the impression that they were the product of a judicious, well-informed and humane physician.

It could have been that Campbell's reticence and scrupulous intellectual honesty combined to prevent his being adept at the art of showmanship, to which neurological practice can prove so well suited. Possibly this, and the inescapable diagnostic limitations of the times, prevented his example from persuading a younger generation of Australians to enter neurology. Campbell left behind him no clinical disciples, and he fathered no Australian school of clinical neurology, despite his apparently outstanding qualifications for doing so. His circumstances, and possibly his retiring personality, may have conspired against him, but that is no criticism of the merits of the man, or of the enduring greatness of his original contributions to neuroscience.

Chapter 2 A W Campbell: Australia's First Neurologist

Campbell – an overview

From an overall point of view, Campbell's career was earlier interpreted on one occasion (Eadie, 1981) as presenting the paradox of a wonderful early scientific flowering which was abruptly and seemingly volitionally cut short, with a brief blooming again, many years later. Subsequent recognition of the existence of his largely unnoticed investigation of the cerebellum invalidates this view. Rather, interpretation now yields the impression of a profuse early flowering which gradually withered with time and relative scientific isolation, the original science gradually being replaced by a mixture of investigational and clinical practice, though the latter did not have quite the impact on his juniors that might have been expected.

But the question still remains as to why the collaborator of Henry Head and the protege of the great Sherrington chose to return to the former colony he apparently had not seen for almost 20 years, and there took up a new, seemingly less intellectually stimulating and satisfactory pattern of professional life? The available written records provide no adequate reason, and in later life it appears that Campbell gave some wistful hints that he would have preferred to remain more heavily involved in scientific work. One might speculate about all manner of possibilities, but the simple answer may lie in the fact that Campbell married a fellow countryman, and their family and financial interests lay in Australia. Campbell, with his sense of responsibility, may have believed that the post he occupied in Britain, whatever the prospects it held for his personal scientific advancement, would not enable him to keep his future wife in the style to which she was accustomed, for she had been able to travel extensively for some years before the marriage. A return to Australia, and clinical practice in that country in a major city, near the family properties (but not on them, for his daughter said her mother hated country life), may have offered much more realistic financial and lifestyle possibilities. If this was the basis of the decision, Campbell's failure to seek some appointment which would have enabled him to carry out neuropathological and neuroanatomical work in Australia still needs explanation. Campbell appears to have been a reticent man and showed himself reluctant to compete against a local applicant for a post in Victoria for which he was well qualified and exceptionally strongly recommended. Therefore one may suspect that when he returned to Sydney and found Flashman and Oliver Latham already ensconced in neuropathology posts in the Mental Health Service in Sydney he again chose to keep at a distance from a situation in which tensions might have arisen, and in which he might have disadvantaged someone else. As it happened, Latham long outlived Campbell and continued to work in neuropathology, so that there was no place for a formal appointment in the specialty in Sydney for Campbell.

Paradoxically, as its first practising neurological clinician Campbell seemed to have had relatively little enduring influence on the course of Australian neurology, yet when his original achievements are set in relation to the circumstances of his times he must stand as arguably the greatest neuroscientist his country ever produced.

Chapter 3

The Founding Generation of Australian Neurologists

As Walter Campbell's career in Sydney drew to its close, and no disciple or successor to his role emerged in that city, another man, Leonard Bell Cox, began to practise in Melbourne as a clinical neurologist. Like Campbell, his career was intertwined to a considerable extent with neuropathology, and his very considerable original achievements lay in this area. As early as 1934, Cox received formal appointment as an Honorary Neurologist to a Victorian teaching hospital, the Alfred Hospital, where his brother-in-law, Hugh Trumble, set about developing the specialty of neurosurgery. In that same year another Melbourne graduate, Edward Graeme Robertson, returned to his home city after several years of clinical neurological training in London, where he had occupied junior consultant posts in neurology at St Bartholomew's Hospital and the Postgraduate Teaching School at Hammersmith. Robertson practised clinically as a neurologist in Melbourne, but his formal appointment at the Royal Melbourne Hospital was that of Honorary Physician to Outpatients. It was to be several years before he was to be accorded the title of Honorary Neurologist to the (Royal) Melbourne Hospital, and to the Children's Hospital. Thus in the years just prior to the outbreak of the Second World War, at a time when the only neurologist practising in Sydney was near the end of his career, two men in Melbourne had begun to practise purely in clinical neurology. In Sydney, at the same time there were then practising two younger general physicians with strong interests in clinical neurology. However, neither of these men ever restricted his practice purely to the specialty. K B Noad was Physician to Sydney Hospital and E L Susman Physician to the Royal Prince Alfred Hospital. In Perth, Gerald Moss, despite appointment as an Honorary Physician to the Royal Perth Hospital, in private practised predominantly, though not exclusively, as a neurologist. At the time, there were no medical practitioners in the other State capital cities of the Commonwealth of Australia who practised purely, or even mainly, in clinical neurology. Thus, at the eve of World War II, there were practising in the whole of Australia two full-time clinical neurologists and three physicians with major neurological interests. Campbell had died shortly before.

It should be mentioned for completeness that there was another man apart from Leonard Cox and Graeme Robertson who practised in Melbourne as a neurologist for a short period after 1939. This man was the Austrian émigré Arthur Schüller.

Arthur Schüller (1874–1957)

Schüller had been born in Czechoslovakia as long before as 1874. He had graduated in Medicine from the University of Vienna in 1895, and had been involved in the specialty of radiology almost from its time of origin. Schüller had been appointed Professor in that subject in the University of Vienna in 1909. He retained his Chair until 1938, when he and his wife fled Nazism in Austria. By 1939 they had made their way to Australia, leaving behind all their possessions, their two sons and their whole previous way of life.

In his time, Schüller was probably the greatest authority on skull radiology in the world, his name being commemorated in the Hand-Schüller-Christian syndrome. He was a prolific writer and, according to Frank Morgan's moving obituary of him (1958), a most admirable and gifted man of very great genius and learning who during his life made contributions to neurosurgical technique as well as to neuroradiology. He also was a competent clinical neurologist.

Schüller's later life brief foray into clinical neurology in Australia seems to have little influence on the development of that specialty even in Melbourne. However, his continuing contacts with St Vincent's Hospital to the end of his life appear to have enhanced that institution's neuroscience and radiology, and also enriched its culture.

During the war years (1939–1945) there was no further recruitment to the ranks of Australian clinical neurologists, but in 1948 a medical graduate from Melbourne, John Billings, began to practise neurology in his home city after neurological training in London. A little later an Adelaide medical graduate, John Game, who had also received postgraduate neurological training in Britain, returned to Melbourne, and commenced full-time neurological practice there. Billings was appointed to St Vincent's Hospital, and Game as junior to Cox at the Alfred Hospital. In addition, and again in Melbourne, the youthful Professor of Anatomy at the University of Melbourne, Sydney Sunderland, who as a student had collaborated in research with Cox, and who during the war years had been responsible for a nerve injury clinic as well as for his University duties, maintained his interest in peripheral nerve disorder. In the immediate post-war years Melbourne certainly was the centre of Australian clinical neurological practice. It was also the only Australian city with a potential critical mass of neurological clinicians which appeared large enough to offer any realistic prospects of neurology developing further in the immediate future. At least in Melbourne, neurology in Australia seemed to have taken root.

Chapter 3 The Founding Generation of Australian Neurologists

With the exception of John Billings, all the men who belonged to this founding generation of Australian neurologists are no longer living. Their obituaries have appeared in print and, together with personal knowledge when it is available, form the basis of the accounts of their careers which follow. In these accounts the emphasis lies on the parts they played in the development of Australian neurology. No attempt has been made to provide complete listings of their publications. In particular, the material which they wrote at various times for publication in the Australian Association of Neurologists' *Proceedings* has rarely been mentioned in the text, though it is listed in Appendix VII.

Leonard Bell Cox (1894–1976)

Leonard Cox (Plate 3), concerning whom information is available in the obituaries written by Russell and Bradley (1977) and Schwieger (1994), and in an essay by Sydney Sunderland (1994), was born in Melbourne, the son of a clergyman. After attending Wesley College, where he formed a lasting friendship with the future Australian Prime Minister, Sir Robert Menzies, Cox graduated in Medicine in the University of Melbourne in 1916. Almost immediately after this he became a medical officer in the Australian Army. After World War I ended, he took the Membership of the Royal College of Physicians of Edinburgh in 1919 (he appears never to have become a Fellow of that College). Cox returned to Melbourne in 1920 to take up the position of Beaney Scholar in Pathology in the University of Melbourne, which awarded him an MD in that year. After a period of illness, he married Nancy, sister of Hugh Trumble, in 1925 and began to build a consultant practice as a neurologist in Melbourne. At the same time he continued to do neuropathological research at the University and at the Baker Research Institute, as well as in his own garage (Billings – personal communication).

In 1934, at the age of 40, Cox became Honorary Neurologist to the Alfred Hospital, and Lecturer in Neuropathology in the University of Melbourne, being appointed Stewart Lecturer there three years later. At the Alfred Hospital a Department of Neurology was opened, where Hugh Trumble, at his brother-in-law's urging, began to develop the specialty of neurosurgery. As well as continuing to be involved in neuropathological work, Cox lectured to medical students in clinical neurology. He became a Foundation Fellow of the Royal Australasian College of Physicians in 1938.

With the growth in the number of neurologists practising in Melbourne in the immediate post-war years, Cox became the driving force in founding the Australian Association of Neurologists. He was its first President, holding that office from 1950 to 1957. After retiring from the Presidency he continued to serve on the Association's Council until 1961. By this time he was in his later sixties, and his days as a clinical neurologist and neuropathologist were coming to their close. It seems that his last appearance at a Meeting of the Association was in Melbourne, in May 1965, at the Ordinary General Meeting held in the building of the Royal Australasian

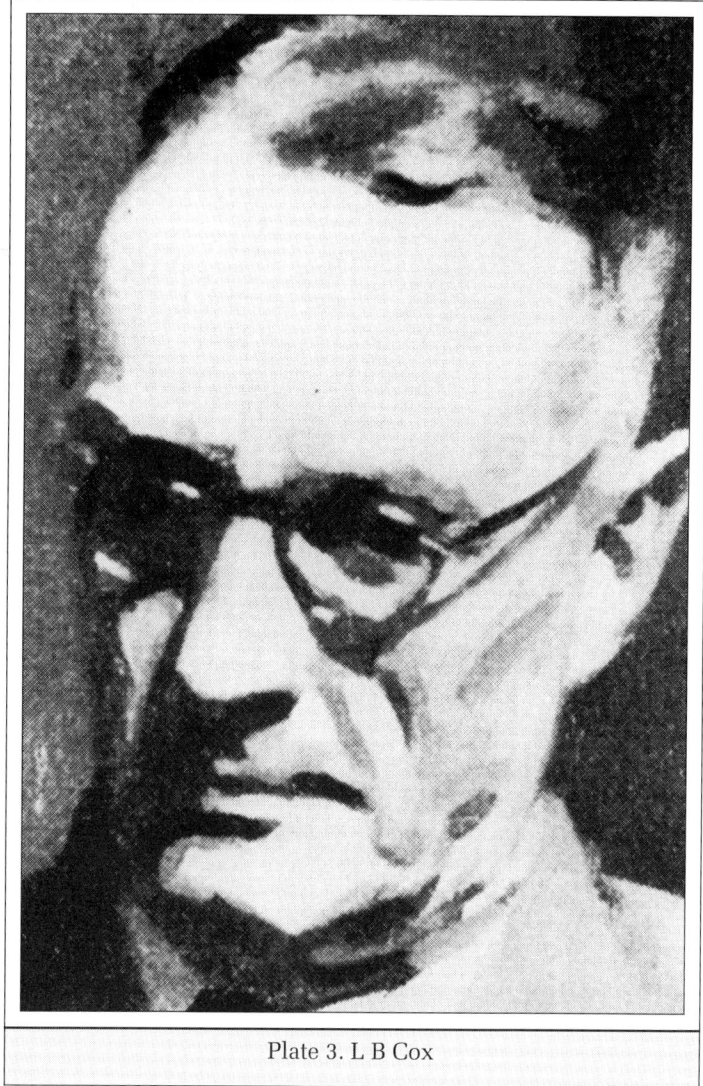

Plate 3. L B Cox

College of Surgeons. In 1968 the Association he had founded elected him an Honorary Member Emeritus.

Well before his retirement from professional practice, Cox had found a consuming interest in collecting Chinese ceramics and art, and also developed an interest in Chinese history. He played a major role in the affairs of the National Gallery of Victoria over a long period, and in later years to some extent sacrificed his neurological practice to serve the interests of the Gallery. This aspect of Cox's life was brought out by Schwieger (1994) in his obituary. It was principally for his contribution to the development of culture in Australia that Cox was awarded a CMG in 1968. He had written a much acclaimed history of the Gallery whose

Chapter 3 The Founding Generation of Australian Neurologists

welfare and advancement had become a major concern of his life: *The National Gallery of Victoria 1861–1968: a search for a collection*.

From the perspective of one who had never spoken with Cox, or indeed recalls seeing him more than once (in Sydney at a Scientific Meeting of the Association of Neurologists held in the Maitland Theatre of Sydney Hospital in June 1963, where Cox sat alone in the front row listening to the papers being presented with the afternoon sun streaming through the stained glass windows and casting a coloured pattern at his feet), it would seem that Cox made four main contributions to Australian neurology. While these contributions are individually identifiable, their effects overlapped harmoniously. Cox's role as founder and first President of the professional association for Australian neurologists was obviously of the greatest importance to the development of the specialty. His vision, organising ability, and professional reputation were crucial for setting the fledgling organisation on a sound footing from which it could grow in a relatively untroubled fashion, as it subsequently did. Secondly, there was the example that his career provided in demonstrating that it was practicable to work purely as a clinical neurologist under the conditions of Australian life of his day. His third significant contribution lay in the fact that he led others to the practice of clinical neurology, and into neuroscience. He saw to it that John Game became first his junior at the Alfred Hospital, and later his successor there. While Sydney Sunderland was still a medical student in Melbourne, Cox perceived his talent and introduced him into the neuroscience research in which he was to make so great a career. There were also men such as the neurosurgeon Kenneth Jamieson and the neuropharmacologist David Curtis whose career directions were at least partly influenced by Cox and his example. A small Australian school of basic and clinical neuroscience emanated from Leonard Cox. His influence was therefore an ongoing one, unlike that of Walter Campbell in Sydney who, though probably a greater genius and no less worthy or likeable a man, for reasons which can no longer be clear was unable to ensure that there was someone to whom he could hand on the torch. Fourthly, as one gets further away from the times when Cox lived, his original investigational work takes on an increasing significance among his numerous achievements. He was not merely a pioneer clinical neurologist or a routine neuropathologist. He did scientific work of international calibre over much of his professional life, and he did it in relative intellectual isolation far away from the research centres and research facilities of the Northern Hemisphere countries. He does not seem to have ever received any extended period of formal training in neuropathological research, or to have obtained special funding to support his studies. Yet from his energy, genius and initiative there came at least three very significant original contributions to neurological knowledge. His work on the cytology and classification of intracranial tumours, guided by the behaviour of their cellular elements in tissue culture, resulted in the publication in 1933 in the American Journal of Pathology of *The cytology of the glioma group with special reference to inclusion of cells derived from the invaded tissue*. This work became a widely used reference source for neuropathologists for a number of years. He also wrote on various aspects of cerebral and spinal tumour for the consumption of a local readership in a series of papers (Cox, 1932a, 1934, 1935, 1939a,b; Cox and Trumble, 1939) which could easily have been reworked into a monograph on tumours of the nervous system. Secondly, Cox investigated the neuropathology of cryptococcal infection of the nervous system, and in collaboration with the microbiologist Jean Tolhurst wrote *Human Torulosis*, a substantial monograph which appeared in 1946 under the imprint of the University of Melbourne Press. Thirdly, his synthesis of his own observations and various data obtained from the literature in the paper *Tumours of the base of the brain: their relation to pathological sleep and other changes in the conscious state*, published in the *Medical Journal of Australia* in 1937, anticipated the post-war interest in the role of the reticular formation of the brain stem in maintaining alertness in higher animals. Had work of such calibre and critical insight, written in clear and cautious language, been published in the medical journal of a more populous and more affluent Northern Hemisphere country, and had its author been better known at a personal level there, he probably would have received much more considerable academic acclamation for his synthesis than Cox did. Early in his consultant career Cox had also had interests in other neurological topics, e.g. Sluder's spheno-palatine neuralgia (Cox, 1931, 1932b), the formation of syringomyelic cavities (Cox, 1938b), whilst after the end of World War II he took up the question of the clinico-pathological correlations of the effects of head injury (Cox, 1949b).

Melbourne's first professional neurologist, and the Australian Association of Neurologists' founder, was also a home-grown neuroscientist of considerable genius, something that succeeding generations of Australian neurologists have sometimes appeared a little slow to appreciate, even if they have not lost sight of the fact entirely.

Edward Graeme Robertson (1903–1975)

A number of accounts of Graeme Robertson's life and career are available. These include the obituaries by Game (1976) and Lance (1988), the recollections of Critchley (1990) in his *The Ventricle of Memory* (which contained a few inaccuracies), and certain preliminary remarks made by some of those who at Meetings of the Australian Association of Neurologists have delivered the annual lecture named in Graeme Robertson's honour, especially that given by his cousin and surgical colleague Reginald Hooper (1978). In addition, in the Preface to the first edition of his work *Pneumoencephalography* (1957) Graeme Robertson wrote almost lyrically of his own neurological apprenticeship and the men and influences that helped shape his career.

Graeme Robertson (Plate 4), like Cox a Victorian, was educated at Scots College Melbourne before undertaking medical studies at the University of Melbourne. He graduated MB BS with honours from Melbourne University in 1927. He spent the next three years in various capacities at the then Melbourne Hospital, where he

Chapter 3 The Founding Generation of Australian Neurologists

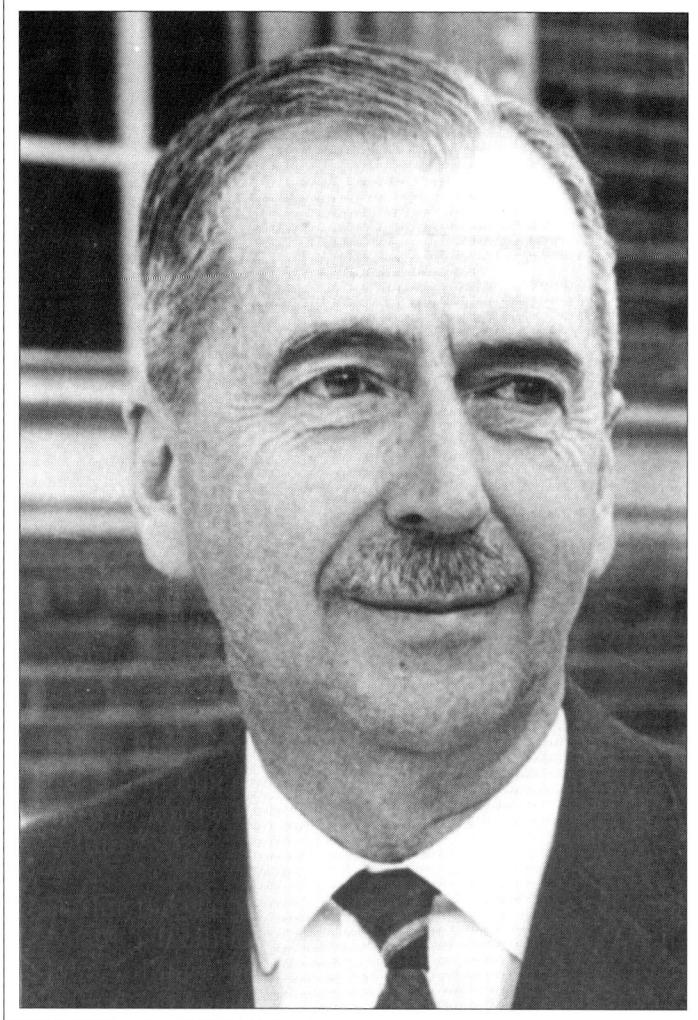

Plate 4. E Graeme Robertson

came under the influence of Sidney Sewell. After taking the Melbourne MD in 1930 Robertson spent several years in London 'on the house' at the National Hospital at Queen Square, during this time becoming a Member of the Royal College of Physicians. During those years he collaborated with the New Zealander, Derek Denny-Brown, later to become the J Jackson Putnam Professor of Neurology at Harvard, investigating the innervation of the sphincters in humans in health and in spinal cord and cauda equina disease (Denny-Brown and Robertson, 1933a,b; 1935; Robertson, 1935). He also published other investigative work during these years in Britain, e.g. on the effects of frontal lobe lesions (Walshe and Robertson, 1933) and on oligodendrogliomas (Greenfield and Robertson, 1933). His period of neurological apprenticeship was followed by appointment to the consultant staff of St Bartholomew's Hospital in London as Assistant to C M Hinds Howell, and also as First Assistant to Francis (later Sir Francis) Fraser at the London Postgraduate Teaching Hospital at Hammersmith. In 1934 Sewell persuaded Graeme Robertson to return to Melbourne, to what it was hoped would be a neurological appointment at the Melbourne Hospital. For some years prior to that time, it appears that neurology at that Hospital had been partly the province of the psychiatrists, notably H F Maudsley (1891–1967), who possessed the qualifications of a physician as well as those of a psychiatrist. As it happened, for a decade Robertson had to work at the Hospital as Honorary Physician to Outpatients before a Department of Neurology was created, at which time he became Honorary Neurologist to the Hospital and also to the nearby Children's Hospital. He also held consultant neurological appointments to various Victorian institutions, to the Royal Australian Navy, and to the Tasmania Government. He was a Foundation Fellow of the Royal Australasian College of Physicians, and became a Fellow of the Royal College of Physicians of London in 1946.

Graeme Robertson engaged in private consulting neurological practise from rooms in Collins St, Melbourne. He was an Originating Member of the Australian Association of Neurologists, and its second President (from 1957 to 1965). From 1965 to 1972 he was the Editor of the Association's annual publication *Proceedings of the Australian Association of Neurologists*, which he saw through the difficult period of its establishment and some rather precarious financial times.

In his later years Graeme Robertson held several prestigious positions, e.g. Vice-President of the Royal Australasian College of Physicians and President of the Second Asian and Oceanian Congress of Neurology which was held in his home city. Throughout his career he travelled frequently, mainly to Britain, where he maintained contacts with his old alma mater at Queen Square and with English neurologists, in particular his old mentor Gordon Holmes. In the 1970s Robertson's health began to fail. His last attendance at an Australian Association of Neurologists' Meeting was at Canberra, in May 1974, and on that occasion his appearances were brief. He died at Christmas 1975, the news of his passing being broadcast over the national radio network as he had become a rather well-known community figure. He had achieved this status not so much because of his neurological achievements as because of the series of books on old cast iron work and Australian colonial furniture which he had authored and illustrated, e.g. Robertson (1984). For many years he had combined his urge for perfectionism, his photographic talents, and his love for old cast iron work in a consuming hobby which produced a number of superbly illustrated books, the final one written in combination with his daughter Joan. These books dealt with the colonial iron work from the early years that was fast disappearing from Australian cities and country towns. In his last years he was also co-author of an illustrated work on old Australian colonial furniture and, from conversation with him, had hoped to take this more recently acquired interest further.

Chapter 3 The Founding Generation of Australian Neurologists

When Graeme Robertson visited another Australian city, it often became the lot of one of the younger neurologists from that city to drive him from site to site to allow him to inspect, and photograph, the local cast iron work. On such expeditions members of the Australian neurological community now in their own twilight years came to know something of the man. He appeared in dress and in manner a highly conservative person, diffident and almost shy. He was invariably courteous and considerate except when any circumstance threatened to interfere with his opportunity to photograph an item of iron work under conditions which he deemed ideal. Then he would suddenly become quite assertive, and almost irascible, though he would soon enough become apologetic for his period of aberrant behaviour. He was happy enough to try to educate his companion about iron work and photographic technique, but he seemed more guarded in talking of neurological matters and the personalities and deeds of neurologists. Possibly he may have behaved differently in the company of his contemporaries.

Among the Australian neurologists of his day, Graeme's Robertson's fame was perceived not so much to depend on his works on ornate cast iron or on his other artistic contributions as on his reputation as the world's greatest living authority on the procedure of pneumoencephalography. This was the radiological technique which, in his day, more adequately than any other, permitted the display of the structure of the brain in the living patient. For his work on this subject he had been elected to Honorary Fellowship of the College of Radiologists of Australasia. He published his experience with pneumoencephalography in a series of amply, indeed almost lavishly, illustrated monographs of increasing size: *Encephalography* (Robertson, 1941); *Further Studies in Encephalography* (Robertson, 1946a); *Pneumoencephalography* (Robertson, 1957, with a second edition in 1967) as well as in a book chapter (Robertson, 1974) and several research papers (e.g. Robertson, 1947, 1949a). It is sad to reflect that, by the end of his life, he must have realised that the technique to which he had devoted so much of his effort was fast being superseded by the much more comfortable and safer method of computed tomography, and was fated to soon disappear entirely from use in neurological practice.

Over the years following his return to Australia, Graeme Robertson published on several topics other than pneumoencephalography, though this was probably the main subject with which he dealt in his later years. There had been aspects of his work on the innervation of the sphincters, and during his period in waiting for a formal neurological appointment at the (Royal) Melbourne Hospital, he did some research on poliomyelitis at the Walter and Eliza Hall Institute (Robertson, 1940), some of it in collaboration with Macfarlane Burnet. There were also writings on topics such as cerebral aneurysm (1936, 1949b), spinal arachnoiditis (Robertson, 1938), toxoplasma encephalomyelitis (Robertson, 1946b), photogenic epilepsy (Robertson, 1954) and other aspects of epilepsy (Robertson, 1937, 1959), the neuropathology of Murray Valley encephalitis (1952), and historical essays on James Parkinson (Robertson, 1955) and on John White, who had been the Surgeon General with the first fleet which came to settle New Holland in 1788 (Anderson,

1933; Jackson, 1926), and who continued to live for several years in the infant colony at Sydney before returning to Britain (Robertson, 1968).

Graeme Robertson played a major role in establishing the stature of Australian neurology not only in Australian eyes, but in the eyes of world medicine. He was thoroughly steeped in the great Queen Square neurological tradition, and had gone a significant way towards establishing himself professionally in the London neurological scene before he elected to return to his homeland. There he attempted to transplant the Queen Square tradition to Australian soil and, by and large, succeeded in doing so. His existence and his personal contacts linked the neurology of the parent institution in Britain with that of its offspring in its former colony. Critchley's (1990) conclusion:

> 'we remember him not only for putting neurology on the map in Australia, but for his unique artistic achievements'

seems a fair summary of the way in which his influence and achievement were perceived internationally. Throughout his career he had continued to publish at a rate at least comparable with that of most of his British and American contemporaries in neurology. As well, he achieved an international reputation for his mastery of a particular diagnostic method. All this was enhanced by his notable contributions to an aspect of non-neurological cultural life in his own country. The Australian neurology of his time saw him as its leading exponent. It could take pride in him, and realise that, through his example, it could appropriate some of that pride for itself. Graeme Robertson was its figurehead and, to a major extent, its inspiration.

There can be little doubt that, a quarter century ago, many Australian neurologists considered him to be a much more significant figure than Leonard Cox. However, with the passage of time there may be occasion for some reassessment of the relative merits of the two men. Australian neurology over the years since Graeme Robertson's death has acquired the maturity and independence which would allow it to appreciate better its comparability to the neurological standards of other advanced countries. It would probably no longer see a single hero figure as so important to it. Although Graeme Robertson did ensure a clinical neurological succession at the Royal Melbourne Hospital, those he trained tended to remain neurological clinicians and did not branch into investigational neuroscience to the extent that Cox's intellectual progeny did. It may be that the Queen Square tradition, so important for establishing embryonic Australian neurology, tended to encourage convention in practice, and to stifle the urge towards innovative curiosity-driven inquiry. Therefore Cox, to a greater extent neurologically self-educated than Robertson, may have been capable of greater original contributions to the knowledge of nervous system disease and to the advancement of Australian neuroscience. Undoubtedly they were both very great men, and in their lives and achievements Australian neurology found a sure foundation on which to begin building.

Chapter 3 The Founding Generation of Australian Neurologists

Eric Leo (Gus) Susman (1896–1959)

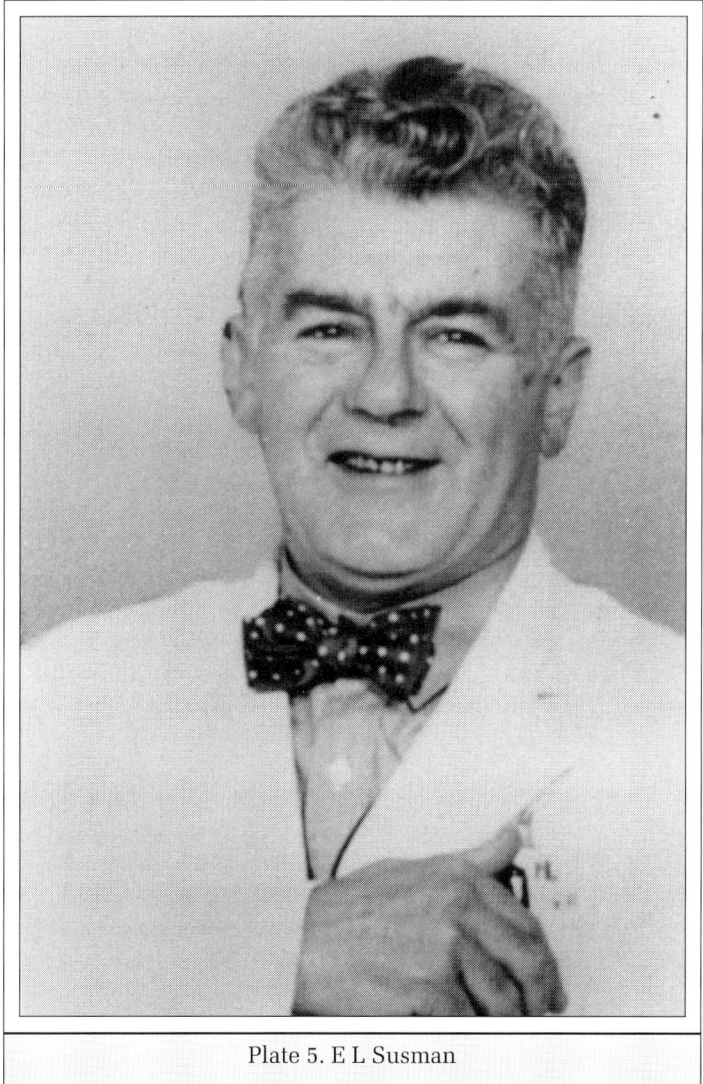

Plate 5. E L Susman

Few are still living and active who knew Susman well, and the following account is based on his obituaries (Kempson Maddox, 1959; Larkins, 1959; Selby, 1988) and on recollections of several conversations with the late George Selby.

Susman (Plate 5) was a Sydney man, educated at the Sydney Church of England Grammar School. His entry into medical school was delayed by service in World War I, where he was wounded at Gallipoli and repatriated to Australia, after which he commenced his medical studies. Susman's medical career was interrupted by war a second time, for he served in the Royal Australian Navy throughout World War II.

After graduating in Medicine from the University of Sydney in 1921, Susman was a resident medical officer at the Royal Prince Alfred Hospital where he was George Rennie's last house physician. He subsequently spent time in London where he took the Membership of the Royal College of Physicians in 1924. After being house physician to James Purves-Stewart at the Westminster Hospital, he worked at the National Hospital at Queen Square before returning to Sydney in 1925. In the following year he became Honorary Assistant Physician to the Royal Prince Alfred Hospital, and from 1945 to the end of his life was Honorary Physician to that hospital. In 1938 he became a Foundation Fellow of the Royal Australasian College of Physicians. Although he never held a formal appointment as a neurologist to the Royal Prince Alfred Hospital there is little doubt that he was, *de facto*, that institution's neurologist. He also provided a neurological consultant service to the nearby Royal Alexandra Hospital for Children, and was involved in the affairs of the Northcott Neurological Centre. Susman was one of the Originating Members of the Australian Association of Neurologists and served on its Council from its inception until his death some nine years later. By all accounts, Susman was a man of some style, wit and character. He was in a position to be able to live largely as he pleased, and his happy qualities of personality and eccentricities endeared him to those with whom he had dealings. During his life he became something of a local legend, and the memories of the man and his influence and generosity still linger in his old hospital and in the Royal Australasian College of Physicians.

Susman was neither a researcher into neurological phenomena nor a prolific writer on neurological matters, though he and Kempson Maddox reported a series of cases of the Guillain-Barré syndrome in 1940, and in 1949, in a racy style, he addressed the question of the treatment of neurosyphilis. His role in neurology was a clinical one, and his contribution to Australian neurology lay in his establishing the specialty in modern times in the main teaching hospital of the University of Sydney, in helping to keep it alive in Sydney after Campbell's death, and in stimulating younger men to enter it, including George Selby, to whom Susman with typical generosity left his Zeiss ophthalmoscope and his collection of classical neurological texts.

Kenneth Beeson (Bob) Noad (1900–1987)

Susman's fellow New South Welshman, K B Noad, outlived him, and also most of his own contemporaries. Noad's death occurred at the time when the *Medical Journal of Australia* had, sadly, ceased to publish detailed obituaries, even those of the great figures of Australian medicine. Fortunately, Wolfenden's account of Noad's life (1994) is available, and a generation is still living which remembers him, at least as he was in his later years.

Chapter 3 The Founding Generation of Australian Neurologists

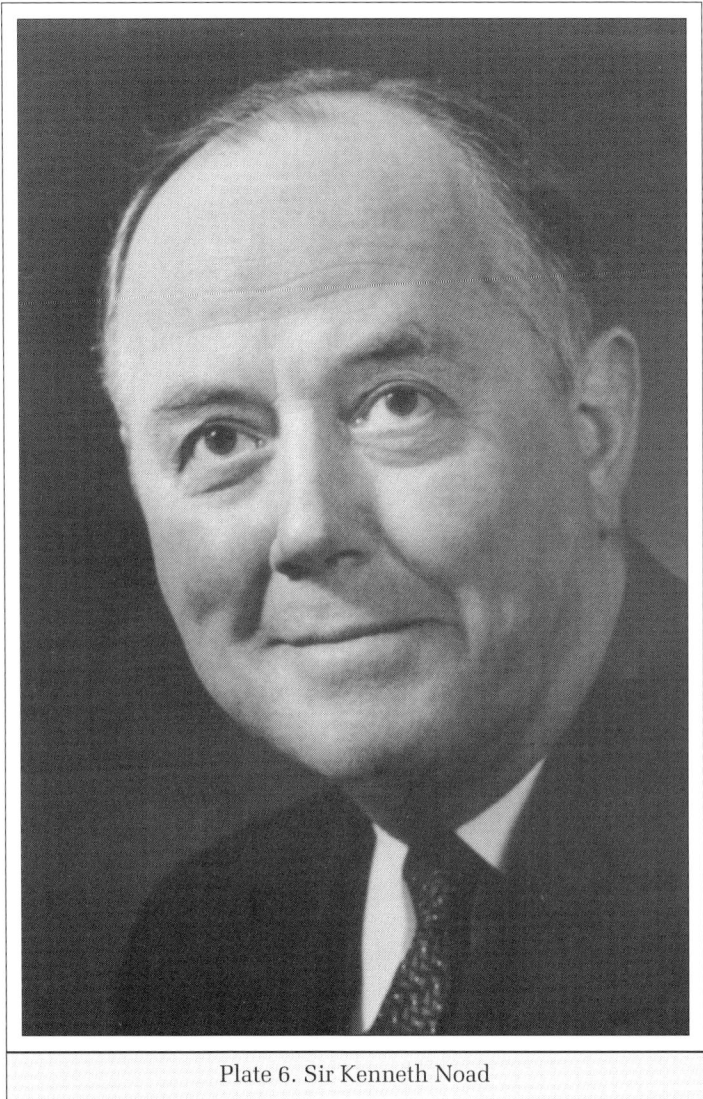

Plate 6. Sir Kenneth Noad

K B Noad (Plate 6) was born at Maitland, in New South Wales, and graduated in Medicine from the University of Sydney in 1924 with the old MB ChM qualification. After residency at the Sydney Hospital, he spent the years 1928 and 1929 in London, where he took the Membership of the Royal College of Physicians. On his return to Sydney he was taken under the wing of the senior physician Alan Holmes à Court. In 1935 Noad became Honorary Assistant Physician to Sydney Hospital, and subsequently became Honorary Physician there. On the eve of World War II he became one of the Foundation Fellows of the Royal Australasian College of Physicians. After war service in the eastern Mediterranean theatre and in New

Guinea he returned to consultant practice in Sydney, becoming a Fellow of the Royal College of Physicians of London in 1948, and being awarded a Doctorate of Medicine by the University of Sydney in 1953 for a thesis dealing with infectious diseases as he had encountered them during his war service in the Middle East. Noad became increasingly involved in the affairs of the then youthful Royal Australasian College of Physicians and in time became its Censor-in-Chief and, soon afterwards, its President (1962–1964). In the latter capacity, he developed an awareness of the possibility of the College playing a major role in postgraduate medical education in South-East Asian countries. Over the subsequent years he expended considerable effort and time in advancing this cause. During the later stages of his career Noad continued to be involved at a high level in many aspects of medical and educational affairs in Australia. He received further academic and professional honours, and a knighthood in 1970.

Noad always remained a general physician at heart and by acknowledgement, though he was responsible for the development of neurology as a specialty at Sydney Hospital. During his time in Britain early in his career he had made neurological contacts and gained neurological experience, and over his career he published a number of observational type studies on various neurological matters including tumour simulating cerebral vascular disease (Noad, 1933), head injury (Noad, 1943), uncinate epilepsy (Noad, 1944), the details of a family with cerebello-olivary atrophy (with Hall and Latham, 1945), the ocular manifestations of carotid artery disease, and the neurological features of tsutsugamushi fever (Noad and Haymaker, 1953). He had been one of the Originating Members of the Australian Association of Neurologists, and served on its Council between 1950 and 1959. He was elected an Honorary Member Emeritus of the Association in 1968, and occasionally after that time was to be seen at its meetings when they were held in Sydney.

As he grew older Noad gradually faded from clinical practice. His last years were blighted by failing health and he once confided that he had become terribly handicapped by the onset of dyslexia, which deprived him of the pleasure he had always found in reading. Despite this, he proposed to pretend to read a long address to a major medico-political meeting in Melbourne, having already committed its entire substance to memory. He got through the occasion without significant apparent difficulty. Noad, despite his distinction and seniority, always appeared kindly and helpful in his relations with younger colleagues, but in his later years may have been lonely for want of contact with professional contemporaries. Some time after he had ceased to appear at Association of Neurologists' meetings I approached him to seek his help in trying to obtain information about Walter Campbell. On more than one occasion after that he went well out of his way to help me, and ultimately presented me with his copies of the two volumes of Haymaker and Adams' massive work on *The Histology and Histopathology of the Nervous System* which he said had been a gift to him from his old friend Webb Haymaker.

Like Susman, Noad played a key role in initiating the development of neurology in one of the two major Sydney teaching hospitals of the day. There it continued to flourish after his time until the hospital itself ceased to exist as a viable entity, because of a Government decision reflecting the consequences of geography and demography. Noad's role in the Royal Australasian College of Physicians, given the circumstances of his time, virtually precluded him from practising purely in neurology, but for a physician he made contributions to neurological knowledge that were at least as substantial as those of many of the neurologists of his time in other countries.

Gerald Carew Moss (1901–1972)

Gerald Moss was the first man to practise neurology in West Australia. Details of his career are available in obituaries written by Gillett *et al.* (1973) and Sadka (1988).

Moss (Plate 7) was educated at Guildford Grammar School and, after commencing medical studies in Perth, completed his undergraduate medical education in Melbourne in 1925 because at that time there was no full medical course in Perth. He then entered general practice in Claremont. Later he went to Britain where, in 1936, he took the Membership of the Royal College of Physicians of London. On his return to Perth he practised in St George's Terrace as a physician with a particular interest in neurology. During the 1939–1945 War he served in the Army Medical Corps in the Middle East and in Australia. He had become a Foundation Fellow of the Royal Australasian College of Physicians in 1938.

Moss was Physician to the (Royal) Perth Hospital for a number of years prior to 1955, when he resigned his hospital appointment to become Neurologist to the Mental Health Service. He had also been Senior Honorary Neurologist to the Fremantle Hospital. At the Perth Hospital he had fulfilled the role of neurologist without receiving a formal appointment bearing that designation, and had functioned as the medical counterpart of the neurosurgeon James Ainslie. He was one of the Originating Members of the Australian Association of Neurologists and a Member of its Council from 1961 to 1970, becoming an Honorary Member Emeritus of the Association in 1971.

In 1956, with his now more easily regulated pattern of professional life, Moss was able to commence part-time studies for a Bachelor of Arts degree at the University of West Australia, and in 1960 graduated with first-class honours in Greek. After this he became interested in matters such as disease and drugs in the ancient world and the mentality and personality of the Julio-Claudian emperors (Moss, 1963). He published original work on these topics, as described in his obituary (Gillett *et al.*, 1973). The latter part of Moss' life appears to have been more concerned with such classical investigations than with clinical neurology, though he maintained some professional interests.

During Gerald Moss' time in practice, travel between Perth and the Eastern seaboard of Australia was neither as easy nor as convenient as it later became. As a consequence, West Australia medicine tended to develop somewhat in isolation from the medicine of the rest of Australia. Moss' importance to the development of

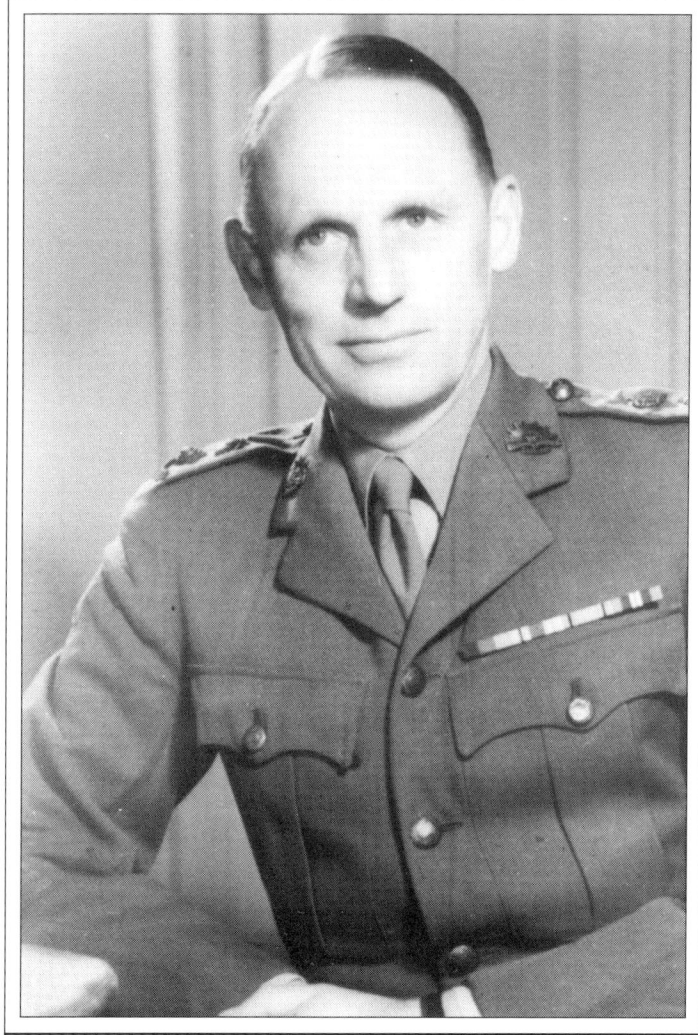

Plate 7. G Moss

Australian neurology would appear to lie more in his being the first to raise the neurological flag in Perth, in the example of professional competence which he set for his contemporaries and juniors in that city, in his qualities of personality and scholarship, and in his providing the link between neurology in West Australia and that in the eastern states, than in any original contributions which he made to neurological knowledge. However, he did publish an account of subacute and chronic meningococcal infection (Moss, 1941), and one on encephalitis and encephalomyelitis (Moss, 1949), though neither broke much new ground. By his presence and activities in Perth he created a situation such that others were not unhappy to try to follow in his pioneering neurological footsteps.

Chapter 3 The Founding Generation of Australian Neurologists

Sir Sydney Sunderland (1910–1993)

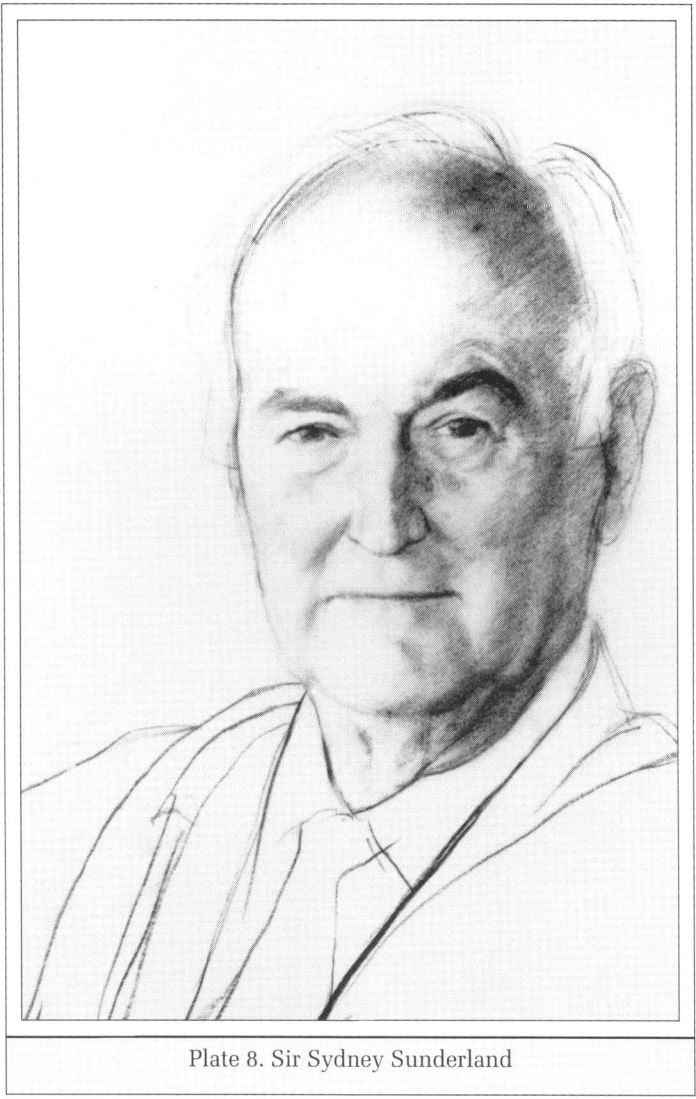

Plate 8. Sir Sydney Sunderland

It could be argued that Sydney Sunderland was an active clinical neurologist (and even then only a part-time one) for no more than a relatively short portion of his long career, so that his life should not merit inclusion in the company of the other men discussed in the present chapter. However, he was one of the eight Originating Members of the Australian Association of Neurologists, and over many years his name was among the few Australian ones that were readily recognised in international neuroscience.

Sydney Sunderland (Plate 8) was born in Brisbane and received his earlier education in that city (Ryan, 1993). He completed the first year of a science degree at the University of Queensland, but because at that time there was no full medical course in Brisbane he then entered on medical studies at the University of Melbourne. As has already been mentioned, during his undergraduate years he was invited by Leonard Cox to collaborate in work on the culture of cerebral tumour tissue, and this brought him to the notice of the Professor of Anatomy, Frederick Wood Jones. As soon as Sunderland graduated MB BS in 1935 he was appointed to a Senior Lectureship in Anatomy in the University of Melbourne. He continued his investigations in the Anatomy Department and in collaboration with Leonard Cox and his neurosurgical counterpart Hugh Trumble at the Alfred Hospital. In 1938 Sunderland worked in the Department of Human Anatomy at Oxford, and from there applied for, and was appointed to, the Chair of Anatomy in the University of Melbourne which had been vacated by Wood Jones. After gaining further experience overseas Sunderland took up his Chair in 1940. During the war years, as well as carrying out his University duties, he was in charge of an Army peripheral nerve injury unit in Melbourne. He became interested in the anatomy and biology of the peripheral nerves and in the surgical repair of severed nerves. This interest continued through his professional life and he wrote two major textbooks on the subject, the massive *Nerve and Nerve Injuries,* first published in 1968 with a second edition 10 years later, and the smaller *Nerve Injuries and Their Repair: A Critical Approach,* which appeared in 1991, when he was already an octogenarian.

From 1939 to 1961, Sunderland remained Professor of Anatomy in the University of Melbourne. His University title then became that of Professor of Experimental Neurology. He continued in the latter position until 1975, maintaining his research whilst becoming increasingly involved in highest level administrative tasks in his own University and in the wider Australian University system and community. During his career he acquired two 'earned' doctorates (in Medicine and in Science) from University of Melbourne, and in addition several honorary doctorates from various Universities and also Honorary Fellowship of the Royal Australasian College of Surgeons. He was also a Fellow of the Royal Australasian College of Physicians and of the Australian Academy. Within the Australian Association of Neurologists he remained an Ordinary Member until elected to Honorary Membership in 1964, one assumes in recognition of his already great distinction and the fact that he had become very much a part-time clinical neurologist, though remaining a very considerable and very active neuroscientist.

Whilst a great deal could be written about Sydney Sunderland's service to medicine and to the Australian academic and scientific communities, in the present context the main interest lies in his place in the development of Australian neurology. Very clearly he was a great authority, probably the greatest authority of his time in the world, on peripheral nerve tissue and its injury. The knowledge that this was the case was important for the self-esteem of Australian neurology and neuroscience. Long after Sydney Sunderland ceased to attend meetings of the Association of

Neurologists one could judge from conversation with him that he maintained a benevolent interest in that body and in local neurological affairs more generally, though his clinical interests had inevitably become more remote as the passage of the years increasingly involved him in the highest levels of academic administration. He remained enviably alert and active well after most men are no longer able to make any intellectual contribution to the life of their communities. Though he trained no clinical neurologists and founded no school of clinical neurology, the Australian neurological community understood that in Sydney Sunderland it could claim that it possessed within its ranks a very great neurological scholar.

John Aylward Game (1913–1995)

John Game (Plate 9), a Tasmanian by birth, received his schooling in Adelaide at St Peter's College and obtained his basic medical qualifications from the University of Adelaide, graduating there in 1938 (Gilligan, 1996). After service in the Royal Australian Air Force during World War II he spent the following two years with the rank of Group Captain as commanding officer at the Heidelberg Repatriation Hospital. During this time he took an MD (presumably by examination) from the University of Melbourne. He then worked for some time at the National Hospital for Nervous Diseases at Queen Square in London, and returned to Melbourne in 1950 to take up a consultant neurological position as junior to Leonard Cox at the Alfred Hospital. He became Honorary Neurologist to that institution in 1955 after Cox retired. After John Game's return to Melbourne he had become a Member of the Royal Australasian College of Physicians, and subsequently was elected to Fellowship of that body. In the years after his return to Melbourne, his publication record suggests an interest in the newly developing field of percutaneous cerebral angiography, and in the general question of cerebral tumour (Game, 1951). Earlier, he had published on polyarteritis nodosa (Game, 1946). Game resigned his appointment at the Alfred Hospital in 1963, to devote himself to private consultant practice. Over the last decade his life, or rather longer, he was increasingly limited by chronic illness which did not maintain a satisfactory response to the available treatments. He struggled to be active for as long as he could, and was cared for with great devotion by his wife Barbara over the many difficult years that followed.

Although he was always very conscious of the importance of research for the advancement of neurology, John Game was neither by nature nor by talent a researcher, and he published relatively little during his career. Rather, he was a fine clinical neurologist and, perhaps as a consequence of his Air Force experiences, an excellent organiser and far-sighted planner. When the Australian Association of Neurologists was founded in 1950 he was the first Honorary Secretary and Treasurer of the body. He continued in the former capacity until 1963, when he became the Association's third President. He occupied that office for a term of nine years, during which he organised a thorough revision of the Association's original constitution and led it patiently through complex negotiations with the governments of the day and with certain outside bodies, in an attempt to establish the status and

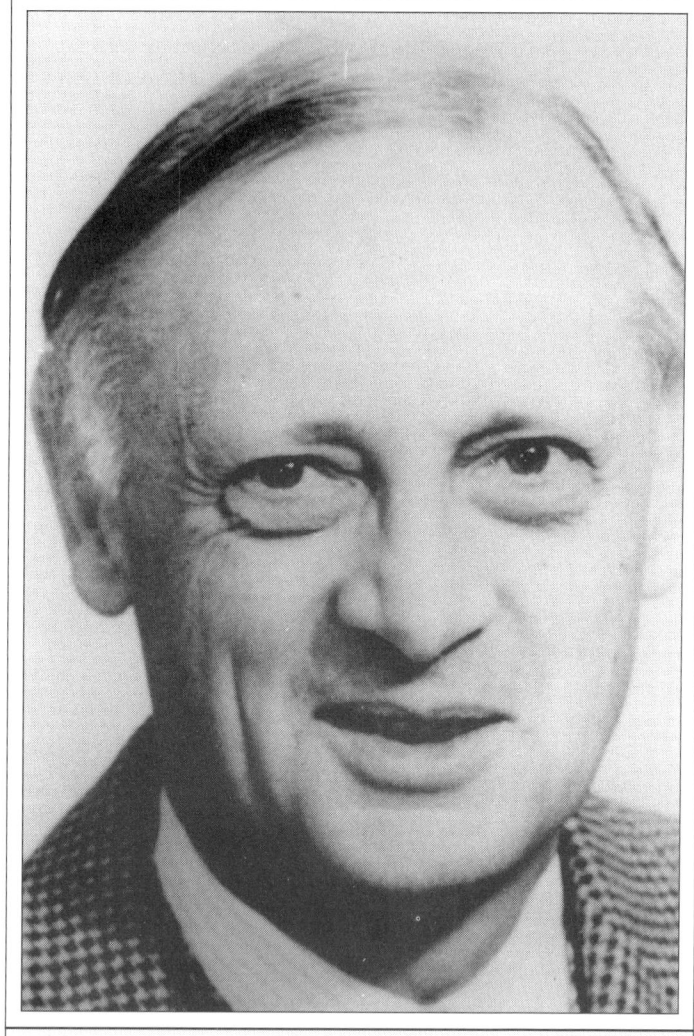

Plate 9. J A Game

improve the financial remuneration of clinical neurologists. During the same period he conceived, and moved to put in place, his vision of an Australian Neurological Foundation. This body was intended to advance neurological education, research and patient care throughout the country. He served as the Foundation's first President from its inception until 1980.

John Game was a man of strong principles, courteous and distinguished in manner, but firm when he considered that he needed to be. Occasionally his sense of principle may have led him into decisions and situations which became a little impracticable in their operation, but his vision played a very significant role in shaping the development and organisation of Australian neurology for some two decades. His memorial is the Australian Association of Neurologists, and the affectionate memory in which he is held by those of a generation fortunate enough to have known him.

John Billings

Melbourne born (in 1918), John Billings (Plate 10) was the youngest of the eight Originating Members of the Australian Association of Neurologists, and is their only survivor at the time of the writing of the present book. He was educated in

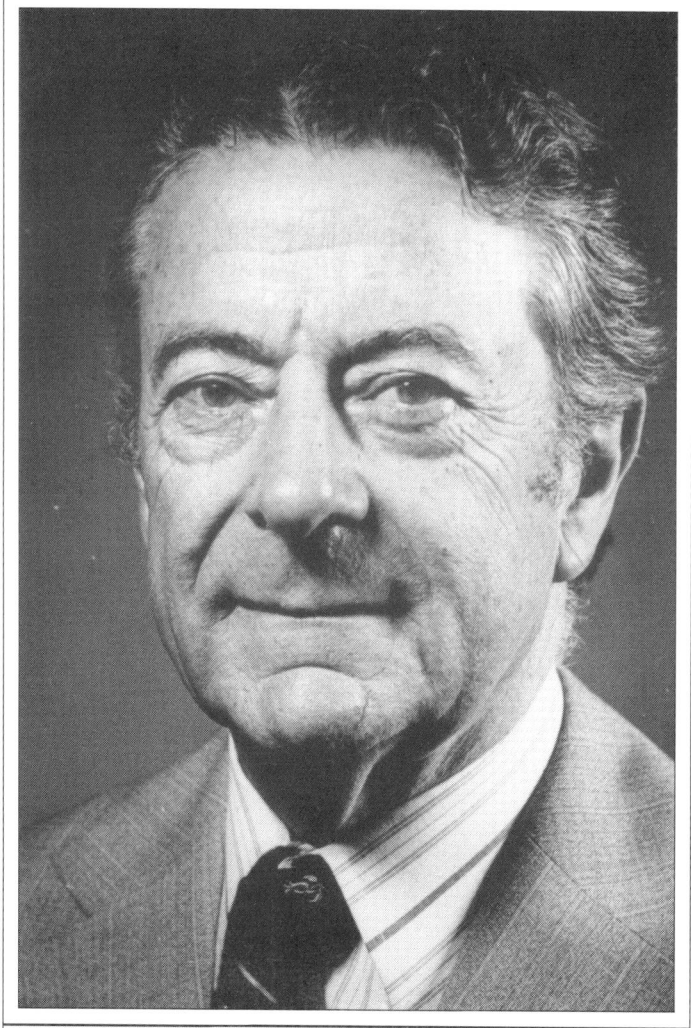

Plate 10. J Billings

Melbourne at Xavier College and the University of Melbourne, from which he graduated MB BS in 1941. After a two-year residency at St Vincent's Hospital in his home city, he spent three years in Papua-New Guinea with the Australian Army before returning to Melbourne to take the local MD and the Membership of the Royal Australasian College of Physicians. He then went for two years to London, to the National Hospital for Nervous Diseases at Queen Square, becoming a Member of the Royal College of Physicians of London during this time. He returned to Melbourne in 1949 and began his long period in the practice of neurology at St Vincent's Hospital. There he worked in collaboration with the neurosurgeon Frank Morgan, over so many years both of them seemingly ageless, whilst younger men came, stayed a while, and seemed to disappear again.

From 1950 to 1984 Billings was Head of the Department of Neurology at his old hospital, St Vincent's, subsequently becoming Consultant to that Hospital where, from 1974 to 1983, he was also Dean of the Clinical School. He had, in the course of time, become a Fellow of both of the Royal Colleges of Physicians of which he had previously been a Member. From 1961 to 1975 he was a member of the Australian National Health and Medical Research Council.

Outside clinical neurology, John Billings, together with his wife Evelyn, herself a medical practitioner, had a close and continuing involvement in promoting family planning achieved by exploiting knowledge of the expected time of ovulation. They advocated what came to be called the 'Billings' method in many countries throughout the world, a service for which John Billings received a Papal Knighthood in the Order of St Gregory the Great and Honorary Doctorates from four Universities.

John Billings as a neurologist was a clinician and not a researcher, though he published a number of articles on neurological phenomenological topics during his career, e.g. paraplegia following chest surgery (Billings and Robertson, 1955). His professional life spanned almost the entire first half-century of the existence of Australian clinical neurology, and his activities played a very significant part in the growth of the specialty. He also played a distinguished role in the wider Australian medical scene. At an age when most men, if they had survived as long, would have felt justified in leisurely and perhaps contemplative inactivity, John Billings has remained energetic and vigorous, his mental capacities undimmed, his physical appearance largely unchanged, and his strong sense of duty toward society undiminished by the passing of the years.

Chapter 4

The Foundation of the Australian Association of Neurologists

The actual time and circumstances of the origin of the idea of setting up a professional organisation to serve the interests of Australian neurologists, and to provide a forum for their scientific and educational activities, will probably always remain somewhat uncertain. The evidence, such as it is, would suggest that the notion arose in Melbourne in the years immediately following World War II, probably either in the mind of Leonard Cox or that of Graeme Robertson. However, perhaps one should not entirely discount the possibility that the then youthful Sydney Sunderland may have planted the seed. He certainly had the vision and intellectual capacity to do so. During an occasion in later life when he talked about the Association's foundation during a private conversation, he gave absolutely no indication that he had played any initiating role, and there was abundant evidence that his memory of the times was very clear indeed, but he was a modest man. John Billings, the only survivor from the eight men who were the Originating Members of what they named the Australian Association of Neurologists, was probably still undergoing neurological training in Britain when the idea of the Association is likely to have first been mooted in Melbourne, and he is now unaware of its exact source. It is, of course, quite possible that with the passing of time even the true originator of the idea may have forgotten how it arose in his mind. No one seems to have claimed the priority for himself, or attributed it to anyone else.

Because of the distances between Australian State capital cities, and the less easy communications in those immediately post-war times, it seems likely that a Melbourne originator of the idea would have consulted his colleagues in that city before approaching Noad and Susman in Sydney, and Moss in Perth. Probably the younger Melbourne men, Billings and Game, were made aware of the possibility later, after they had returned from overseas. Apparently the matter was taken as far as setting up an *Ad Hoc* Council for the proposed association, even before the first formal meeting to constitute the association took place. This interim council comprised Cox, Robertson, Noad and Susman. Whatever the actual course of events may have been, it seems likely that there would have been a considerable period of preparatory work, one which may have lasted for many months, before the arrangements were sufficiently advanced for the relevant neurologists to come together to set up the association. Perusal of the Minutes of the first meeting of the body which was to be named the Australian Association of Neurologists (Appendix I) suggests that Leonard Cox was the driving force in guiding the emerging organisation through the period of its gestation, and conducting it into the world. In doing this Cox would have had available the examples of at least two comparatively recently formed professional medical specialist organisations in his own country, viz. the Royal Australasian College of Physicians and the Neurosurgical Society of Australasia.

The former had been constituted in the years immediately prior to the outbreak of World War II. As well as providing a focus for the scientific and professional interests and aspirations of consultant physicians, it was intended to function as an examining body to determine those medical practitioners who were worthy of the status of physician. From the outset, the College had a reasonably sized corpus of Foundation Members. It seems unlikely that the handful of neurologists then in practice in Australia, almost all of whom had relatively recently been accepted into the Australasian College of Physicians, at that time would have had any serious thoughts about setting up a rival examination mechanism to determine suitability to practise clinical neurology. The small group of neurologists probably considered that their situation was much closer to that of the eight neurosurgeons who, in 1940, had set up an Australasian body which was to become the Neurosurgical Society of Australasia (Simpson *et al.*, 1974; Curtis *et al.*, 1980). Both the College of Physicians and the Neurosurgeons had included New Zealanders within their ranks from the outset, but the neurologists did not do this. It seems a curious course of action when, for some years after 1931, Ivan Allen had practised in New Zealand exclusively as a neurologist, the only one in that country (Burns, 1963). Allen had received a thorough neurological training in Britain at Queen Square and had a significant record of personal neurological publication, e.g. on aseptic meningitis (Allen and Spencer, 1935), reflex epilepsy (Allen, 1938) and grasping and tonic innervation (Allen, 1939) which had appeared in the *Medical Journal of Australia*, so that it is most unlikely that the Australian neurological community was unaware of his existence. It seems possible that the Originating Members envisaged that their Association, unlike the Royal Australasian College of Physicians, would be required to play a medico-political role and not mainly a scientific and educational one in the future. If so, an Association that was Australian rather than Australasian may have seemed better suited to dealing with an Australian government.

The first gathering of the Australian neurologists took place on 25 October 1950. The venue could be regarded as having been on comparatively neutral ground in

Chapter 4 The Foundation of the Australian Association of Neurologists

Melbourne, in Sydney Sunderland's Department of Anatomy, rather than in the professional rooms or homes of one of the Melbourne neurologists. However, the site of the meeting may really have been determined by the fact that it was to be followed by another meeting, a scientific one, which probably required a more public and larger venue. The original meeting and its attendance have been described by Game (1975), though Sydney Sunderland in private conversation once gave a slightly different account of the meeting. From the Minutes, it seems that originally six people were invited, and that these six constituted the proposed 'Originating Members'. Of this six, Gerald Moss was absent on the day and he apologised for his inability to be present. However, Sunderland and John Game were also in attendance at the meeting, presumably by invitation, and were there also admitted as Originating Members. Thus the original meeting involved seven members physically present, plus the absent Gerald Moss. Cox opened the meeting, and Graeme Robertson, seconded by Noad, proposed that he be elected President. Cox then suggested that the posts of Honorary Secretary and Honorary Treasurer be combined, and Robertson and Noad nominated John Game for that combined office. There was obvious convenience in this arrangement, as Game was the junior to Cox at the Alfred Hospital. The two would be likely to see a considerable amount of each other in the course of their ordinary work. Once the office bearers were in position, the newly appointed President submitted a draft Constitution of the Association for discussion. The name suggested for the association was the Australian Association of Neurologists. However, Susman suggested the alternative title 'The Association of Australian Neurologists', but it was pointed out to him that this title would have excluded from the Association's membership neurologists who were not Australians. Otherwise the draft Constitution appears to have been accepted without difficulty, and with some alacrity. It was realised that the Constitution might later require modification after it underwent legal scrutiny, and that this was a necessary preliminary to the Association's being registered.

A Council comprising Cox, Robertson, Noad, Susman and Game was decided on at the Meeting, the initial annual subscription was set at one guinea, and plans were made concerning the principles to be applied in meeting the costs of future social functions of the new Association. Susman raise the important question as to whether the terms of membership of the Australian Association of Neurologists might make it too exclusive of general physicians with some interest in neurology. However, Cox and Robertson took the view that the membership needed to be reasonably exclusive, and of high standard, to allow the objectives of the Association to be achieved.

The first Meeting commenced at 10 a.m., and concluded some 55 minutes later. Clearly there had been some very careful and thorough preparation beforehand, and a good measure of prior agreement. Whilst the philosophy underlying the Association's aims needs to be examined further, a potentially important issue had already arisen at the initial Meeting, viz. the question of the exclusivity of its membership.

Those present at the Meeting then seemed to have moved on to the initial Scientific Meeting of the Australian Association of Neurologists, also held in the Anatomy Department of the University of Melbourne. It appears that certain guests were present at the Scientific Meeting for, beside papers by Sunderland, Susman, Robertson and Cox, a paper was read by the Melbourne anatomist and neurosurgeon Keith Bradley, and a joint paper by Game and Luke, the latter a Melbourne radiologist. The details of the programme are shown in Appendix II.

The original Constitution of the Association

The full text of the original Constitution of the Australian Association of Neurologists is reproduced in Appendix III. Those possessed of a legalistic turn of mind may find interest in perusing it in its entirety, but certain aspects of the document appear to hold the key to how the Association was intended to function and to the role in Australian medicine that was envisaged for it.

The stated 'objects', i.e. objectives, of the Association were to bring together neurological clinicians and neurological scientists with the broad aim of facilitating their interaction and thereby advancing knowledge of the normal and diseased nervous system. The document defined four classes of membership of the Association and provided for members of all classes to attend the Annual General Meetings and Scientific Meetings of the Association but gave voting rights only to Ordinary Members. The criteria for the various classes of membership were not very tightly defined at that stage, but it was made very clear that the Council had the right, and responsibility, to determine the class of membership to be offered to any person. The criterion for Provisional Membership, viz. to practise neurology but not to hold a senior neurological appointment to an approved hospital, and in the opinion of the Council to possibly not adhere to the practice of neurology, may seem somewhat contradictory at first sight. However, in practice it seems that persons who would have been qualified to practise neurology but who, by virtue of their professional circumstances, were not yet committed fully to its practice were admitted to this category of membership. The status of each provisional member was to be reviewed after three years in that category of membership. By this time it would have been expected that the person concerned would either have demonstrated a commitment to practise fully as a neurologist, or would have moved into some other area of medicine. In the latter case there would not have been much point in his or her maintaining a relationship with the Association. The powers of Council were clearly defined and were considerable, and the composition of its membership was made explicit. In effect, the Council controlled the Association, and it was only the Ordinary Members who had the power to elect the Council. As a result, the Association was to be very much a body controlled by professional clinical neurologists. Those with an interest in clinical neurology, but who did not appear to have made a commitment to make their dominant or exclusive pattern of practice in the specialty, could only with difficulty reach even the fringes of the Association, though non-clinical neuroscientists had a place in it. In being an association

Chapter 4   The Foundation of the Australian Association of Neurologists

dominated by clinical neurologists, rather than being a body which embraced on a more or less equal footing all those in the country who had some neurological interest, the Australian Association of Neurologists differed from most of the other bodies which were later set up to cater for the interests of those in other sub-specialties of internal medicine. Its exclusivity made the Association of Neurologists numerically smaller than other sub-specialty bodies for a long time, but simultaneously made it very much more cohesive and internally stronger. Its smaller numbers tended to cause its members to make friendships and alliances across State boundaries and to develop more easily a national rather than a more parochial attitude.

In a generally far-sighted document such as the original Constitution was, even though the initial membership of the Association was so small, one wonders at the seemingly strange formula of having the quorum for the Ordinary General Meeting, which was to be held once each year, comprise at least 30 per cent of the Ordinary Members present in person or by proxy. There was no comma between the words 'members' and 'present'. If a comma was intended, there was risk that insufficient numbers of members might be present to constitute a quorum on some future occasion, yet if no comma was intended there seemed little point in mentioning the 30 per cent figure. In fact, the Third General Business Meeting of the Association, which was to have been held in March 1953, lapsed for want of a quorum.

At the Second General Business Meeting of the Association held in the Boardroom of Sydney Hospital on 10 April 1951, only six of the Originating Members were present (Sunderland and Moss being absent). At that time the draft Constitution was still with the lawyers. The Constitution had achieved its definitive form and was then signed by the members of Council in October 1954, though no actual day, but only the month of signing was shown on the document itself (Plate 11). However, the Fourth Ordinary General Meeting of the Association was held in the Boardroom of Sydney Hospital on 12 October 1954, and the Minutes of that meeting indicated that the final draft of the Constitution was to be confirmed by Council later on that day. Hence this probably was the date of the signing.

The original Constitution remained in force over the first decade of existence of the Australian Association of Neurologists, but some modification was put into effect in 1961. The main change was that the mechanism for nomination of new members was made very much more specific. Each prospective member was to be nominated by two Ordinary Members of the Association, and a Council Member, briefed by one of the nominating members, was to sponsor the application for its consideration by the Council. The academic and professional training, and the qualifications, required for Ordinary and Provisional Membership were set out in detail. Basically the possession of a medical degree from a recognised University was required, plus Membership or Fellowship of the London or the Australasian Colleges of Physicians, or of one of the other Royal Colleges of Physicians, together with at least one year of approved neurological training and, in the case of Ordinary Members, at least three years' experience in a consultant neurological role. For Provisional

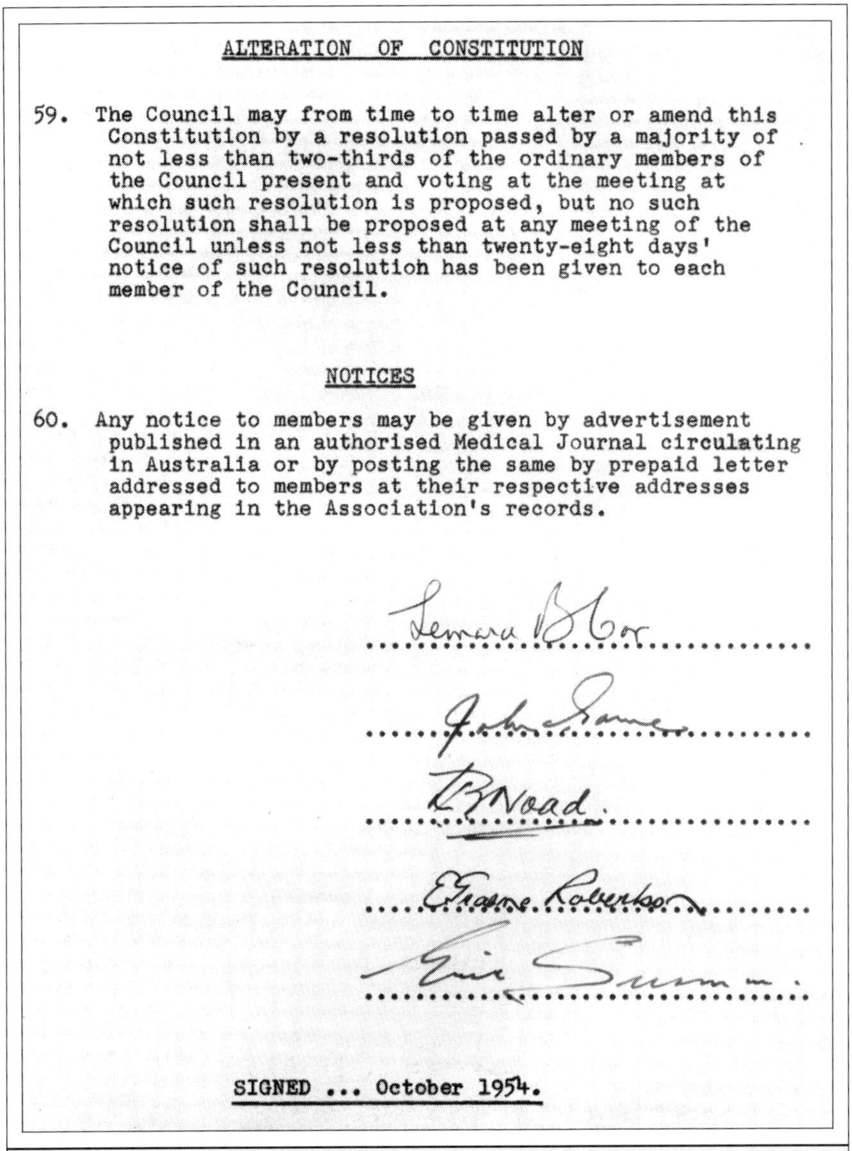

ALTERATION OF CONSTITUTION

59. The Council may from time to time alter or amend this Constitution by a resolution passed by a majority of not less than two-thirds of the ordinary members of the Council present and voting at the meeting at which such resolution is proposed, but no such resolution shall be proposed at any meeting of the Council unless not less than twenty-eight days' notice of such resolution has been given to each member of the Council.

NOTICES

60. Any notice to members may be given by advertisement published in an authorised Medical Journal circulating in Australia or by posting the same by prepaid letter addressed to members at their respective addresses appearing in the Association's records.

[signatures]

SIGNED ... October 1954.

Plate 11. Signatures on the original Constitution of the Australian Association of Neurologists

Members the latter requirement was not necessary, but in practice if it had not been met within the next three years the Provisional Membership was likely to be allowed to lapse. The specific criteria are reproduced in Appendix IV. For many years they have in practice determined who would, and who would not, be likely to be admitted to the Association. They also have tended to define, in the eyes of

Chapter 4   The Foundation of the Australian Association of Neurologists

the Australian Government, those persons in the country who were to be regarded as clinical neurologists.

The first decade of the Association

During the period between 1950 and 1954 the Minutes of the Annual General Meetings (sometimes called Business Meetings) of the Australian Association of Neurologists and those of its Council suggest that there was very little activity within the Association. However, the tempo had increased by 1954.

Membership

At the Council meeting held in April 1951 at Sydney Hospital, Drs Fisher (of Perth), Rail and Selby (both of Sydney) became Associate Members of the Association, and the neuropathologist Dr Oliver Latham and the then Professor of Anatomy at the University of Sydney, Norman Birkett, were elected the Association's first Honorary Members. The reasoning behind Fisher, Rail and Selby being elected to Associate rather than Provisional Membership is unclear. At the Council meeting held in March 1953 in the Anatomy School of the University of Melbourne, Dr Macdonald Critchley of London was elected to Honorary Membership, thus becoming the Association's first overseas Honorary Member. At the following Council meeting on 12 October 1954 there was still more activity. Drs Rail and Selby were appointed Ordinary Members of the Association after their periods of Associate Membership, whilst W G Burke (of Sydney), J Gordon (of Adelaide) and A Schwieger (of Melbourne) were appointed directly to Ordinary Membership without any qualifying period in Provisional or Associate Membership. Why Selby and Rail had been required to go through the preliminary period of Associate Membership whereas their three colleagues had not, is unclear from the Minutes. Possibly Selby and Rail were victims of the lack of clear definition of the membership criteria in the original Constitution. It may be that realisation of this led to the constitutional changes referred to above which came into operation a few years later. These changes clarified the whole matter for the future. At the same 1954 meeting the Melbourne neuropathologist Ross Anderson and John Tyrer, Professor of Medicine in the University of Queensland, who had received neurological training under Russell Brain at the London Hospital, were appointed Associate Members, and Sir Charles Symonds of London was given Honorary Membership. Thus by late 1954 the eight original Ordinary Members had increased to a total of 13 members in this category. The number of Ordinary Members then remained stationary until 1957, when a further Ordinary Member, A Fisher, was appointed from the ranks of Associate Membership and the first batch of Provisional Members, nine in total, was added to the Association. From the time that the Provisional Membership category began to be employed, it is probably meaningful to think of the total of Ordinary plus Provisional Members as being the measure of the clinical neurological component of the membership of the Association, since the Provisional Members were potential career neurologists who after three years in the category nearly always moved into the Ordinary Member category. If this interpretation is accepted, by the end of 1960 the Association had a total of 26 members, of whom 18 were Ordinary Members. That is, the number of neurologists in Australia had a little more than trebled over the decade since the inauguration of the Australian Association of Neurologists.

In the first decade of the existence of the Association, Council meetings were nearly always held in conjunction with Ordinary General and Scientific Meetings. The composition of the original Council was unaltered until 1957, when Graeme Robertson succeeded Leonard Cox as President, the latter reverting to being a Council member. At the same time Billings was added to the Council as Honorary Treasurer, Game relinquishing this component of his previous dual office. Two years later there were further changes in the composition of the Council, Rail and Selby becoming members, replacing Susman, who had died recently, and Noad, who had become overburdened in his office as Censor-in-Chief of the Royal Australasian College of Physicians. With the new appointments, there were still two Council members from New South Wales, though there is no suggestion in the Minutes that considerations of State representation were involved in the appointments.

Scientific Meetings

Until 1959 all the Scientific Meetings of the Association were held in Melbourne or Sydney, tending to alternate between the Anatomy School of the University of Melbourne and the Maitland Lecture Hall of Sydney Hospital. In 1959 the Meeting was held at the Medical School of the University of Adelaide and, later in that year, in conjunction with a session of the Royal Australasian College of Physicians, there was a Meeting in the Australian Academy conference chamber in Canberra. The Scientific Meeting in 1960 returned to the Anatomy School in the University of Melbourne. The programmes for these meetings, and several subsequent ones, are contained in Appendix II. It is interesting to note that, between 1950 and 1957, the number of papers presented at each meeting varied between five and seven, but for the next three years averaged 10 per meeting. The Council meeting in October 1958 discussed the possibility of tape recording the proceedings of the Scientific Meetings. Two years later there was a proposal to have a stenographer record the papers given at future scientific meetings. The prospects of publishing these papers was subsequently discussed, and the possibility considered of seeking from the Royal Australasian College of Physicians an agreement to allow the papers to appear annually as one of the issues of the College's journal *The Australasian Annals of Medicine.* The possibility of publishing the papers in conjunction with the Psychiatrists was also raised, as well as that of the Association publishing the papers in its own right. At that time, only a decade after the inauguration of the Association, Council found itself needing to discuss the possibility of extending the length of the Scientific Meeting from one to one and a half days, with the individual papers to be of 30 minutes duration, each to be followed by 20 minutes of discussion.

Thus over the first decade of the Association's existence one can see evidence that an increased amount of scientific material had become available for presentation by its members, and that a feeling had developed that this material was worth preserving in the form of some durable record. From the nature of the material presented at the Scientific Meetings it is clear that, from the outset, the presentations tended not to deal with individual case reports so much as with the consideration of particular neurological topics. This is reflected in the fact that, in 1958, the Council decided that no case reports would be presented at Annual Scientific Meetings unless they were of 'unusual interest'.

Financial affairs

After mention that the original annual subscription for Ordinary Members was set at one guinea, the Minutes of the Ordinary General Meetings were silent about financial matters until 1954 when the Association had a credit balance of £3–12–9. By 1958 the credit balance was £38–1–2 and two years later the balance had grown to £46–11–0. Two years after that the credit balance was reported as about £60. In 1958 the annual subscription had been increased to £2–2–0.

Other matters

In 1957 the Council had discussed the possibility of including New Zealanders in the membership, but did not seem to reach any decision. By the end of the decade increasing amounts of time at Council and Ordinary General Meetings were being spent in discussing the relationships between the Association and outside bodies such as Government departments, lay groups interested in specific neurological disorders and the Royal Australasian College of Physicians, as well as the British Medical Association in Australia. Clearly the Association was becoming recognised, and influential, in the Australian medico-political arena.

At the 1954 Ordinary General Meeting the President drew the attention of those present to a wooden gavel which had been presented to the Association as a gift from Macdonald Critchley. The gavel had been made from wood salvaged from the area of the National Hospital, Queen Square, which had been bomb-damaged during World War II. The gavel was inscribed:

> 'To the Australian Association of Neurologists from the President of the Section of Neurology, Royal Society of Medicine, London, 1953'.

The first decade of the Australian Association of Neurologists' existence had seen it grow in membership, begin to establish itself financially, start to have influence within and beyond the Australian medical profession, expand its academic activities and commence thinking about enlarging its educational role, at least within its country of origin.

Chapter 5

The Decades of Growth – Australian Neurology

By 1960, the efforts of the founding generation of Australian clinical neurologists had provided the specialty with a reasonably sure footing on the Australian medical scene. The ensuing four decades have seen Australian clinical neurology grow in a relatively steady and largely untroubled fashion. The number of those practising it has increased and they have distributed themselves more widely over the centres of population throughout the continent. The specialty has increased in academic status and senior academic appointments in neurology have been made in most of the larger Australian medical schools. Australian neurological research has developed in magnitude and sophistication. It began with simple, though very valuable neuropathological studies and largely observational-type investigations into unusual clinical phenomena which were carried out by occasional individuals. Such studies have increasingly given way to a number of nationally competitive self-sustaining investigative programmes carried out by research groups which have used advanced technologies to probe several major issues in basic and applied neurobiology. Nonetheless, at times, smaller-scale studies at levels ranging from the largely clinical to the technologically complex have continued to be carried out. Paralleling the growth in academic research activity in Australian neurology, publication of original journal papers, monographs and neurological textbooks has increased. Overall, a sense has developed that contemporary Australian neurology can hold its own in the international scene, both in relation to the quality of its clinical practice and the standards and achievements of its scholarship and its research.

Clinical neurology

As can be inferred from some of the data in the previous chapter, by 1960 there were full-time neurologists practising in all the Australian State capital cities apart from Hobart, though there was none in the national capital of Canberra, itself situated only a comparatively short distance from Sydney. There was no neurologist in the Northern Territory. Since that time the number of neurologists has increased in all of these places, with the exception of the Northern Territory. As well, neurologists have gradually come to provide intermittent services to the major Australian provincial cities, followed in many cases by one or more neurologists settling in those cities and making them their main or exclusive places of practice. In like manner, new and for the most part increasingly elaborate neurological investigative facilities have first appeared in the more populous State capital cities (Sydney and Melbourne), then spread to the other State capitals and, if there were sufficient demand, to larger provincial cities. In essence, demographic and economic factors have determined the expansion of Australian neurological services over the latter half of the 20th century, though there have been certain exceptions. Thus, as result of local initiatives, computed tomography became available in Perth earlier than in the larger Eastern State capital cities, and plasma anticonvulsant drug monitoring services were first developed in Brisbane.

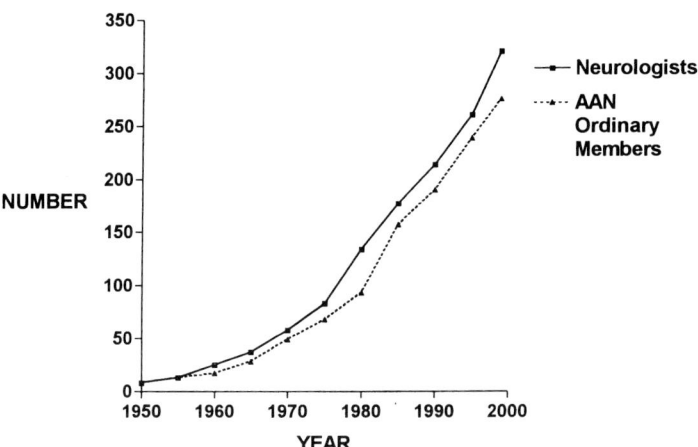

Figure 1. Growth in numbers of neurologists in Australia and in Ordinary Membership of the Association.

For practical purposes, the combined categories of Ordinary and Provisional Membership of the Australian Association of Neurologists coincide with the clinical neurologists who practise in Australia (after excluding the relatively few New Zealanders who have chosen to become members of the Association). Hence a plot against time of the number of Australian members of the Association in these two categories provides a useful measure of the numerical growth of the specialty in Australia (Figure 1). Similar plots on a State-by-State basis reveal the growth of numbers of neurologists in each Australian State over the past 50 years (Figure 2). Contemporary information on the distribution of neurologists and the available investigational facilities within the individual States (and the areas of research strength and expertise that have developed), at least in the major centres, is available in the publication of Morris (1994a). Although the present book attempts to preserve a national perspective throughout, there is some logic (and convenience) in dealing with the growth in Australian clinical neurology on a State-by-State basis.

New South Wales

Allsop (1994) has described the development of neurology in New South Wales. The following account is dependent both on his material, and on other sources.

As already mentioned, at the time of the foundation of the Australian Association of Neurologists in 1950, there was no full-time neurologist practising in Sydney. In 1951 George Selby commenced exclusive private consulting practice as a neurologist in that city. However, his major hospital appointments, first, and but briefly

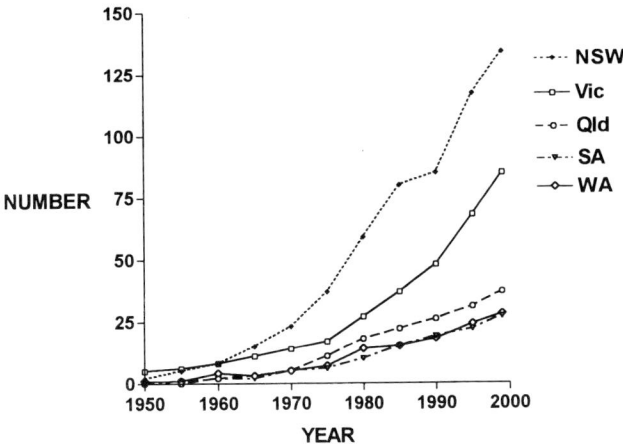

Figure 2. Growth in numbers of neurologists in the larger Australian States.

held, as a Clinical Assistant at the Royal Prince Alfred Hospital, and subsequently over many years at the Royal North Shore Hospital, were as a physician. Under this designation he provided a consultant neurological service to the latter institution. This was a pattern of professional practice within the New South Wales hospital system similar to that which K B Noad had followed at Sydney Hospital, and E L Susman at the Royal Prince Alfred Hospital. Soon after Selby, William Burke was appointed as an Assistant Physician to the Department of Neurosurgery at St Vincent's Hospital in Sydney. From this position he provided the medical neurological input to the Neurosurgical Clinic which Douglas Miller (later Sir Douglas) had established. A little while later John Allsop received an Assistant Physician appointment at the Royal Prince Alfred Hospital, where in time he was to inherit the role left vacant by the death of Eric Susman in 1959.

The Children's Hospital and some of the smaller Sydney hospitals had created consultant neurological appointments at rather earlier stages of their developments, prior to World War II, e.g. for Walter Campbell at the Coast and the Children's Hospital, for John Irvine Hunter at the Lewisham Hospital (though the latter may have been more or less a token one), and Selby later was to hold a designated consultant neurology appointment at the Hornsby Hospital. However, it was to be rather a long period before formal consultant neurological appointments and departments of neurology appeared at the major senior University of Sydney teaching hospitals of the day (the Royal Prince Alfred Hospital, Sydney Hospital, St Vincent's Hospital, and the Royal North Shore Hospital). The Sydney physicians, including those who played a very influential role in setting up the Royal Australasian College of Physicians, seemed to see little necessity, or even desirability, in openly acknowledging neurology as a discrete sub-specialty within the general province of the physician. The notion that the consultant physician should be competent in every area of internal medicine appeared slower to disappear in Australia's oldest city that in much of the remainder of the country.

During the past four decades, the first designated neurological unit that was set up in a major Sydney teaching hospital was that created in the Prince Henry Hospital. The unit was in a sense the resurrection and expansion of Campbell's old position at the Coast Hospital which, re-named in the interval, had become a principal teaching hospital of the newly inaugurated University of New South Wales. In 1961 a Department of Neurology within the Division of Medicine of the University was sited at the Prince Henry Hospital, and James Lance took charge of it. Other appointments to this Department soon followed (Fine, Preswick, Lethlean, Anthony), and there were further ones as time passed (e.g. Gillies, Burke, Mellick). The history of this particular Department has been described in some detail in the book *Mind, Movement and Migraine* (Lance, 1987).

The Royal Alexandra Children's Hospital, which had appointed Campbell as its neurologist well before World War II, had used Susman as a *de facto* neurologist in the years immediately following the war. The late Donald Hamilton subsequently conducted a Seizure Clinic there, but Don Hamilton never would have wished to regard himself as a neurologist. Leonard Rail, a neurologist with a major interest in electro-encephalopathy, developed the latter facility at the Hospital after the untimely death of Geoffrey Trahair in 1950. It was to be 1968 before Robert Ouvrier was appointed as Staff Neurologist to the Hospital, followed in 1973 by a similar post for Peter Procopis. Additional neurologists subsequently received appointment to the institution (Jane Anthony, Elisabeth Fagan, and P Grattan-Smith). At the Prince of Wales Children's Hospital, affiliated with the University of New South Wales, Graham Wise became the first paediatric neurology consultant, and other appointments followed.

The status of William Burke's *de facto* neurological unit at St Vincent's Hospital became formally acknowledged by the hospital in 1962. The unit's consultant staff grew to include O'Sullivan, Coffey, O'Neill, Darveniza and Brew. A neurological unit was established at the Royal North Shore Hospital in 1964, George Selby being appointed to its charge. Over the ensuing years its staff numbers increased (Davis, Williamson, Terenty, Herkes). At Royal Prince Alfred Hospital, John Allsop's neurological activities were finally legitimised in a titular way in 1970, his general medical unit then becoming purely neurological in its pattern of practice. A formal Department of Neurology was established at the Hospital in 1978, with Professor James McLeod as its head. Allsop continued his activities within this unit, and a number of neurologists came to be associated with it, e.g. Walsh, Pollard, Halmagyi, Leicester. Neurology at the venerable Sydney Hospital was never able to achieve its apparent growth potential, or formal independent titular status. Demographic considerations resulted in that institution's development being curtailed and then its size being scaled down as the needs of the growing population in the western part of Sydney required the development of the local Westmead Hospital as another major teaching hospital of the University of Sydney. In the 1960s and 1970s a number of neurologists worked at Sydney Hospital (Wolfenden, Lorenz, McLeod), but they had to transfer their allegiances elsewhere as the Hospital progressively closed down. From the outset, Westmead Hospital had its own Department of Neurology, headed by John Morris. Smaller neurological units also opened at the Concord Hospital, and at the Lewisham and St George's Hospitals, all within the city of Sydney.

Soon after the end of World War II, the Northcott Neurological Centre was opened in Sydney to provide neurological facilities for ex-servicemen. The existence of this Centre openly acknowledged the status of neurology as a medical specialty at a relatively early stage in Australia and, beginning with George Selby, several neurologists worked as its Director. However, with the expansion of neurological services in the Sydney teaching hospitals and the increasing recognition of neurology within the local medical community, the role of the Northcott Centre progressively diminished in importance.

Within the State of New South Wales, Newcastle was the first city outside the metropolis at which neurology developed. There by 1965 Adrian Dawson had begun to provide a neurology service to the Royal Newcastle Hospital. He was later joined at that Hospital by Terence Holland, who continued to head the Hospital's neurological services when it moved in 1991 to the new John Hunter Hospital, which by 1994 had on its staff a total of six neurologists. As well, by the 1990s, within the State of New South Wales there were neurologists living and practising in certain major country towns, for example Orange, Tamworth and Goulburn.

Victoria

By 1960 in Melbourne there were well-established neurological units at the Alfred Hospital, where Leonard Cox was already beginning to fade from the clinical scene, though John Game was active, at the Royal Melbourne Hospital, where Graeme Robertson had been joined by Arthur Schwieger, and at St Vincent's Hospital, where John Billings worked. Neurologists seem to have been accepted as a respectable species by their physician colleagues in Melbourne at a rather earlier stage than in Sydney. In 1963 John Game resigned from the Alfred Hospital to practise purely as a private consultant, though he continued to play a major and ongoing role in the affairs of the Australian Association of Neurologists. Cox came back for a short time to cope with the neurological situation at the Alfred Hospital. Then, in 1965 Bernard Gilligan, after completing neurological training at Queen Square, returned to Melbourne and thereafter provided the Alfred Hospital with its consultant neurological service. As time passed, he was joined at the Hospital by others, beginning with Richard Stark. At the Royal Melbourne Hospital, Peter Ebeling joined Robertson and Schwieger and on Robertson's retirement became head of the Hospital's Department of Neurology. Schwieger moved to Prince Henry Hospital where he undertook responsibility for the development of the neurology service. At Prince Henry Hospital he was joined by John Balla. However, the latter subsequently became interested in educational questions and for a time moved to Hong Kong. Ultimately the unit at Prince Henry Hospital was closed down. That institution, and the Queen Victoria Hospital, situated almost in the centre of Melbourne (where Barrie Morley had become neurologist), met the fate of Sydney Hospital, and for the same reason, viz. the need to shift hospital facilities to areas of population growth nearer to the periphery of an expanding city.

At the Royal Melbourne Hospital, Robert Hjorth had joined the Department of Neurology as Ebeling's junior, and he was followed successively by John King, Stephen Davis and Christine Kilpatrick. By 1994 the numerical strength of the Department at that Hospital included nine neurologists, with Ebeling in an honorary consultant role.

In the 1960s, Peter Bladin was appointed as junior to John Billings at St Vincent's Hospital, but before the end of that decade had moved to the Austin Hospital to found a neurological unit there. As John Billings grew older, and increasingly devoted his energies to the non-neurological activities in which he has served the local and international community so long and so well, St Vincent's Hospital moved to import Edward Byrne, who was subsequently appointed Professor of Neurology in the University of Melbourne. Under his leadership, at the time of writing, neurology appears to be in a phrase of expansion at St Vincent's Hospital.

Bladin spent several years establishing neurology at the redeveloping Austin Hospital, and devoted much energy to developing programmes directed towards the management of stroke and epilepsy. As the result of his initiatives, neurological staff numbers increased, with Frank Vajda, followed by Merory, Symington, Donnan and Berkovic, becoming members of the Department. On Bladin's retirement in 1994, Donnan became his successor, with Berkovic developing the epilepsy area. Both were subsequently appointed to Chairs in Neurology within the University of Melbourne. Vajda transferred to St Vincent 's Hospital in the late 1990s to take up a Professorial Fellowship and the Directorship of the new Australian Centre for Clinical Neuropharmacology which was established there. Heidelberg Hospital, close to the Austin Hospital, developed its own neurology service which came to be staffed mainly by those with a background in Austin Hospital neurology (Chambers and Merory).

The Monash Medical Centre was developed in proximity to Monash University. In a sense this Centre replaced, on a different site, the inner-city Melbourne hospitals closed down by the Victorian State Government, as mentioned above. At first, the Monash Medical Centre absorbed some of the neurological consultants displaced by the closure of the older hospitals, but with the passage of time a new generation of neurologists has come to provide its staffing. Malcolm Horne, who now holds a Chair of Neurology at Monash University, currently heads the unit.

For a time, the Royal Children's Hospital in Melbourne obtained its neurology consultant service from the nearby Royal Melbourne Hospital, but in the 1960s Ian Hopkins was appointed to it as its first paediatric neurologist. Subsequently he was joined at the institution by Lloyd Shield and Kevin Collins.

Unlike the situation in New South Wales, there was much less tendency, or need, for Victorian neurologistists to reside and practise outside the State capital. By Australian standards, Victoria is a comparatively small State, and much of its population is concentrated in and around Melbourne. Hence the demography and economic geography of the State tended to make dispersion of neurological personnel unnecessary, when it was practicable to provide neurological services to rural centres from a base in the State capital.

Queensland

During the 1950s a Queensland medical graduate, Peter Landy, returned from neurological training in London to be appointed as neurologist to the Mater Hospital in Brisbane, but this was a relatively small institution at the time. For several years Landy also held appointments at Royal Brisbane Hospital, but as an Outpatient Physician rather than a neurologist. Prior to his return to the city, neurology in Brisbane had been within the province of the psychiatrists, notably Vincent Youngman. Ellis Murphy (later Sir Ellis), a physician, had some neurological experience in the United Kingdom but never attempted to practise exclusively in the specialty in Brisbane. Shortly after Landy returned, John Tyrer took up an appointment as the first full-time Professor of Medicine in the University of Queensland. Tyrer had received neurological training at the London Hospital, under the then Sir Russell Brain, but the demands of his academic post, and the fact that he at first had no academic colleagues in his Department, precluded his practising purely as a neurologist. In fact, he had to devote much of his time and energy for many years to building up his Department rather than to advancing neurology in the Queensland hospital system. However, in late 1956 he appointed John Sutherland as a Senior Lecturer in Medicine. Sutherland had been trained in neurology at Glasgow under Douglas Adams, and soon began to provide a neurological consultant service at the then Brisbane General Hospital, where he collaborated with the recently appointed neurosurgeon Kenneth Jamieson. When

Sutherland resigned his University position in 1960 to enter private practice as a neurologist, an appointment was created of Senior Visiting Neurologist at the Brisbane General Hospital, soon to be the Royal Brisbane Hospital. Sutherland received the appointment. Originally the neurological beds were in the neurosurgical unit, but later separate neurological beds were allocated. In 1961 Eadie was appointed as junior to Sutherland, and with Sutherland also supplied neurological consultant services to the adjacent Children's Hospital.

Within the city of Brisbane, on the south side of the Brisbane River, the large Princess Alexandra Hospital began to open from 1956 onwards, and Landy was among the former Royal Brisbane Hospital consultants staff who in stages transferred to the new institution. There he was at first nominally a physician, though formally appointed as its Neurologist in the early 1960s. He was also, for some years, Neurologist to the Repatriation Hospital at Greenslopes in the inner southern suburbs of Brisbane.

The two large hospitals, the Royal Brisbane and the Princess Alexandra, became the main sites of development of neurology in Queensland. John Sutherland continued to head the neurological unit at the former institution until 1977. He then moved to the country city of Toowoomba to semi-retirement, though continuing some private neurological practice. At almost the same time Eadie accepted a full-time academic research appointment in the University of Queensland, whilst remaining as Neurologist to Royal Brisbane Hospital. By this time younger neurologists had been appointed to the Hospital and they continued the neurology services (Edwards, Mann, Ohlrich, Banney, Bradfield and Lander, and for a time John Corbett). Later two academic appointees to the University Department of Medicine joined the Hospital's neurology service (Michael Pender, subsequently to be Professor of Medicine, and Pamela McCombe). Sutherland and Eadie had continued to serve as neurological consultants to the Royal Children's Hospital in Brisbane until 1972, when both resigned, making way for a trained paediatric neurologist Barry Appleton, who was subsequently joined at the Hospital by Christopher Burke and James Pelekanos.

At the Princess Alexandra Hospital, Peter Landy built up his Department of Neurology, coming to be joined in it by a number of colleagues as his own activities diminished to some extent with the passage of time (Boyle, Cameron, DeWytt, Reid, Sandstrom and Staples, and later Silburn).

After some years of working at the Mater Hospital, Landy resigned from its staff, being replaced there by Noel Saines, later to be joined by Daniel Maclaughlin.

Unlike Victoria, and even New South Wales, Queensland is a very large State. Along its east coast and in the south-east corner there are scattered, often at a considerable distance from one another, a number of population centres, each containing upwards of 50,000 people. From the 1960s, Peter Landy had provided an intermittent visiting neurology consultant service to Toowoomba, some 100 km west of Brisbane. Other neurologists from Brisbane later provided the same type of service to that city until John Sutherland moved into residence there in 1977. J Barrie Morley, displaced from the Queen Victoria Hospital in Melbourne when it closed, moved to Toowoomba in the early 1990s. After being trained in neurology in Melbourne, Gamini Jayasinghe in the later 1970s and the 1980s provided a consultant neurological service in north Queensland, based in Townsville. In the 1990s he moved to Brisbane and was replaced in Townsville by John Reimers, whilst Geoffrey Boyce from time to time based his neurological services in Cairns, even further north. Three neurologists (Adams, Corbett and Maxwell) came to live in various parts of the Gold Coast, south of Brisbane, and to practise in the local area with its rapidly growing population. Vivian Edwards moved to Ipswich from Brisbane, relinquishing his neurological appointment at Royal Brisbane Hospital, and continues to practise in that city at the time of writing. Various Brisbane neurologists visit the so-called Sunshine Coast area a short way north of Brisbane and one neurologist (Schapel) resides there. Thus as time has passed, the distribution of neurologists and neurological services in the State has followed the distribution of the major centres of population, as has been the case in other parts of Australia.

South Australia

In 1953, after several years of postgraduate training at Guy's Hospital with Sir Charles Symonds and at the National Hospital at Queen Square, John Gordon returned to Adelaide to practise neurology. Prior to this time, except for the short period between 1920 and 1924 when H V Fry had been appointed Honorary Assistant Physician in Neurology at the Royal Adelaide Hospital (Rischbieth, 1994), neurology had been the province of the general physicians and the Adelaide neurosurgeons (Lindon and Dinning). Gordon's consultant career at the Royal Adelaide Hospital began with appointment as a Physician, though he also acted as Clinical Assistant to the Neurosurgical Unit. In 1959 his appointment was changed to that of Honorary Neurologist to the Hospital. He held a similar appointment at the Adelaide Children's Hospital until 1969. As well, he provided an electro-encephalography service to both of these institutions.

Just before John Gordon received his formal neurological appointment at the Royal Adelaide Hospital, Rischbeith returned to Adelaide from Queen Square to become Consultant Neurologist to the Queen Elizabeth Hospital. Richard Burns, after neurological training at Cleveland in the United States, joined Gordon in the Department of Neurology at the Royal Adelaide Hospital in 1967. In the mid-1970s there was some turnover among the Royal Adelaide Hospital neurologists. The Medical Centre attached to the new Flinders University opened, and Burns moved there in 1977 as its Associate Professor of Neurology. In the following year John Gordon himself resigned and moved to the United Kingdom to pursue his musical interests. Peter Rice took over responsibility for neurology at the Hospital, being joined there by Jeremy Hallpike. Subsequently Burrow, Kneebone and Heather

Waddy received consultant neurological appointment to that institution. Later Thompson took up a Chair of Neurology there.

In the meanwhile, the number of neurologists at the Queen Elisabeth Hospital grew, Paul Hicks (in 1972) and Andrew Black (in 1975) joining Rischbeith. Later Purdie (1983) also became a member of the unit, and further consultant neurological staff were recruited, whilst Rischbeith and Hicks retired with the efflux of time.

John Gordon's resignation in 1969 from his neurology post at the Adelaide Children's Hospital was quickly followed by the appointment to that institution of its first paediatric neurologist, James Manson. Later Abbott and Harboard joined Manson as the neurological consultant staff of the Hospital.

At the Flinders Medical Centre, Burns developed a neurological unit which came to include John Willoughby and William Blessing, both neuroscientists as well as clinical neurologists.

As is the case in Victoria, the South Australia population is concentrated on the State capital of Adelaide. As a result the entire neurological workforce of the State is based in that city, and provides for the State's neurological needs from that site.

Western Australia

Like Victoria and South Australia, the population of the vast State of Western Australia is mainly concentrated in one region, in the south-west around the State capital of Perth and its neighbouring port of Fremantle. The reminder of the State remains sparsely settled, and nowhere is there a sufficient number of persons to warrant the continuing presence of a neurologist.

In the account of the career of Gerald Moss (Chapter 3) it was pointed out that, though he provided the Royal Perth Hospital with a neurology consultative service both before and after World War II, he never received the title of neurologist to that institution. However, after his resignation in 1955 to become Neurologist to the West Australian Mental Health Service, the Hospital began to develop neurology as a medical specialty, though slowly. Ernest Beech became Senior Honorary Neurologist in 1957, with Anthony Fisher, a Melbourne graduate, as Assistant Honorary Neurologist. Beech also functioned as a Physician to the Hospital. In the latter capacity he retained his general medical beds in which the neurological patients were accommodated. In 1959 Mercy Sadka, Australia's first female neurologist, returned to Perth after training in Boston to take up a position of Clinical Assistant Neurologist at the Hospital and to establish an electroencephalography service there. She also developed a rehabilitation service which became one of her great and continuing professional interests.

When the Sir Charles Gairdner Hospital opened in 1963, there was some redistribution of the neurological personnel in Perth. Mercy Sadka moved to the new institution as Honorary Consultant Neurologist. In 1968 Beech abandoned neurology to pursue other professional avenues. Fisher replaced him as Senior at the Royal

Chapter 5 The Decades of Growth – Australian Neurology

Perth Hospital, Sadka became Assistant Neurologist there and Sonny Gubbay was appointed Clinical Assistant Neurologist. Frank Mastaglia, after training under John Walton (later Lord Walton) at Newcastle-upon-Tyne, returned to a Senior Lectureship in Medicine at the Sir Charles Gairdner Hospital in 1971. During the next two years the West Australian neurologists and neurosurgeons came to an arrangement whereby they all had dual appointments to the two major adult hospitals in Perth. This led to the need for some readjustment in affiliation, especially since University units transferred from the Royal Perth to the Sir Charles Gairdner Hospital at much the same time. In effect Sadka and Fisher changed places, Gubbay succeeding the former as head of neurology at the Royal Perth Hospital in 1977, there being joined by Stewart-Wynne and Edis, and later by Dunne after Sadka retired in 1987, and subsequently by Hankey. In 1978 the University of Western Australia appointed Frank Mastaglia to a Personal Chair in Neurology which he held at the Sir Charles Gairdner Hospital. There the neurological consultant staff over time came to include Scopa, Grainger, Carroll, Day, Stell and Kermode, with Anthony Fisher, after his official retirement in 1989, continuing to maintain an interested role.

After 1981, at the Repatriation Hospital in Perth a Senior Lecturer in Medicine at the University of Western Australia, Louis Herzberg, was responsible for providing a general neurological service, with a minimal quota of visiting sessions being provided by Fisher and later by Day.

From around 1960, paediatric neurology in Perth was in the hands of Peter Silberstein who worked at the Princess Margaret Hospital. Harvey Sarnat was appointed to the neurology staff of that Hospital in 1976, but left after a little more than one year. A few years later Walsh joined the neurological consultant staff of the institution.

For a time neurology consultant services were provided to Fremantle Hospital by Anthony Fisher on a visiting basis. Subsequently Bajada and later Knezevic and Goodheart became that institution's neurologists.

Tasmania

In Tasmania until comparatively recent times, Hobart was the only city large enough to sustain the practice of a clinical neurologist (in the form of Keith Millingen). However in 1981, Siejka began practice in the specialty in Launceston, and P T Yeo received the second neurological appointment at the Royal Hobart Hospital, as Clinical Assistant in Neurology. Prior to 1952, neurological services in Tasmania had been provided from Victoria, principally by Graeme Robertson, who would visit the island from time to time.

The late Keith Millingen, after obtaining neurological experience at the National Hospital at Queen Square, commenced practice in Hobart in 1952 and was later appointed Neurologist to the Royal Hobart Hospital. In time he accepted a Senior Lectureship and subsequently a Readership in the University of Tasmania's

Department of Medicine, but continued to work as a neurologist at the Hospital until his retirement in 1987.

Australian Capital Territory

Prior to 1973, neurology in Canberra either was handled by the local general physicians or by referral to neurological specialists in Sydney. Then Colin Andrews, who had recently taken a Doctorate in Medicine from the University of New South Wales whilst working in James Lance's unit, moved to Canberra to practise neurology. He became Consultant Neurologist to both the Royal Canberra Hospital and the Woden Valley Hospital. Soon afterwards Gytis Danta joined the staff of the Woden Valley Hospital as a full-time neurologist, and continues to head the unit there, with Roger Tuck later joining the neurological consultant staff. With the closure of the Royal Canberra Hospital, neurology in the Australian capital came to be centred on the Woden Valley Hospital.

As one looks at the development of clinical neurology services in the Australian States over the past 40 years, it becomes clear that neurologists have tended to enter practice where there were sufficient numbers of people who lacked neurology services, and where the neurologists could obtain consultant appointments to local hospitals. Survival without such appointments appears to have often been difficult, though certainly not impossible. In the longer established hospitals, neurosurgical demand for congenial and effective neurological support to deal with the non-operative aspects of surgical practice often proved a significant stimulus to making the initial neurological appointment to the institution. Once that appointment was put in place the addition of one or more neurological colleagues usually proved desirable to maintain continuity of service and to cope with demand. Under Australian conditions of relative geographical isolation except in the larger cities, the solo neurologist practising at a distance from colleagues functioned under difficult conditions professionally, and tended not to be as productive as those who were able to work in proximity to others with similar interests. When new hospitals have been opened in Australia in recent times it has nearly always been recognised that neurology and neurosurgery should be developed side by side, intellectually and, as far as feasible, physically.

These factors, plus population growth and movement, increasing community affluence and the quality of Australian clinical neurological practice, have over half a century allowed the number of neurologists in the country to grow from seven (Sydney Sunderland being excluded from the original count because clinical neurology was not his dominant mode of activity), to some 45 times that number.

Academic neurology

Half a century ago, when neurology was first becoming established in Australia as a clinical specialty, academic clinical medicine was not itself at all well developed. There was a long-established Chair of Medicine in the University of Sydney, a more

Chapter 5 The Decades of Growth – Australian Neurology

recent one in the University of Adelaide, and a half-time Chair in the University of Queensland, whilst the University of Melbourne had its Stewart Lectureship in Medicine. In the eyes of clinicians, this latter post was equivalent in status to that of a professorship, but in University eyes it lacked the titular recognition accorded to a Chair. In general, the occupants of these four positions were expected to be first and foremost clinicians and teachers – research (if any) and a role in University politics were very much subsidiary requirements at that time. In such a situation it is not surprising that the founding generation of Australian neurologists at first appeared to see little advantage, or practicability, in having academic aspirations for the specialty. Rather, the eyes of at least some of them tended to become fixed on a vision of transplanting not only the Queen Square neurological culture to Australian soil, but of creating a Queen Square-like physical facility somewhere on that soil. That vision, probably never explicitly and publicly enunciated, though mentioned in the Minutes of the 1970 Annual General Meeting of the Australian Association of Neurologists, took many years to fade away completely, yet it would never have appeared to be realisable. The Australia of that time did not have the total population to sustain such an institution. Moreover, the smaller population of the country was scattered over a very much greater land mass than that of the total area of Britain, there was no single incontestably predominant population centre, and neither of the country's two major cities was the national capital. Nor was there at all well developed any tradition of private charity such as that which instigated and supported the development of the National Hospital at Queen Square. At the time in question, Australia was still recovering from the effects of a recent major war. Sydney possessed the only institution in the country specifically dedicated to neurology, the Northcott Neurological Centre, but by virtue of the purposes for which it had been set up access to that Centre was open only to a limited section of the community. On the other hand, Melbourne had much more experience of established neurological practice, but that practice was subdivided between two, and arguably three, major hospitals, without any one institution clearly being the preponderant centre.

As the possibility of an Australian Queen Square became increasingly unlikely, some Australian neurologists began to visualise another, probably more achievable, goal, that of a Chair (or Chairs) of Neurology in one or more of the Australian universities of the time. By 1960 the Australian University system was expanding. Staff numbers, particularly at the sub-professorial level, in the academic clinical departments were increasing, Queensland and Melbourne had recently created full-time Chairs in Medicine, research was being done in the university departments and research funding was becoming available in increasing amounts. At least in the mind of a few of the more senior neurologists of the day, notably John Game, there seems to have arisen the idea that neurology might find its way to a place in the sun through being acknowledged academically (specifically in the form of at least one professorial appointment in the area). By this means neurology might also gain access to funding to conduct its own research (though the particulars of that research were always left nebulous). Certainly such ideas were recorded in the

Minutes of the Australian Association of Neurologists' Annual General Meetings on at least two occasions (1969, 1970), though to the present-day reader the concepts always seemed to lack particularity. Nonetheless, these ideas did ultimately come to realisation through a variety of processes, and in the end probably did achieve something of what had been hoped of them.

Whilst such notions were beginning to form, John Tyrer in 1954 had been appointed to the Mayne Chair of Medicine in the University of Queensland. Although the research for which he had obtained his MD from the University of Sydney had been in the cardiovascular area he had subsequently spent a year at the London Hospital with Russell Brain acquiring neurological knowledge. Thus, almost before the idea dawned of having a Chair of Neurology created somewhere in Australia, a person with neurological training had come to occupy one of four chairs of Medicine then existing in the country. It could, of course, be argued that at that time in the person of Sydney Sunderland the Australian University system already possessed someone with a professorial level appointment and considerable neurological knowledge. However, Sunderland was primarily a neuro-anatomist, and a very great one, and the Australian neurologists of the times regarded him in that light. For some years, rather than being considered a neurologist, Tyrer was perceived as a physician who probably would have been a neurologist if he did not also, by virtue of his academic appointment, have to take responsibility for the teaching and clinical practice of internal medicine as a whole. It was only after his department had built up sufficient academic staffing, with expertise in other areas of medicine, that he achieved conditions in which he was able to practise more exclusively in clinical neurology. However, well before that time, Tyrer had imported to Brisbane in 1956 a Scottish-trained neurologist, John Sutherland. However, Sutherland also had to function clinically outside his specialty for a few years until he resigned from his University position to enter full-time consultant neurological practice. He then received a part-time appointment as Lecturer and Research Consultant in Neurology in the University of Queensland, his appointment perhaps constituting the first recognition in a titular sense of clinical neurology as an academic discipline in an Australian university.

James Lance resigned a neurological consultant appointment at Sydney Hospital in 1961 to become Senior Lecturer in Neurology in the University of New South Wales. As mentioned earlier, this new University had from the outset created a Department of Neurology, though as a section within its Division of Medicine. Lance, by virtue of his scholastic and research achievements, not only built up the Department, but was promoted first to Reader, and in 1976 was appointed to a Personal Chair in Neurology. By this time his Department also contained academic appointees in neurology at sub-professorial level. With Lance's appointment to a designated chair in neurology the two-decade-old dream of the founding generation of Australian neurologists first became a reality.

Prior to this time, another academic neurologist in Australia had come to hold a professorial level appointment, though in Medicine, not Neurology. James McLeod, a former Sydney Rhodes scholar, had returned to his home city to a Senior Lectureship in the Department of Medicine at Sydney University in 1960, and worked as a neurologist at Sydney Hospital. He later became the second Professor in the University of Sydney's Department of Medicine. In this position, unlike Tyrer more than a decade earlier, he was in the situation where his Department contained a sufficient range of professional expertise for him to be able to continue to practise predominantly as a clinical neurologist. At a later date McLeod was also able to combine his Chair of Medicine with the newly created Bushell Chair of Neurology in the University of Sydney. However, shortly before this happened the second Australian professorial level appointment in neurology had occurred, this time in Brisbane. There Sutherland had first become part-time Reader in Neurology and Eadie was appointed to the part-time Lectureship in that discipline which Sutherland had vacated. In 1972 Eadie's appointment was changed to that of a half-time Readership and in 1977 to a half-time Professorial Fellowship in Neurology. Later in the same year he was appointed to a named Chair in Clinical Neurology and Neuropharmacology in the University of Queensland.

In 1983 Frank Mastaglia, who had held an academic appointment in medicine in the University of West Australia, and who had recently deputised for John Walton in the Chair of Neurology in the University of Newcastle-upon-Tyne, was appointed to a personal Chair in Neurology in his home institution.

Thus the decade 1975 to 1984 saw the creation of professorial appointments in neurology in four of the Australian medical schools, with Richard Burns being appointed to an associate professorship in the discipline in the new Medical School at Flinders University in 1976. John Game had the satisfaction of knowing that his goal had been reached within Australia, not once, but four times and in four separate places, over a comparatively short period. And the medical schools of his home city of Melbourne were to follow suit later, with Chairs in Neurology being created at St Vincent's Hospital (for Edward Byrne), at the Austin Hospital (for Geoffrey Donnan), where Peter Bladin previously had held a Professorial Fellowship, at the Royal Melbourne Hospital (for Stephen Davis) and at the Alfred Hospital (for Elsdon Storey) and at the Monash Medical Centre (for Malcolm Horne), with Samuel Berkovic later (1998) being appointed to a Personal Chair in Neurology at the Austin Hospital, and Frank Vajda to a Professorial Fellowship at St Vincent's Hospital. Sydney too was not idle in making further professorial appointments in neurology. David Burke was appointed to a Chair in the University of New South Wales and later John Pollard to a Personal Chair in the University of Sydney at Royal Prince Alfred Hospital, whilst John Morris received an Associate Professorship at Westmead Hospital. The University of Adelaide appointed Phillip Thomson to a Chair of Neurology there, and John Willoughby became the second Associate Professor in Neurology at Flinders University. As well, two neurologists were appointed to Chairs in Geriatrics, Robert Helme in Melbourne and Anthony Broe in Sydney. Thus in Australia, from 1976 onwards, professorial appointments in neurology, and academic neurology itself, expanded more rapidly than the development of the remainder of the specialty. But did this luxuriant growth achieve what John Game and his generation had hoped would flow from the creation of senior academic appointments in neurology?

The answer is probably a mixture of 'yes' and 'no', though predominantly 'yes'. There can be little argument with the assertion that the research done by many of the academic neurological appointees, both prior to their formal appointments and subsequently, has contributed more than any other single factor to making Australian neurology known internationally for its achievements and its quality. The existence of the academic appointments has meant that Australian medical students have learned their neurology from neurologists rather than from physicians, and this has tended to bring home to them early in their professional lives the stature and the importance of neurology within the discipline of internal medicine. It has also provided neurology with a platform on which to build within a community which is more wide-ranging intellectually and less restricted in its vision, and less service-orientated, than the hospital one. It is also a community in which neurology's influence is more readily perceived internationally. Where the effect of the academic appointments in neurology has probably fallen short of the earlier expectation is that, when the idea of chairs of neurology was first mooted, it was anticipated that such chairs would be associated with the headships of established university departments of neurology. That is, it was expected that the chairs of neurology would be so-called establishment ones. Instead, over the intervening years the circumstances of professorial appointments have changed somewhat within universities in Australia. Nearly all of the chairs of neurology that have been created have in essence been personal ones, or ones based in hospitals and funded by them, rather than being primarily university based and funded. As such, the chairs of neurology may have become subservient to other academic or hospital considerations to a greater extent than would have been envisaged a generation or more ago. It is easier for a university to suppress, or leave unfilled, a personal chair than it is to treat an established chair, or a department, in the same way. Therefore, the changed basis of the foundation of many university chairs over recent years has meant that neurology still does not have as sure a home in the academic world in Australia as might appear at first sight, despite the fact that so far neurology certainly has not been made unwelcome in that world.

Neurological research and scholarship

As has already been pointed out, prior to 1950 much neurological research in Australia was prompted by local problems for which appropriate overseas answers were not available so that local solutions had to be sought. There were, however, some attempts to set up investigational programmes into unsolved, or unsatisfactorily understood, global problems, e.g. the Hunter and Royle work on spasticity, Campbell's studies on cerebral and cerebellar architectonics. By the time of the founding generation of Australian neurologists, investigation of the known peculiar local neurological problems in Australia had become a fairly well-tilled field, though a few new problems were to arise in the subsequent decades and to become the objects of research.

With the relative exhaustion of local neurological problems as research topics, Australian neurological research in the past 40 years has moved increasingly in the direction of studying more global problems, in doing so usually in competition with investigators from elsewhere in the world. Such studies have often involved the activities of research groups rather than the solo investigator, and increasingly have required sophisticated and expensive facilities likely to be available only in universities, research institutes or larger and more amply funded hospitals. Rather than discuss such research over the past 40 years on a purely chronological basis, which must inevitably lead to discontinuity in tracing the progress of the understanding of particular matters, it has seemed better to discuss it topic by topic. It should be pointed out that the work to be mentioned is much less than the sum of all the Australian investigations carried out in the relevant areas. The account that follows merely attempts to pick out the major themes that have been studied, commencing with two disorders which were, in a sense, discovered by Australian medicine, before proceeding to consider the various fields of research which have attracted the attention of Australian neurological scholarship over the years.

New diseases

Kuru

From the viewpoint of neurobiology, the recognition of kuru was an event of immense importance. It provided the stimulus for the set of investigations which led to the realisation that there was a new class of human infective disease, that due to prions. This was a concept which brought together, and explained, a number of hitherto ill-understood nervous system disorders.

Kuru occurred on Australia's northern doorstep, its presence being restricted to the Fore people who inhabited an isolated area of the eastern highlands of Papua-New Guinea. At the time when the existence of kuru became known to the world, Papua-New Guinea was an Australian protectorate. There is no question that the major discoveries in the area of kuru were made by Americans, notably the Nobel Laureate Carleton Gadjusek. Therefore the propriety of associating Australian medicine with the kuru research may at first sight appear doubtful. However, the fact that the existence of kuru was first recognised by a medical officer employed by the Australian authorities should not be forgotten. This man was Vincent Zigas. He became aware of the presence of kuru and, soon after, in December 1956, reported the existence of the disorder to his local medical seniors. Zigas also persuaded Gadjusek to study the matter (Gajdusek, 1981), and thereafter collaborated in its investigation in the field.

The whole set of correspondence and field notes relating to the investigation of kuru was published in a volume under the editorship of Farquhar and Gajdusek in

1981. Zigas, after coming to live in Brisbane near the end of his life, gave the present author his own copy of the volume, one bearing Gadjusek's signature.

Zigas' report dated 26 December 1956, directed to his superior in Port Moresby, read:

> 'I have to inform you that on 22/10/56 I left station for Moke area to investigate a form of encephalitis amongst the Okapa people – returned on 12/11/56 with preliminary brief report which reads below.
>
> A number of people were found suffering from a probably new form of encephalitis attributed by inhabitants to sorcery and called 'kuru', the prominent clinical symptoms of which are as follows:
>
>> Disease originally started with fever, somnolence, muscular pain and weakness, headache (mostly occipital), vertigo, occasional vomiting. As course progresses condition becomes far more pronounced giving the well-known condition of Parkinsonism with its mask-like face, flexed arms and wrists, and unsteady walk, ocular disorders such as diplopia, strabismus, nystagmus, tremors of fingers and hands giving a cigarette rolling movement. In the late stage – no control of sphincters, increased W.B.C. and C.S.F under increased pressure. Duration of disease approximately from seven to nine months, slowly progressive and usually ends in death.
>>
>> During my stay at Moke no more than 27 cases were under my close observation for three weeks, during which time two cases died in coma. I also visited surrounding villages and found another 11 cases. I observed that no age is immune, female more affected than male and I would say in ratio 3 to 1. I sent 22 samples of blood sera and a brain to Dr Anderson of Eliza Hall Institute in Melbourne and am anxiously awaiting the results of tests.'

Zigas had come from the Baltic states as a post-war refugee and his medical qualifications were considered not adequate to allow him to be registered to practise in Australia, though they were deemed sufficient for him to work as a medical officer in Papua-New Guinea. He appeared to be a very modest, indeed humble, man who was extraordinarily cheerful and who, after he left New Guinea, worked at the Queensland Institute of Medical Research in Brisbane for a time prior to his death.

Australians were also involved in some of the earlier laboratory investigations on kuru, though the critical studies were later carried out in the United States. Anderson, of the Walter and Eliza Hall Institute in Melbourne, was responsible for the earlier virological studies which failed to reveal any organism. Graeme Robertson provided the initial neuropathological data with subsequent reports by Ross Anderson, and with electroencephalographic studies being carried out by Leonard

Rail, of Sydney. The New Zealand neurologist Richard Hornabrook at a slightly later stage played a role in documenting the clinical neurology of the disorder.

In retrospect, the Australian contribution to the investigation of kuru was more in the nature of opportunistic research than of a deliberately planned investigational programme. However, had the disorder not been recognised when it was the understanding of a new factor in the pathogenesis of nervous system disease would have been delayed, and possibly might not have happened.

Reye's syndrome

In 1963, the pathologist Douglas Reye (1912–1977) and certain of his colleagues from the Royal Alexandra Hospital for Children in Sydney described an apparently novel illness which they had observed in 21 children between 1951 and 1962. The disorder comprised a fairly rapidly progressing illness which proved fatal in 17 of the sufferers. It involved increasing depression of consciousness, convulsions, vomiting, a disturbed respiratory rhythm, and altered muscle tone and reflexes. There was hypoglycaemia and biochemical evidence of disturbed liver function during life. At autopsy, the brain was swollen, the liver a little enlarged with a bright yellow colour, and the renal cortex pale and a little widened. Microscopically, the brain showed evidence of neuronal abnormality, and the glia were swollen. There were extensive fatty changes in the liver.

Reye *et al.* (1963) remarked on the similarity between the condition they described as 'Encephalopathy and fatty degeneration of the viscera' and Jamaican vomiting sickness, though they did not then consider the two disorders identical. The illness has usually been referred to as Reye's syndrome since the original description. As experience of the disorder accumulated, it became clearer that a failure of mitochondrial metabolism was involved, and that it was a syndrome with a number of possible causes, e.g. inherited metabolic defects, exposure to various toxic substances including a chemical in the Jamaican akee fruit, salicylates and the antiepileptic agent valproic acid, and that sometimes infections seemed to precipitate it.

Reye's syndrome stands as an example of a neurological and metabolic disorder first described in Australia, and to which an Australian's name is attached.

Research fields

Headache

James Lance seems to have taken the decision to involve himself in headache research at a relatively early stage in his postgraduate career, and to have remained in the area throughout his professional life. He had worked in Boston after the traditional (for a would-be Australian neurologist) period of training at the National Hospital at Queen Square in the mid-1950s. In Boston he was probably influenced by Graham, one of the Americans who took up the legacy of headache research which remained from Harold Woolf's pioneering studies in the 1950s. Lance returned to Australia and received an academic appointment to the University of New South Wales. There he took up two main lines of clinical and laboratory investigation into headache. The first was a neuroanatomical one with which he seems to have maintained a close association over the years. The second was a biochemical one in which he was soon joined by Michael Anthony and, for a time, by the biochemist Herta Hinterberger. The overall attempt developed into a broad-ranging and sustained programme of investigations into the basis of headache, and in particular into the basis of migraine. It yielded a series of publications and has received very considerable international recognition.

Before such studies began to pay dividends Lance, in collaboration with George Selby, his predecessor at the Northcott Neurological Centre, published a detailed analysis of the clinical features of migraine (Selby and Lance, 1960). Selby, though his main research and clinical interests lay elsewhere, later produced a monograph on migraine, one with a dominant clinical orientation. Lance also produced his own book, though one on the more general topic of *The Mechanism and Management of Headache* (Lance and Goadsby, 1998). This work ranged over a broader territory than merely that of migraine, and the text was based on a more detailed scientific background. The first edition of Lance's book appeared to provide, relative to the bulk of the second edition of Wolff's classic *Headache and Other Head Pain* (1963), a concise but competent account of the subject. With Wolff's death and the later and smaller multi-authored editions of the book still bearing his name, the subsequent editions of Lance's monograph, each a little larger than its predecessor and the most recent, the sixth, co-authored by Peter Goadsby (1998), increasingly took on the stamp of final authority. Throughout its evolution, the book retained its characteristics of clarity, balance and thoroughness, and a sense of homogeneity produced from being written by a single author who had made himself into a great authority on his subject. It would probably not be unfair to regard the book as, in the eyes of many, the world's leading text on the subject of headache, the symptom which provides the bread and butter of clinical neurological practice. Lance's own pre-eminence in the headache field has itself been recognised internationally in the number of other ways, but his book stands as a consistent reminder to the world of an Australian's contribution, and that of his colleagues, to a major global neurological problem.

The studies on the neuroanatomical background to headache carried out under Lance's leadership attempted to trace the central connections of the pathways whereby pain impulses from various structures in the head and neck reach the levels of the brain at which they are responsible for the experience of pain. The studies were linked to investigations of cerebral vascular behaviour and its response to various forms of stimulation and treatment. The associated biochemical investigations stemmed from Sicuteri's observation of increased 5-hydroxyindoleacetic acid excretion in urine during migraine attacks. Lance with his colleagues defined the changes that occurred in whole plasma concentrations of serotonin, the metabolic precursor of 5-hydroxyindoleacetic acid, around the time of migraine episodes. The work on serotonin later moved to cluster headache, where the role of histamine was also explored. Under Lance's supervision, Brian Somerville probed the relation between female sex hormonal changes and migraine attacks. These laboratory and patient-based investigations were difficult to carry out because of logistic problems in obtaining patient co-operation at appropriate times. Bogduk took up a rather unfashionable and previously largely ignored aspect in examining the role of neck structures in the pathogenesis of headache. Associated with these investigations into headache mechanisms, there were clinical trials of the efficacy of various drugs in particular varieties of headache. Such studies may perhaps not be perceived as constituting highly innovative science, but nevertheless they have been of considerable value to clinicians grappling with the difficulties of treating headache sufferers.

The multifaceted headache programme initiated and directed by James Lance at the University of New South Wales has considerably enhanced the international standing of contemporary Australian neuroscience, and has also been to the real benefit of patients. It provided the venue for Michael Anthony's own headache studies and enabled the training in medical research of a number of younger Australian neurologists, of whom at least two have arrived at the stage of building up their own empires in headache studies, Andrew Zagami at St George's Hospital in Sydney and Peter Goadsby at the National Hospital for Nervous Diseases at Queen Square in London.

Apart from the Lance group, there has been relatively little headache research in Australia over the past four decades though a monograph considering *The Biochemical Basis of Migraine* emanated from Brisbane (Eadie and Tyrer, 1985), and an investigation into the absorption of orally administered aspirin during migraine attacks, and the effect of orally administered metoclopramide on this, was carried out in that city (Ross-Lee *et al.*, 1982).

Epilepsy

Epilepsy, like headache, is a frequent neurological problem, and research into it has gone on in a number of centres in Australia during the past four decades. As early as 1905, George Rennie in Sydney had chosen to ventilate the question as to what was epilepsy, and whether it could be cured, though he dealt with the matters more at a philosophical than at an investigative level. After an interval of 40 years, N V Youngman (1945), a Brisbane psychiatrist, returned to the question of the curability of epilepsy. He concluded that epilepsy could not be cured because it was the expression of a tendency inherent in the sufferer. However, he considered that it could be controlled, as it was in some 50 per cent of his patients treated with the then available antiepileptic agents. It should be noted that, to him, 'control' of epilepsy could be present though epileptic auras continued to occur. Cade (1947), famous for his discovery of the efficacy of lithium in the prophylaxis of mania, reported a personal investigation in which he showed that creatinine protected against pentylenetetrazole-induced seizures in experimental animals.

In the early 1960s Peter Bladin at the Austin Hospital in Melbourne began to develop a clinical investigative programme into the disorder of epilepsy, associated with certain laboratory studies which were carried out under his aegis. The work, which had its major emphasis on improving patient management, flourished. Others joined the investigations and, as Bladin increasingly moved towards retirement, one of his protégés, Samuel Berkovic, after gaining experience in epilepsy research at the Montreal Neurological Institute, took over the direction of the Austin Hospital epilepsy programme, and continued to expand its horizons, partly by virtue of international collaborations.

To the outsider, the original main thrust of the Austin Hospital programme would appear to have been the attempt to relieve medically intractable epilepsy by surgical procedures. This attempt made it necessary for the Austin Hospital neurologists to assemble the equipment to allow them to investigate the presence of epileptic seizures and to determine the site of epileptogenesis in their patients undergoing assessment for surgery. Beginning with video-EEG monitoring, they developed and then utilised single proton emission computed tomography scanning, depth electrode studies and neuropsychological assessment to help locate the site of epileptogenesis. At the time of writing, positron emission tomography is coming into use there for the same purpose. Over many years, the concentration of patients with epilepsy, and often difficult-to-control epilepsy, at the Austin Hospital permitted the study of the features of particular epileptic syndromes, e.g. tonic seizures, the Lennox-Gastaut syndrome, the myoclonic epilepsies. It also permitted the delineation of at least one new epileptic syndrome, nocturnal frontal lobe epilepsy. Underlying the epilepsy work at the Austin Hospital appears to have been a continuing awareness of the social implications of the disorder, and this aspect has been studied sympathetically in a variety of ways. As well, Berkovic examined the genetic basis of various epileptic syndromes by a number of means, including twin studies. In collaboration with overseas investigators, he and local colleagues defined the molecular abnormalities in the nicotinic acetylcholine receptor which are present in nocturnal frontal lobe epilepsy (Bertrand et al., 1998). The Austin Hospital epilepsy programme also provided the initial medical impetus for the formation of the Epilepsy Society of Australia, which as it grew came to provide a forum for discussion and action in relation to numerous matters connected with the disorder. The earlier scientific meetings of this Society took place at the Austin Hospital. Members of Bladin's Department edited the proceedings of these meetings into a series of small volumes which reflected the contemporary Australian thinking about various aspects of the disorder.

Other Melbourne teaching hospitals, often in collaboration with the Austin Hospital, subsequently developed their own epilepsy programmes, all with the primary purpose of achieving control of medically refractory epilepsy, principally by means of surgery. Considerable interest has developed into studying the anatomy and volume of the hippocampus and other temporal lobe structures by means of magnetic resonance imaging (and in correlating these volumes with matters such as the prognosis after epilepsy surgery). Similarly motivated epilepsy programmes have also been developed at the Adelaide Children's Hospital and at several Sydney hospitals. Unquestionably, the Austin Hospital investigation clearly holds priority in the area in Australia, and the research done there has been more innovative and has received more international notice than that carried out in the Australian centres which entered the area later.

In Adelaide, at Flinders University during the early 1990s, John Willoughby abandoned his previous research area of neuroendocrinology and took up the experimental study of the generalised epilepsies, in particular absence seizures, in animal models. There has not yet been time for the impact of his work to have achieved its potential.

In Sydney for some years Beran has paid attention to the population and social aspects of epilepsy, and to the legal implications of suffering from the disorder. Eadie (1994), in Brisbane, published an analysis of the clinical features of some 1900 patients with epileptic seizures who presented to a neurological consultant practice over a 30-year period. Earlier, he had collaborated with Sutherland and, originally also with Tait, to produce a small student level textbook on epilepsy *(The Epilepsies. Modern Diagnosis and Treatment)* which ran to three editions (Sutherland and Eadie, 1980).

The clinical pharmacological approach to the management of epilepsy was opened up in Brisbane in the late 1960s and early 1970s in the wake of the investigation of an outbreak of phenytoin intoxication which will be described later in this chapter. Vajda shortly afterwards began utilising the same therapeutic drug monitoring approach in Melbourne. It has since been applied throughout the country and has led to research of some practical significance. This topic will be described further in relation to the section on neuropharmacology research, though logically it could have been dealt with in the present context.

Involuntary movement disorders

Reports of instances of, and of families afflicted with, Huntington's disease had appeared in the pages of local Australian medical journals by the turn of the century. Brothers (1964) traced the history of the disorder in the comparatively enclosed population of the island State of Tasmania, and in Victoria. Several workers examined aspects of the disorder in various other Australian communities (e.g. Parker, 1958; Wallace, 1972; Pridmore, 1990) without breaking ground of any fundamental importance. In comparatively recent times a very unusual Queensland family was reported in which biochemically-proven Wilson's disease was present together with clinically diagnosed Huntington's disease in other family members (Parker, 1985). In at least one such member without evidence of abnormal copper metabolism the movement disorder was more suggestive of a torsion dystonia.

As mentioned earlier, Parkinsonism was reported in the wake of the outbreak of encephalitis lethargica in Australia though, with a possible solitary exception (Burnell, 1922), it did not follow Australian 'X' disease. There was relatively little interest in Parkinson's disease in Australia until the various types of basal ganglia and thalamic stereotaxic surgery came into vogue for its treatment in the late 1950s and early 1960s, following Cooper's serendipitous discovery of the benefits obtained from surgical injury to the inner part of the globus pallidus in patients suffering from the disorder. Parkinsonian patients with inadequate responses to the then relatively ineffective medical therapies began to accumulate in neurosurgical clinics, where they became available for investigation. In Brisbane, Eadie studied the medullary pathology of the disorder in such patients, and the contribution these brain stem changes might make to the alimentary tract dysfunction present in Parkinson's disease. Selby, at the Royal North Shore Hospital of Sydney, carried out his own stereotaxic procedures to alleviate the symptoms of Parkinsonism after his neurosurgical colleague Mr John Grant had made appropriately placed burr holes in the patient's skull. Over the years Selby amassed a considerable number of Parkinsonian patients, and quantified matters such as the clinical features of the disorder, the presence of cerebral atrophy in patients suffering from it, and the long-term prognosis following therapy with dopaminergic agents. At a later date, John Morris at Westmead Hospital in Sydney, undertook the study of involuntary movement disorders in general, using quantitative methodologies, and also took an interest in the therapeutics of these conditions. There have, in recent times, been several large-scale collaborative trials of various agents in the treatment of Parkinson's disease. Blessing and colleagues at Flinders University re-examined aspects of the brain stem pathology of the disorder, using more refined investigational techniques than those employed in earlier studies of this brain region, but came to conclusions similar to the earlier ones.

Demyelinating disease of the central nervous system

The early history of multiple sclerosis in Australia was described in Chapter 1.

There was relatively little Australian interest in the disorder in Australia until the second half of the decade 1950–1960. Then John Sutherland emigrated from Scotland, fresh from the research he had done in his homeland into the aetiology of the disease and its prevalence in Scots people of different racial backgrounds, e.g. Celts, Norsemen. This was work which had obtained for him the degree of Doctor of Medicine from the University of Glasgow and which was responsible for the subsequent recognition that he had been the first to demonstrate evidence of a genetic basis for susceptibility to multiple sclerosis. Sutherland, whose life story is recounted in his autobiography *A Far-off Sunlit Place* (1989), proposed carrying out epidemiological studies in Queensland similar to those he had already done in Scotland. His main aim was to see if the increasing prevalence of the disease with increasing distance from the equator which had been demonstrated in the Northern Hemisphere also applied in the Southern. This he proposed to do in a State where the general belief at the time was that the disorder of multiple sclerosis did not occur in native-born Queenslanders. Sutherland, with co-investigators, proceeded to carry out a field survey of the main population centres along the lengthy eastern coastline of Queensland (Sutherland *et al.*, 1966). He demonstrated not only that multiple sclerosis did occur in Queenslanders, but that it became more prevalent the further south one went within the State. Heartened by the outcome of this study, he then proceeded to organise a prevalence study of the disorder throughout the whole Australian subcontinent. This investigation, carried out in conjunction with colleagues in the other States surveyed, confirmed the increasing prevalence of the disorder with increasing south latitude (McCall *et al.*, 1968, 1969). After this came some smaller investigations into the relationship between multiple sclerosis and certain factors which correlated with latitude, viz. the prevalence of poliomyelitis and sunlight exposure and various geophysical factors, the latter carried out in collaboration with a geologist, William Layton (Layton and Sutherland, 1975).

Peter Landy, the other neurologist who began practice in Queensland at much the same time as John Sutherland, also had a continuing interest in multiple sclerosis and clearly recognised that it did occur within the State. His particular interest lay in the relation of optic neuritis to the disorder.

Sutherland's work on the epidemiology of multiple sclerosis in Australia was later developed further by James McLeod of Sydney. With a team of co-investigators he carried out a more detailed survey of the prevalence and clinical features of the disorder throughout Australia. The conclusions from the study (published in stages in a number of places) proved to be reasonably similar to those of the earlier work, though the prevalences were found to be roughly 50 per cent greater (Hammond *et al.*, 1987, 1988a, 1988b, 1989; McLeod *et al.*, 1994). This was possibly in part due to more thorough case ascertainment, and in part to a greater medical awareness of the disorder which had been prompted by the earlier survey. A therapeutic trial of the effects of transfer factor on the progress of the disease was also carried out under McLeod's aegis, and suggested that this substance did indeed have disease-modifying properties (Basten *et al.*, 1980; Frith *et al.*, 1984).

Following on from Weston Hurst's studies in Adelaide in the years around 1940, work on the pathology and pathogenesis of central nervous system demyelination and its animal model experimental allergic encephalitis has been carried out in Australia by research groups in Canberra (Willenborg and Danta), in Melbourne (Bernard, and Carnegie, though the latter subsequently moved to Perth) and in Brisbane by Michael Pender. There was controversy over a possible feline virus found in central demyelinative lesions in multiple sclerosis brains by Cook, from Perth (Cook *et al.*, 1981, 1986). Many of these various studies on demyelination mechanisms still continue at the time of writing, and it as yet seems difficult to know how significant they will ultimately prove to be.

Spino-cerebellar degenerations

This now somewhat outmoded nosological category provides a convenient designation under which to discuss work carried out in Australia on a number of progressive central nervous system disorders of genetic or uncertain aetiology. It probably would be fair to say that none of the Australian work on these conditions has achieved more than to add further descriptive data to the world stockpile of such information. No major contribution to the understanding of their natures has been made on Australian soil.

As mentioned in Chapter 1, quite convincing clinical descriptions of Australian families afflicted with Friedreich's ataxia were recorded late in the 19th century and subsequently. The neuropathological changes in an instance of the disorder were described by Lichfield *et al.* (1917), though the two neuropathologists associated with this particular publication (Latham and Campbell) appeared to have had reservations about the precise classification of the pathological abnormality that was present. Hall *et al.* (1945) recorded a family with the uncommon degenerative disorder formerly designated cerebello-olivary atrophy (Greenfield, 1956), and Lambie *et al.* (1947) a family with the manifestations of olivo-ponto-cerebellar atrophy.

Tyrer and Sutherland (1961), in Brisbane, documented a substantial case series of the various spino-cerebellar degenerations as they could be traced in Queensland. They also analysed the mechanisms involved in the production of pes cavus when it occurred in these disorders. Later, each of these authors, and also Eadie, wrote as individuals on particular varieties of cerebellar and spino-cerebellar degeneration for Volume 21 of the Vinken-Bruyn *Handbook of Clinical Neurology* (1975).

In more recent times a peculiar form of progressive neurological disorder involving a bilateral neo-cerebellar degeneration was described as occurring in the Arnhem Land region of the Northern Territory. Originally this condition was suspected to be a manifestation of manganese poisoning. Ultimately, after further data had accumulated and genetic studies had been carried out, it proved to be due to the Machado-Joseph disease. Presumably it was a legacy from the voyages of Portuguese navigators more than two centuries earlier and of their contacts at those times with the local Australian aboriginal women (Burt *et al.*, 1993, 1996).

Cerebral vascular disease

In Australia, the specialist management of stroke has usually remained within the province of the general physician. In more recent times neurologists have increasingly made inroads into the territory, bolstered by knowledge of the research that some of their members have carried out into the phenomenology of the disorder.

Over the past half-century cerebral aneurysm, ruptured or unruptured, and cerebral vascular malformation have largely been the clinical territory of the neurosurgeon, who is in the position of being able to offer potentially definitive management for these disorders. More effective therapy for arterial hypertension in the hands of general practitioners and physicians has reduced the frequency of intracerebral haemorrhage, and once such a haemorrhage has occurred the treatment options continue to be rather limited. Systematic Australian research into cerebral ischaemia and infarction began in the hands of Peter Bladin in the 1960s, initially at St Vincent's Hospital and then at his unit at the Austin Hospital in Melbourne. Bladin instigated an attempt to diagnose varieties of stroke more reliably and to trace their natural histories and devise better management strategies to mitigate their consequences. He recruited more junior colleagues to his investigations and organised collaborations with specialists in other relevant areas of medicine, e.g. neuroradiologists, neurosurgeons and vascular surgeons. As a consequence of his type of work, some of the old syndromes of occlusion of the various individual cerebral arteries which were written about in textbooks of neurology, and which seem to have been defined more on the basis of theoretical expectation than clinical actuality, began to disappear from neurological thinking in Australia. They have been replaced by a smaller number of syndromes which could be recognised empirically and correlated with arteriographic and neuroimaging studies in the patient (Donnan et al., 1991, 1993; Read et al., 1998). One of Bladin's protégés, Geoffrey Donnan, became increasingly involved in the field, and took over the area, and Bladin's former Department, when Bladin reached his date of retirement. Donnan had already organised, and conducted, a number of studies attempting to define risk factors for various stroke syndromes in the hope of identifying targets for the prevention of ischaemic stroke (You et al., 1995). In particular he showed for the first time the role of tobacco smoking in increasing the hazard of such events (Donnan et al., 1989; You et al., 1995), although the role of smoking in coronary and peripheral arterial disease had been established earlier, by others. Donnan formed collaborations with Stephen Davis, of the Royal Melbourne Hospital, and others in Melbourne to expand the stroke studies, Davis' interest seeming to lie mainly in stroke outcome and cerebral blood flow studies.

In Perth, Hankey and Stewart-Wynne in the past decade devised and carried through a programme of investigations into stroke, including a stroke survey of the city of Perth intended to define the demographics and other features of the condition (Stewart-Wynne et al., 1987).

Multi-centre Australian trials of various interventions in stroke, e.g. thrombolysis, have been carried out or are in progress at the time of writing.

The cerebral vascular disease research carried out by Australian neurologists has been mainly directed towards defining the phenomenology and risk factors for the disorder, or else has been therapeutic in its intention. However, a good deal of work in vascular biology has also gone on in Australia, carried out by non-neurological investigators in various research groups in institutions throughout the country.

Peripheral nerve disease

The development of clinical neurophysiological techniques and nerve and muscle biopsy opened up the area of peripheral nerve and muscle disease in the decades following the end of World War II. Although Peter Ebeling was probably the first to bring electromyography and clinical neurophysiological studies back to Australia, it was James McLeod in Sydney who initiated the first large-scale programme of investigation into peripheral nerve disorder in the country. By progressively accumulating sufficient numbers of cases and studying them by electrophysiological and biopsy techniques, including electron microscopic examination, he and those who worked in his research group at various times (e.g. Pollard, Tuck, Fitzsimons, McCombe, Walsh, Nicholson) made a series of contributions to the knowledge of various types of peripheral polyneuropathy (e.g. the Guillain-Barré syndrome, chronic inflammatory demyelinating polyneuropathy, alcoholic, lepromatous and autonomic neuropathies). McLeod's interests extended to the neuromuscular junction and myasthenia gravis and its treatment, particular treatment by plasmapheresis or immunoglobulin therapy. John Pollard was involved in many of the studies and in time instigated his own programme of investigation of the peripheral neuropathies, particularly those with an immunological basis. His work enhanced the understanding of some of the mechanisms involved in demyelination, particularly the complementary roles of antibody and T-cells in targeting the inflammatory processes involved. Nicholson, whose research orientation was biochemical, worked on the genetic basis of the hereditary neuropathies, particularly Charcot-Marie-Tooth disease (Ouvrier and Nicholson, 1995; Nicholson *et al.*, 1998).

Muscle disease

When muscle biopsy first began to come into common use, Byron Kakulas, in Perth, commenced a series of investigations into muscle disease in animals and humans which continued over some three decades or longer. The main thrust of the work has been directed towards the muscle dystrophies and other myopathies. It began with morphological and electron microscopic studies, and later moved into genetic aspects. A clinical interface was maintained throughout the course of the investigations. Mastaglia, an academic clinician in the same city, became involved in the investigations but expanded his interest to muscle disease more generally, including the inflammatory and drug-induced myopathies. Mastaglia produced, in collaboration with John Walton of Newcastle-upon-Tyne, a monograph upon the pathology of the subject.

In contrast to the predominantly morphological approach taken to muscle disease by this group of West Australian collaborators, Edward Byrne at St Vincent's Hospital in Melbourne embarked on a series of studies on muscle disease in the 1980s, with emphasis on the biochemical aspects of these disorders, particularly the mitochondrial ones. His work extended to other neurological syndromes which involved disordered mitochondrial functioning, e.g. Leber's optic atrophy, and subsequently he also moved into the area of their genetics.

Neuropharmacology

In recent decades a number of Australian scientists have investigated various aspects of neuropharmacology. One, David Curtis, after a short period soon after graduation under the influence of Leonard Cox at the Alfred Hospital in Melbourne, made his whole career in research neuropharmacology, whilst continuing to maintain links with Australian clinical neurology from his base in Canberra. At the Australian National University, Curtis was for many years a member of the Physiology Department (then under J C Eccles), but subsequently was appointed to a Chair in Neuropharmacology, later changed to one in Pharmacology itself. Curtis' long series of painstaking studies into the pharmacology of synaptic neurotransmission, mainly within the spinal cord of experimental animals, brought him Fellowship of the Royal Society of London and the knowledge that he was one of the pioneers in the recognition of the role of amino acids, and particularly γ-aminobutyrate and glutamate, as neurotransmitters.

Post-war clinical neuropharmacology in Australia began in Brisbane where, in 1968, an outbreak of intoxication with the antiepileptic drug phenytoin was investigated. This outbreak occurred throughout the country, but did not occur simultaneously in the Northern Hemisphere. It was possible to show that, prior to the time of the outbreak, calcium sulphate, the excipient in the marketed Australian phenytoin capsules, had caused some 25 per cent of the oral phenytoin dose to be lost in the faeces. Replacement of the calcium sulphate by lactose (the excipient in the phenytoin capsules marketed in other countries) enabled the full dose to be absorbed. This change caused a significant number of patients taking the drug to become overdosed (Bochner *et al.*, 1972). From the pharmacologist's standpoint, this remains the best documented example existing of a clinically important interaction between a drug and an excipient in a drug preparation. As a by-product, the work also showed that a substantial number of patients taking phenytoin were not being adequately dosed with the drug, and that readjustment of their drug dosages, guided by pharmacokinetic principles, could produce improved control of their epilepsies, and also fewer adverse effects of the therapy. When this was realised, a programme of systematic investigation of the pharmacokinetics and metabolism of the available antiepileptic drug evolved in Brisbane. After a time the approach was extended to other drugs used in neurology, e.g. dexamethasone in the treatment of raised intracranial pressure, aspirin in migraine and stroke prophylaxis, and ergotamine in migraine attacks. The anticonvulsant clinical pharmacology work was also taken up in other Australian cities, notably by Vajda and Kilpatrick, separately, in Melbourne. During the last two decades of the 20th century several monographs on various aspects of clinical neuropharmacology were written or edited by Australian authors, viz. Eadie and Tyrer (1980): *Neurological Clinical Pharmacology*; Eadie and Tyrer (1989): *Anticonvulsant Therapy*; Eadie (1992): *Drug Therapy in Neurology*; and Eadie and Vajda (1999): *Antiepileptic Drugs: Pharmacology and Therapeutics*.

Neurotoxicology

Since the end of World War II Australians have been involved in reporting and sometimes in investigating several patterns of chemically-induced neurotoxicity.

Thallium poisoning. Thallium was introduced into Australia as a rat poison in 1937. Instances of thallium poisoning in humans followed. Allsop (1954) described 18 instances of such poisoning admitted to Royal Prince Alfred Hospital in Sydney and provided a very thorough review of the topic. The poisoning produced a polyneuritis which could involve the cranial as well as the peripheral nerves, and sometimes caused a retrobulbar neuritis and an encephalopathy with depressed consciousness, delusions, hallucinations and involuntary movements. There was also gastro-intestinal disturbance, severe tachycardia and, if the sufferer survived long enough, alopecia.

Bismuth subgallate encephalopathy. Burns *et al.* (1974) encountered five patients who developed a novel and characteristic neurological syndrome involving confusion, tremulousness, clumsiness, myoclonic jerking and gait difficulty. All had undergone abdomino-perineal resection of the rectum and were taking bismuth subgallate as a deodourising agent for their colostomies. The disorder resolved when bismuth subgallate intake ceased. The clinical picture was not that hitherto associated with bismuth toxicity.

Ciguatera poisoning. Outbreaks of a toxic food poisoning associated with the eating of tropical fish have occurred in Queensland coastal communities over more than half a century. A similar toxicity has been reported in other tropical countries. The topic was reviewed in some detail by Gillespie *et al.* (1986). The first report in the Australian medical literature was probably that of Cleland (1942). The symptoms usually commence within 18 hours of eating the contaminated fish. At the outset, paraesthesiae and numbness occur around the lips and tongue and there is a gastro-intestinal disturbance lasting up to 24 hours. However, the sensory symptoms may be present for several days and less well defined ill health may persist for months. The toxins responsible for the condition are thought to originate in a dinoflagellate which has been eaten by fish. Investigators, including Lewis, in Brisbane, one of the co-authors of the review cited above, have shown that ciguatoxin produces its effects by prolonging the opening of voltage-dependent sodium channels in cell membranes. The Brisbane neurologist, John Cameron, carried out clinical neurophysiological investigations on patients and experimental animals affected with the toxicity (Cameron *et al.*, 1991; Cameron and Capra, 1993).

Clioquinol neurotoxicity. Instances of clioquinol-associated subacute myelo-optic neuropathy occurred in Australia (Selby, 1972) at much the same time as they occurred elsewhere in the world. As well, Ferrier and Eadie (1973) added to the mere handful of reports in the world literature two further instances of an acute amnesic syndrome which followed the ingestion of a single large oral dose of clioquinol. Interestingly, after an interval of several years, both the Australian cases developed partial epileptic seizures of temporal lobe origin, an event not previously recorded (Ferrier *et al.*, 1986).

Chapter 5 The Decades of Growth – Australian Neurology

Neurophysiology

Patently, the most eminent figure in Australian neurophysiology since World War II has been the late Sir John Eccles, in his academic youth one of Sherrington's group at Oxford and later the first Professor of Physiology at the Australian National University in Canberra. Eccles' earlier work in Australia was on denervated voluntary muscle (1941) and subsequently extended to the study of the cerebellum and its connections and the functional organisation of the different types of neurons in the cerebellar cortex. Later, and during the years of his long retirement, his thought extended to wider topics, e.g. neuronal plasticity, the physiological bases of consciousness, of memory, of motor control, of the emotions, before it finally spilled over into philosophy and the basis of the self.

Whilst of general relevance to the background of clinical neurology, the work of Eccles, and that of a number of other Australian neurophysiologists (e.g. McIntyre, Bishop, Pettigrew) was directed more towards obtaining basic knowledge than bettering the understanding of human disease mechanisms. Both psychiatry and psychology could have made claims on such work equal to those of neurology. However, particularly in Sydney in recent decades, neurophysiological investigations have also been carried out in which the basic knowledge obtained was almost incidental to the understanding of the disordered human nervous system function that was sought. This work also had a quite different motive from the purely diagnostic clinical neurophysiological studies which have become part of the day-to-day practice of clinical neurology. The more basic work began with James Lance, in parallel with his headache studies. In patients, he investigated the neurophysiological basis of spasticity, of Parkinsonian rigidity and tremor, of myoclonus and other involuntary movement disorders, and aspects of reflex activity. In collaboration with James McLeod, also of Sydney, in 1981 he wrote a book relating to the subject *(A Physiological Approach to Clinical Neurology)*, which later went to more than one edition and was directed mainly towards the interests of postgraduate students in the area of clinical neurology. McLeod himself, early in his own career, had also done some experimental physiological work.

Gradually Lance's own active participation in the area of neurophysiology, though not his interest in it, as judged from his publication record, began to lessen. Increasingly he bequeathed it to David Burke in his own Department. Burke, often in association with Simon Gandevia, gradually tended to move his interest from the basis of diseased to that of normal human neurophysiology. He involved himself in a very substantial series of studies which continue at the time of the writing of this book. The studies have investigated human fusimotor function and the afferent, cerebral and efferent components of the pathways involved in movement, and the effects of a number of factors, e.g. vibration, posture, cutaneous afferent input, on these various elements of the motor mechanism. However, a clinical aspect has been retained in the work, issues such as paraesthesiae and myotonia having also been addressed.

Also in Sydney, in the Neurological Department of the Royal Prince Alfred Hospital, Michael Halmagyi, in collaboration with Ian Curthoys from the Department of Psychology of the University of Sydney, has for some years studied vestibular mechanisms in animals and humans. In this case, the physiological work has merged into the actual practice of clinical neuro-otology.

Neuroanatomy

There have in earlier years been Australian anatomists with a major interest in the nervous system, e.g. Hunter, Wilkinson and Abbie, all referred to earlier, and in Melbourne Berry, Sydney Sunderland (also discussed above) and the anatomist-neurosurgeon Keith Bradley, and there were the great cytoarchitectonic and comparative neuroanatomical studies of Walter Campbell almost a century ago. However, in the past 40 years which saw so much growth of neurology in Australia, the single major original neuroanatomical contribution has probably come from Nicholas Bogduk, another product of the Lance stable. Bogduk found for himself an interest in the applied anatomy of the spine, a hitherto relatively neglected area. Currently holding the Chair of Anatomy in the University of Newcastle, Bogduk combined careful dissection studies of the spine and its ligaments and associated structures with nerve block studies in headache sufferers. In this way he has tried to elucidate the contribution neck disorder may make to the production of headache. Thus he has carried forward Lance's initiatives on another front.

Neuropathology

In the pre-war British Queen Square tradition, neuropathology was often the responsibility of the man earmarked for the next vacancy on the consultant staff of the National Hospital. This pattern continued until J G Greenfield, having received the appointment, chose to remain in it as pathologist to the Hospital throughout his working life. In other places neuropathology was sometimes carried out by neurological clinicians with an interest in the area, or by pathologists who became increasingly interested in the nervous system as their careers progressed. From relatively early times in Australia there have been pathologists with neurological or predominantly neurological interests, though they have always collaborated with neurologists to obtain the material they subsequently studied.

The roles of men such as Flashman and Latham in Australian neuropathology prior to World War II have already been mentioned, and also the neuropathological studies of Walter Campbell, and the contribution in relation to glioma cytology and biology and to cryptococcosis made by Leonard Cox.

The Nazi invasion of Poland brought from Warsaw to Australia the 1911 Moscow medical graduate **Jacob Mackiewicz** (1887–1966), who though a neurologist in his own country, worked in Melbourne as a neuropathologist in the Mental Health Department. In Australia he studied the histological effects of antidepressant drugs and tranquillisers on the brain of the guinea pig, and investigated the pathology of the senile brain. He died before the latter work was published (Stoller, 1966).

Brian Turner (1926–1974) took up the role for so long occupied by Oliver Latham in Sydney, and worked in the laboratory named in Latham's honour. Turner, a Sydney graduate who had been trained in Greenfield's department at Queen Square (Selby, 1974), was initially interested in alcoholic cerebellar degeneration. Whilst never abandoning old-fashioned morphological neuropathology, before his untimely death he had moved progressively into early neurogenetic and neurometabolic work in relation to mental retardation in children.

Ross Anderson (1913–1988), a quiet, gentle man, was a medical graduate of Melbourne University, who subsequently trained in London with Godwin Greenfield and Dorothy Russell. He inherited the neuropathology mantle previously worn by Leonard Cox in Melbourne. Over many years, and continuing into his time of formal retirement, he not only provided a neuropathology service to the Alfred Hospital and to the city more generally, but investigated a number of matters, e.g. kuru, Murray Valley encephalitis, cerebral vascular disease.

In Perth, Byron Kakulas carried out the muscle investigative studies mentioned above, but also conducted, and at the time of writing continues to conduct, investigations into other aspects of pathology, e.g. spinal cord trauma. Those whom he has trained over the years have come to occupy neuropathologist positions in most of the Australian State capital cities, Harper in Sydney in particular contributing to knowledge of the neuropathology of alcoholism, and Colin Masters, in Melbourne, to that of Alzheimer's disease.

Neurological training

Once the stage was reached when at least one neurologist had begun to practise in each Australian city with a medical school, it became possible in theory for universities to have their undergraduate medical students taught neurology by professional neurologists. Such a state of affairs had been achieved by 1960, and the subsequent appointment of academic neurologists simply enhanced the opportunity for undergraduate medical education in neurology to be carried out in the hands of those practising solely in the specialty and having particular knowledge of it.

In the earlier years after the foundation of the Royal Australasian College of Physicians, postgraduate training for practice as a clinical neurologist involved acquisition of the Membership of the College (in general medicine). This was followed by at least one and usually more years of supervised, exclusively neurological, practice with some exposure to neuropathology and neuroradiology, and experience in the common investigational techniques then carried out by neurologists, mainly lumbar puncture, electroencephalography and clinical neurophysiological studies. However, in 1970 the Royal Australasian College of Physicians formalised a pattern of medical sub-specialty training such that Membership of the Royal Australasian College of Physicians was replaced by an examination for the first part of a Fellowship of the College. Success in this was followed by what was in essence a three-year apprenticeship in the specialty, undergone in at least two specialist centres somewhere in the country. If desired, one of these three years could be spent in research appropriate to the specialty. Following that, and subject to satisfactory reports from supervisors, Fellowship of the College was conferred, so that specialist status could be attained.

The customary pattern of Australian neurological training in the 1950s and 1960s involved the trainee in spending one or more years in neurological posts overseas, usually at the home of British neurology, the National Hospital at Queen Square, London. During this time the Membership of the Royal College of Physicians of London was often taken. The trainee then returned home, with admission to the Membership of the Royal Australasian College of Physicians having occurred either before or after the time overseas. There was in those times a perception that Australia could not offer an aspiring neurologist full training in his homeland, if it could offer any adequate training at all. There simply was not a sufficient number of neurologists available in any one centre, or a sufficient number of neurological training positions, for the possibility of a sufficiently varied experience of neurology to be obtained in a single city. The time spent overseas, preferably whilst undergoing Queen Square training, was in those days seen as being virtually obligatory by a profession not yet confident enough in its own educational capabilities.

This situation could change only when one or more of the major Australian cities contained a sufficient number of practising neurologists to provide variety in training, when there was adequate local neurological research underway to allow exposure to the research ethos, if not actual participation in research activity, and when Australian neurology had become convinced of its ability to train its own people. From a purely minimal numerical point of view, Melbourne had probably reached this state by 1950, though the research options there at the time were relatively limited. Brisbane probably achieved this situation next, because of the university connections and the research activities of Tyrer and Sutherland. Sydney did not appear to reach it until a little later when James Lance's research became established. However, in practice, achieving these minimalist criteria did not mean that Australia began to produce its own totally home-grown neurologists in the early 1960s. Greater numbers of practising neurologists and a great diversity of research in the major cities seem to have been needed, but more than this a realisation that Australian neurological research and scholarship in at least several areas had achieved international respectability. Such a situation probably began to apply by 1970. From about that time some neurologists who met Australian accreditation criteria began to practise in Australia prior to, or without ever, receiving overseas neurological training experience. However, the tendency to complete neurological training overseas, or to gain overseas experience after completing neurological training in Australia, persists even at the time of writing.

The increased maturity of academic neurology and of its training capacity meant that, in recent years, young Australian neurologists, or would-be neurologists, tended to go overseas relatively later in their careers than in the past. Therefore they have sometimes been rather too senior for some of the available training posts

Chapter 5 The Decades of Growth – Australian Neurology

there. Because of this, they have tended to find their way into overseas neurological research positions. Accordingly, they have returned to Australia with acquired research skills and with research publications to their names. Although this experience may have been of considerable educational value to them, it has sometimes proved to have been wasted from the point of view of advancing Australian neurological research. The type of research they had been trained to do overseas did not fit into the patterns of, or with the facilities available for, neurological research that were extant in Australia on their return. Overall, by recent times, Australian neurological research has come to cover a reasonably wide spectrum of activity, with the conspicuous absence of neurochemistry. However, in a city where a clinical opportunity for a neurologist may have existed, research possibilities and facilities compatible with a given individual's overseas research training often did not. The expense and the difficulty of setting up the required facility then often proved prohibitive. Clearly it would have been desirable to have achieved better co-ordination of local Australian neurological research with research training opportunities overseas, or else to have organised for prospective appointees to neurological posts in Australia to begin to obtain research experience in their own country before going overseas. With such experience, they should have been in a better position to understand what types of overseas research would be practicable for them to undertake on their return to Australia. The largely makepiece arrangements that have applied in the past appear to have wasted some of the potential to be obtained from overseas research training.

The situation was reached during the 1980s where a clinical neurologist could be fully trained locally in any of the major Australian State capital cities which contained a medical school. As well, one could also be trained in many aspects of neurological research somewhere in the country. Obviously overseas experience remained desirable to add polish and a wider cultural basis and perspective to that which could be acquired locally. In 1993 the Australian Association of Neurologists established a Core Training Committee, chaired by W M Carroll, to review neurological training in the country, and three years later, despite initial opposition from the Royal Australasian College of Physicians, decided to set up a committee in each State to co-ordinate neurological training and the accreditation of training posts in that State. The situation had become such that Australia was also in a position to train prospective neurologists from overseas countries. However, the Australian pattern of training, under the constraints of the formal Royal Australasian College of Physicians' requirements, possibly would have been regarded by overseas graduates as unnecessarily cumbersome for their needs and their country's registration standards. Hence there has been a tendency for overseas graduates, intending to practise neurology in their home countries, to make use of the educational capacities of Australian neurology more as a finishing school than as a full training facility.

By the end of the 20th century Australian neurology had come of age in its clinical, educational, scholarly and research capabilities and achievements.

Some Australian neurologists

A number of the neurologists whose names have been mentioned above, and who belonged to the generation subsequent to the founding one in Australia, had died by the time of the writing of this book. A brief account of their careers, with emphasis on their contribution to the development of neurology in the country, follows.

Ernest Beech (1908–1976)

To a generation accustomed to think of a medical life in specialist practice as involving a steady progression in a single area of medical activity with, at the most, only a single alteration in direction, the course of the career of Ernest Beech must seem something of an uncomfortable aberration. His obituary (Cohen, 1994) gave an account of his professional life. A graduate in Medicine from the University of Adelaide in 1932, Beech spent his first two postgraduate years in Perth, and then another two years in London. There he gained experience in neurology and respiratory disease and took the Membership of the Royal College of Physicians. From 1936 to 1945 he worked in general practice near the outskirts of Perth, where he became increasingly engaged in the practice of anaesthesia. In the latter capacity he worked with the neurosurgeon James Ainslie, and also came to do Ainslie's medical neurological work. In 1938 Beech received an appointment to the (Royal) Perth Hospital as Clinical Assistant to one of its senior physicians. Beech himself became a Physician to the Hospital in 1950, after having been appointed Senior Physician to the Fremantle Hospital in 1946. During this period of simultaneous specialist practice as an anaesthetist, a physician and a neurologist, Beech was appointed President of the Australian Society of Anaesthetists in the immediate post-war years. He resigned his position as Anaesthetist to the Royal Perth Hospital in 1950 and in the following year became Neurologist to the Children's Hospital in that city, and soon afterwards Neurologist to the Royal Perth Hospital after Gerald Moss resigned from the staff of that Hospital. As late as 1961 Beech sat for, and passed, the examination for Membership of the Royal Australasian College of Physicians, of which he became a Fellow a decade later. After Beech retired as Senior Neurologist of the Royal Perth Hospital in 1968 he worked as co-ordinator of the Department of Radiology at that Hospital, and later as its Assistant Neuropathologist. He had become a Provisional Member of the Australian Association of Neurologists in 1957, but resigned from the Association in 1964, before his neurological appointment to the Royal Perth Hospital had expired.

Thus Beech's professional career comprised a most unconventional sequence and admixture of activities in a variety of medical specialties. His contribution to Australian neurology lay in the fact that he filled the potential vacuum and provided consultant neurological services to the major hospitals in Perth from the time Gerald Moss retired until the next generation of dedicated neurologists, Anthony Fisher and Mercy Sadka, had time to become established in practice in Western Australia. Beech does not seem to have become well-known to Eastern

States neurologists, or to have made significant original contributions to neurological knowledge, though he occupied an important place in the development of the specialty in his own State.

William J G Burke (1913–1994)

A Sydney medical graduate (in 1946), Bill Burke's entire professional career was centred on St Vincent's Hospital in that city, except for the period 1950 and 1951 which he spent in London at the National Hospital at Queen Square and at the Maida Vale Hospital for Nervous Diseases. He became a Member of the Royal College of Physicians in 1950, having in the previous year taken the Membership of the Royal Australasian College of Physicians (of which he became a Fellow in 1961). By the time Burke returned to Sydney in 1952, Douglas Miller, later Sir Douglas, had established neurosurgery at St Vincent's Hospital. Miller seems to have arranged for Burke to become Assistant Physician to the Neurosurgical Department there. Burke was also appointed Honorary Neurologist to the Mater Misericordiae and Lewisham Hospitals in Sydney and shared private consulting rooms with Miller. Burke's appointment at St Vincent's Hospital was converted to that of Neurologist to the Hospital and Head of its Department of Neurology when that Department was established in 1962. He continued to occupy this position until his retirement in 1988.

As a neurologist, Bill Burke was first and foremost a clinician and a teacher. He made little original contribution to neurological knowledge. Nor did he publish a great deal, though he delivered a memorable Graeme Robertson Lecture in 1970 on the topic of myasthenia gravis, which testified to his extensive clinical experience with this particular disorder. Burke served his various hospitals in a number of leadership roles over the years. In 1954 he had become an Ordinary Member of the Australian Association of Neurologists and was a Council Member and the Association's Honorary Treasurer from 1963 to 1971. His memorial is the Neurology Department at St Vincent Hospital in Sydney, and the men he trained and who over the years came to be appointed to that Department, later named in Burke's honour.

(Lionel) Adrian Dawson (1921–1994)

Born in the Hunter region, Adrian Dawson was educated at Knox Grammar School, Sydney and became a Sydney medical graduate in 1944. After a year at Royal Prince Alfred Hospital he spent almost his entire subsequent career in Newcastle. He went to Britain in the 1950s, and became a Member of the Royal College of Physicians in 1954 (and a Fellow of that College in 1972) and took the Membership of the Royal Australasian College of Physicians. He was Senior Physician to the Newcastle Mater Hospital from 1955 to 1990, and in 1965 became Senior Consultant in Neurology at the Royal Newcastle Hospital. He retired from the latter position in 1991, and died three years later.

Dawson was the first neurologist to practise in Newcastle. He was a successful and admired consultant in that city, and a very pleasant and well liked man. His interests within medicine were predominantly clinical. He did have some involvement in John Sutherland's epidemiological survey of the prevalence of multiple sclerosis in his home city (McCall et al. 1968), but otherwise seems to have had little record of research productivity.

John Vivian Gordon (1919–1999)

John Gordon graduated in Medicine from the University of Adelaide in 1942, and received a Doctorate in Medicine from that University in 1949. He became a Member of the Royal Australasian College of Physicians in 1947 and a Member of the Royal College of Physicians of London in 1950.

During a period of neurological training at the National Hospital at Queen Square in London, Gordon, like his friend George Selby, came under the influence of Sir Charles Symonds. When Gordon returned to Adelaide in 1953 he was appointed as Clinical Assistant to the Neurosurgical Unit at the Royal Adelaide Hospital, the consultant physicians to that institution at the time being reluctant to accept the desirability of a formal neurological appointment to the staff. In 1955 or 1956 he became Assistant Physician to the Hospital, and in 1960 was appointed Honorary Neurologist to the Royal Adelaide and the Adelaide Children's Hospitals and to the Repatriation Department in South Australia (Rischbieth, 1994).

John Gordon developed a specialist neurological practice in Adelaide, as a private consultant and at the various Adelaide hospitals to which he held appointments. He also induced younger men to take up the specialty, particularly Richard Burns. He did publish some clinical report type material, but he was not a researcher. In fact, as the years passed, his interest became increasingly directed towards music rather than medicine, and in 1977 he left Adelaide to live in London where he pursued his cultural interests. In 1994 he became an Honorary Member Emeritus of the Australian Association of Neurologists, to which he had been elected to Ordinary Membership in 1954. He had served on the Association's Council in its earlier days as its Honorary Treasurer (from 1974 to 1977).

Gordon was a rather large-framed, benign, genial and seemingly gentle man who established neurology on a secure basis in South Australia and inspired considerable affection in those he trained and in those with whom he was associated. His premature departure from the Australian neurological scene was a source of considerable regret to his colleagues in the national neurological community.

Keith S Millingen (1922–1994)

Keith Millingen was a New South Welshman who made his professional career in Hobart. He was educated at the Sydney Church of England Grammar School and the University of Sydney, from which he graduated in Medicine. After spending the years 1945 and 1946 on the resident staff of Sydney Hospital, he moved to

Hobart where he worked for the remainder of his career, except for several periods of study overseas. He became a Member of the London, Edinburgh and Australasian Colleges of Physicians, and subsequently was elected to Fellowship of all of these bodies.

Millingen was appointed Honorary Physician to the Royal Hobart Hospital in 1952, and became Neurologist to that Hospital from 1977 to 1987, when he retired with the title of Consultant Physician to the institution he had served for more than a third of a century.

At first, Millingen worked in private consultative practice in Hobart, but later he became a member of the academic staff of the University of Tasmania, first as Senior Lecturer and later as Reader in Medicine, though continuing in his consultant appointments to the Royal Hobart Hospital.

As mentioned earlier in this chapter, for many years Millingen was the only neurologist working in the whole of Tasmania and it fell to his lot to develop the neurology and clinical neurophysiology services of the State. His publication record indicates that his neurological interests ranged over several areas, e.g. multiple sclerosis, Parkinsonism, epilepsy. In addition, he formed collaborations with members of the Department of Pharmacy of the University of Tasmania which resulted in his co-authorship of papers on the clinical pharmacokinetics of several drugs used in neurology, and on the issue of compliance with prescribed medication in the management of epilepsy.

George M Selby (1922–1997)

Vienna-born, George Selby (Plate 12) emigrated to Australia with his parents in 1938, shortly before Nazi Germany annexed Austria. His secondary schooling was completed at Scots College, Sydney. He then studied medicine at the University of Sydney, from which he graduated MB BS in 1946. After spending a year on the resident staff of the Royal Prince Alfred Hospital and another year in neurological research in Sydney, he went to Europe and the United Kingdom. There he worked for two years at the National Hospital at Queen Square, coming under the influence of, in particular, Sir Charles Symonds. Selby returned to Sydney holding the Memberships of the Royal Colleges of Physicians of both London and Edinburgh, and soon afterwards took the Membership of the Royal Australasian College of Physicians.

At some stage around this time, if not earlier, he seems to have been taken under the wing of E L (Gus) Susman, despite their holding consultant appointments at different hospitals. As already mentioned, Susman later left George Selby the unusual Zeiss ophthalmoscope which he had owned, and also part of his library, including a volume of Gowers' *Manual* which George Selby passed on to the present writer much later.

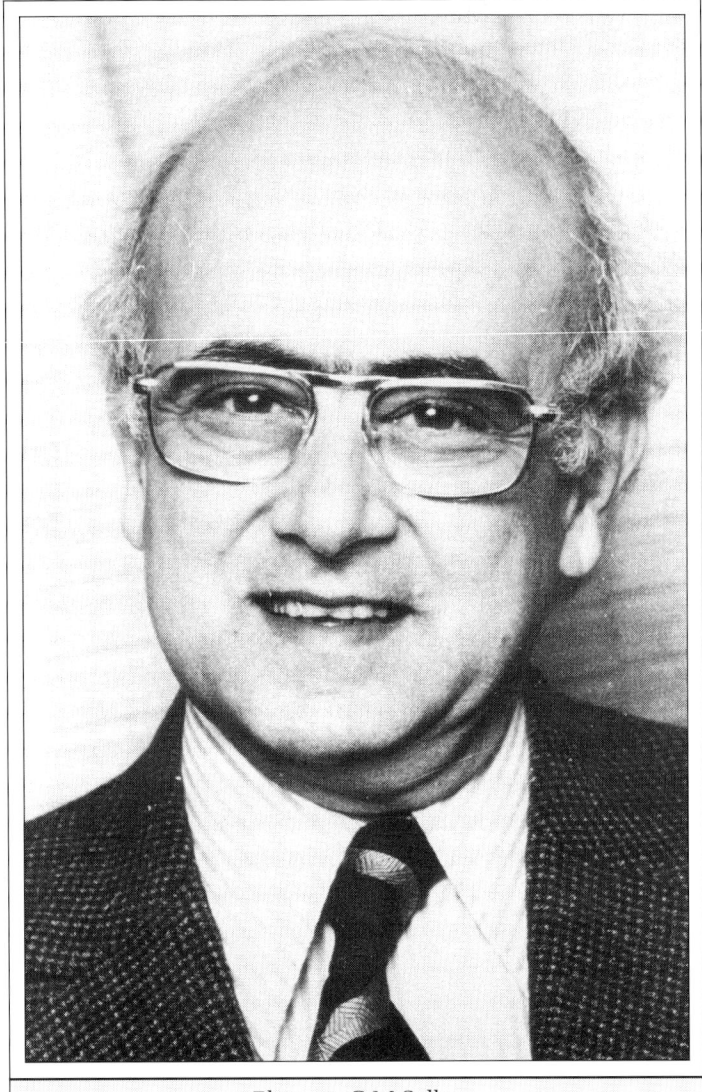

Plate 12. G M Selby

In Sydney, Selby appears to have been the first man since Walter Campbell half a century earlier to attempt to practise in private exclusively in clinical neurology. From 1951 to 1954 he was Neurologist-in-Charge of the new Northcott Neurological Centre, and in 1953 became Honorary Assistant Physician responsible for Neurology at the Royal North Shore Hospital of Sydney. In 1964 his appointment was converted to that of Honorary Neurologist to the Hospital, with charge of its Department of Neurology. After 23 years in that position he became Consultant Neurologist to the Hospital, a position he held to the time of his death. Selby also was Neurologist to the Mater Misericordiae Hospital and the Hornsby Hospital in Sydney. In the fullness of time his Memberships of the various Royal Colleges of Physicians became converted to Fellowships of those bodies, and in 1968 the University of Sydney conferred on him a Doctorate of Medicine for his thesis into research on Parkinson's disease.

George Selby was a great servant to the Australian Association of Neurologists. He became an Associate Member in 1951, when that category of membership was more or less tantamount to what became shortly afterwards Provisional Membership. In 1954 he moved to Ordinary Membership of the Association and was a Council Member from 1959 to 1969, and again from 1971 to 1978, being the Association's President between 1974 and 1978. In later years he was the Association's Honorary Archivist, and after his term of Presidency the Association appointed him an Honorary Member Emeritus. He was honoured by appointment as a Member of the Order of Australia in 1995, in recognition of his services to neurology.

The later years of George Selby's life were clouded by illness. Despite increasing handicaps he remained active as long as he could and bore with great dignity and courage the closing off of one after another of the aspects of life in which he had found his fulfilment in better times. Over those long sad years he was cared for devotedly by his wife Deirdre with the support of professional colleagues, notably Peter Williamson. He died on 28 April 1997, on the day when the Australian Association of Neurologists was meeting in his own home city with the Association of British Neurologists.

George Selby was not only a fine clinical neurologist with gracious European manners who was ever careful to preserve the feelings of other people. He was also an excellent clinical teacher and a lucid lecturer who created an active neurological department at the Royal North Shore Hospital where he trained a succession of juniors. But he was much more than this. He was an active clinical researcher throughout much of his professional life who was well aware of research approaches and statistical techniques and their places in collecting and analysing original data. Parkinson's disease was his great intellectual hobby. His careful longitudinal analysis of a large case series of this disorder was the basis of his MD degree. However, during his career he published over a wider range of neurological topics, e.g. parietal lobe syndromes (Selby, 1956), subacute myelo-optic neuropathy (Selby, 1972). He also wrote an monograph on *Migraine and its Variants* (Selby, 1983) whose contents reflected his extensive clinical experience.

George Selby played a number of very significant professional roles in the evolution of Australian neurology. He was the pioneer of modern-day exclusive neurological consultant practice in Australia's largest city, and he made a long and influential contribution to advancing the affairs of the Australian Association of Neurologists. But above all, he was an example of that uncommon and important phenomenon, a clinical neurologist who was also a clinical researcher, both in attitude and in achievement. His career constitutes a notable bridge between clinical and academic neurology in Australia. Had he lived at a slightly later date it seems highly probable that his attainments would have received fitting academic titular recognition.

John Mackay Sutherland (1920–1995)

John Sutherland was a Highlander, a Caithness man, educated at the Glasgow High School and the University of Glasgow, from which he graduated MB ChB in 1943. After naval service during World War II, he took the Membership of the Royal College of Physicians of Edinburgh and trained in neurology under Douglas Kinchin Adams at the Western Infirmary of Glasgow. The investigation he then carried out into multiple sclerosis, which resulted in his MD from the University of Glasgow, has been mentioned earlier in this chapter. Later, as a senior registrar based in Inverness, he provided a *de facto* neurological service to the north of Scotland and the Hebrides. However, the queue of time-expired senior registrars that then developed in Britain caused him to accept an academic appointment in Brisbane and to emigrate to Australia, also as described earlier in this chapter. He became Senior Visiting Neurologist at the Royal Brisbane Hospital from 1959 to 1977, and then retired, to practise in the quieter professional environment of the country city of Toowoomba, where he died in 1995.

Scientifically, John Sutherland's main achievements were the multiple sclerosis studies already outlined above, but he also obtained very considerable local fame in Brisbane as an expositor of clinical neurology. He took a major interest in medico-legal aspects of the specialty. He co-authored a set of educational case studies for medical students (*Exercises in Neurological Diagnosis*) with John Tyrer and later also with Eadie (Tyrer *et al.*, 1981), and wrote a co-authored work *The Epilepsies – Modern Diagnosis and Treatment* (Sutherland and Eadie, 1980), referred to earlier. As well, in retirement, he produced a small textbook of neurology in note form (Sutherland: *Fundamentals of Neurology*) which appeared in 1981. He was the first man to practise in Queensland purely as a neurologist. He brought the Scottish neurological tradition, different in some ways from the Queen Square one, and more therapeutically conscious, to Queensland soil, and he also made Australian neurology aware of the possibilities of neuro-epidemiological research.

John D Bergin (1921–1995)

Though a New Zealander, Jack Bergin was a long-standing Ordinary Member of the Australian Association of Neurologists. He graduated in Medicine from the University of Otago in 1943, and after war service held training positions in Wellington, becoming a Member of the Royal Australasian College of Physicians in 1947. Between 1950 and 1955 he worked in the United Kingdom, at the Hammersmith Hospital and the National Hospital at Queen Square, and took the Membership of the Royal College of Physicians in 1951. Soon after his return to Wellington in 1955 he succeeded Ivan Allen as Neurologist to the Wellington Hospital. He further developed the neurology service there, and trained a generation of New Zealand neurologists, as time passed being elected to Fellowship of the Australasian (1957) and the London (1969) Colleges of Physicians. Bergin worked at the Wellington Hospital until his retirement date, and then continued on in private consulting practice.

Jack Bergin was a clinical neurologist whose talents were thought of highly by his Australian contemporaries. He was a tall, erect, spare man with a quiet manner, who was capable of taking a firm line on matters which he considered important, but who otherwise did not seem to put himself forwards very often. He published occasionally in the medical literature, though more often on the topic of abortion than on any single neurological theme. As well as serving his profession, he served his community and his Church in a variety of ways, and was appointed to a Papal Knighthood in the Order of St Gregory the Great in 1990.

Chapter 6

The Decades of Growth – the Australian Association of Neurologists

The last four decades of the 20th century have seen the Australian Association of Neurologists grow in financial strength, in organisational maturity, and in influence within the local medical profession, the wider community and at a governmental level. At the same time the Association has continued to serve the needs of Australian neurologists and to provide them with a national voice and with a forum. The various aspects of this growth may be more easily traced if dealt with individually.

Organisational matters

The Association's Constitution

Over the years there have been a number of revisions of aspects of the Australian Association of Neurologists' Constitution. The initial revision, occurring some 10 years after the founding of the organisation, was discussed in Chapter 4. The principal purposes of that revision were to define the Association's membership categories more precisely, and to set a timetable for members to retire from the Australian Association of Neurologists' Council as the years passed and the pool of persons available to serve on the Council increased in size. Subsequent revisions of the Constitution arose from a need to refine the membership categories still further as circumstances changed with the passage of time, or to otherwise advance the interests of the Association or those of its members. Each change in the Constitution usually had a gestation period of one to three years. This allowed time for the alteration to be approved at an Annual General Meeting following the one at which it was first mooted, and for the subsequent necessary legal drafting to be done to allow the Constitutional change to be put into operation. None of the alterations changed the basic organisational structure or the philosophy of the Association. The changes were intended to serve what were seen to be desirable purposes at the times they were made. None caused the Association to deviate from the directions envisaged, and legislated for, by its founders.

The Constitutional changes described in Chapter 4, more clearly defining the various membership categories, came into effect in1961. In 1966, the Constitution was modified again to allow the Association's fiscal year to coincide with the community financial year, and the possibility of termination of membership for non-payment of the annual subscription was stated explicitly.

In 1968, a mechanism was sought to honour the Association's first and second Presidents, Leonard Cox and E Graeme Robertson, respectively. Council, without referring the matter to an Ordinary General Meeting of the Association, created a new category of Honorary Member Emeritus to accommodate these men. The name of K B Noad was added to the category at the time it was first utilised. Later the names of Gerald Moss, John Game, David Curtis, George Selby, John Gordon and John Sutherland were added, and in more recent times those of J W Lance and M J Eadie.

During a period of prolonged and delicate negotiation to set up the Australian Neurological Foundation, and to seek Governmental acceptance of a differential fee for a neurological consultation, the Australian Association of Neurologists in 1971 suspended Article 45 of the Constitution. This made it possible for the then President, John Game, to serve an additional two-year term in office, which permitted him to progress the negotiations in which he was already heavily involved. At the same time provision was made for an additional member to be added to the Council, or, if the Honorary Secretary and Honorary Treasurer happened to be the one person, for two extra members to be added. It was specified that no Associate, Honorary or Provisional Member could be elected to the Council, though an Honorary Member Emeritus could be.

During the latter part of John Game's eight-year term as President, a detailed general revision of the Association's Constitution was carried out. This culminated in 1976 in a series of Constitutional changes which specified that a Council Member could serve no more than two consecutive three-year terms in that office, that after an initial three-year term the President could be re-elected annually for up to a maximum of a further three consecutive years, so long as he or she had not already spent a total time on Council in excess of nine consecutive years. Honorary Secretaries or Honorary Treasurers could occupy these offices for up to six consecutive years. Provision was made for the position of an Honorary Assistant Secretary who would attend Council meetings but not have voting rights there. There would also be an Executive of the Council comprising the President, Honorary Secretary and Honorary Treasurer. In the same revision it was specified that non-medically qualified persons could become Associate Members, and that the Australian Association of Neurologists' Constitution could not be modified without the approval of an Ordinary General Meeting of the Association.

Chapter 6 The Decades of Growth – the Australian Association of Neurologists

In 1975 the Constitution was again altered to create a new membership category of Affiliate-in-Training, intended to accommodate medical practitioners, generally ones possessing an appropriate postgraduate level of qualification, who were undergoing training as neurologists.

In the following year Provisional Members were accorded voting rights at Ordinary General Meetings of the Association, and also the right to nominate Association members for positions on the Council. In 1977 Associate Membership was made open to consultant physicians who had an interest in neurology but were not practising on a full-time basis in that specialty.

After this there were no changes in the Constitution for almost a decade. The possibility of incorporating the Australian Association of Neurologists as a company limited by guarantee was raised in 1977, as it offered certain advantages. The necessary Constitutional changes were put in place a year later. At the same time a new category of Retired Member was created, and the quorum for an Ordinary General Meeting of the Association was set at 30 members instead of 30 per cent of the membership. The term in office for the Honorary Treasurer and Honorary Secretary was set at three years, following which they could serve one further three-year term if re-elected.

In 1991 a new category of Overseas Membership was created for neurologists living overseas who wished to have a relationship with the Association. It was determined that such Overseas Membership would terminate if the holder commenced residence in Australia. The annual subscription to the Association for Overseas Members was to be the same as that for Ordinary Members of the Association who resided overseas. Five years later, in 1996, the Constitution was altered again, to allow for the position of President-elect of the Association. This appointment was to be made in the penultimate year of the term of office of the current President, to ensure a smooth transition to the next Presidency. Categories of Corresponding Member and Corresponding Affiliate Member were created in 1997, the latter category to take in overseas graduates who were undertaking neurological training in Australia but who intended to return to practise neurology in their home countries on completion of their training.

Subsequently, the Constitution was revised to convert its language to a gender neutral form. At the time of writing it is intended that the category of Provisional Member will cease to exist. Persons who would in the past have been appointed to that category will in the future become Ordinary Members of the Association immediately.

As one looks at the Constitutional changes made over half a century it can be seen that their effect has been to broaden the range of persons with neurological or neuroscience interests who could become members of the Australian Association of Neurologists, and to include trainees in neurology within its embrace. However, the alterations still preserved the ability of dedicated clinical neurologists to have the major influence within the Association. Thus the Association would remain the voice of, and the meeting point for, Australian clinical neurology. The Association would continue to serve as a *de facto* register of Australian clinical neurologists, which could rapidly be transformed into a *de jure* one if such a register became necessary at some future time. Any other changes made in the Constitution were to facilitate its workings and to enhance the Association's security and stability.

Membership growth

Over the period of almost 50 years since the Australian Association of Neurologists was founded, its membership has grown from the eight Originating Members, who could be regarded as equivalent to present-day Ordinary Members, to, in 1999, a total of 323 Ordinary Members, 57 Provisional Members, 69 Associate Members, 28 Honorary Members, 3 Honorary Members Emeritus, 29 Affiliates-in-training and several Overseas Members and Corresponding Members. Of course, over the half-century a number of members in various categories of Membership have left the Association, by reason of death, or resignation. Therefore the total number of persons who have held membership of the Association is rather greater than the total membership at the time of writing. Although in 1964 the Ordinary General Meeting of the Association rejected a proposal to include mention of New Zealand in the Association's name, some 22 New Zealand neurologists have been elected to its Ordinary or Provisional Membership over the years.

The main interest in these membership statistics probably lies in the growth of the numbers of Ordinary and Provisional Members as time has passed. These two classes of member, plus the occasional Honorary Member Emeritus who continued in practice, provide a reasonably complete measure of the total Australian neurological workforce at a given time. The growth since 1950 in the numbers of Australian-based Ordinary plus Provisional Members, and in Ordinary Members only, is plotted against time in Figure 1, and the growth in numbers of Ordinary plus Provisional Members, on a State by State basis, is plotted against time in Figure 2. Figure 3 shows the time-course of the growth in all the major categories of Membership of the Association (unlike Figures 1 and 2, Overseas Members are included in Figure 3). The number of Provisional Members has tended to remained relatively constant over time whilst the number of Ordinary Members has increased progressively. This simply reflects the fact that after a period of three years in the category, Provisional Members have normally moved on to Ordinary Membership; new Provisional Members have entered that category at much the same rate as older ones have left it.

Office bearers

The names of the Presidents of the Association, and the dates of their terms of office, are shown in Table 1. The names of the members of the Association's Councils over the half-century of the Association's existence (Presidents, Honorary Secretaries, Honorary Treasurers, and other Council Members), are set out in Appendix V.

Chapter 6 The Decades of Growth – the Australian Association of Neurologists

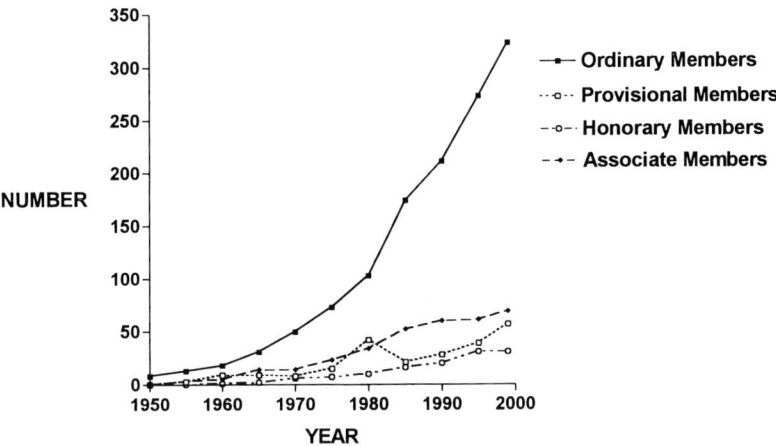

Figure 3. Growth in the main categories of membership of the Association.

Photographs of the Presidents of the Association appear in Plates 3, 4, 9, and 12 to 20.

Following the six-year terms of each of the first two Presidents, Leonard Cox and E Graeme Robertson, the eight-year term of John Game, and the subsequent four-year term of George Selby (cut short by health considerations), it became the norm for the President of the Association to remain in office for a single term of three years duration. Simply as a matter of convenience, the Honorary Secretary was always based in the same city as the President, as this expedited the day-to-day management of the Association. The terms of office of the Honorary Secretaries tended to coincide with those of the Presidents. In contrast, it proved quite practicable for the Honorary Treasurers to work in different cities from those where the President and the Honorary Secretary resided. Further, no disadvantage seemed to follow from the Treasurer's term of office not coinciding with that of the other two members of the Council's Executive.

Table 1. Presidents of the Australian Association of Neurologists and the dates of their terms of office

1950–1957	L B Cox	1984–1987	B S Gilligan
1957–1965	E G Robertson	1987–1990	J P Rice
1965–1974	J A Game	1990–1993	J King
1974–1978	G M Selby	1993–1996	J G L Morris
1978–1981	J W Lance	1996–1998	R Burns
1981–1984	J G McLeod	1998–	W M Carroll

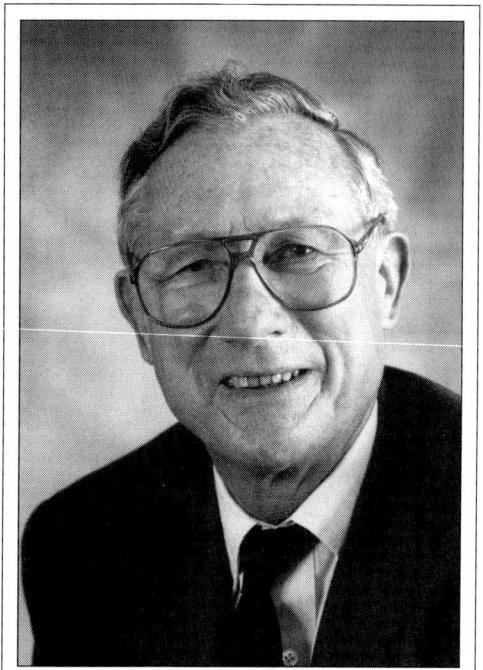
Plate 13. J W Lance

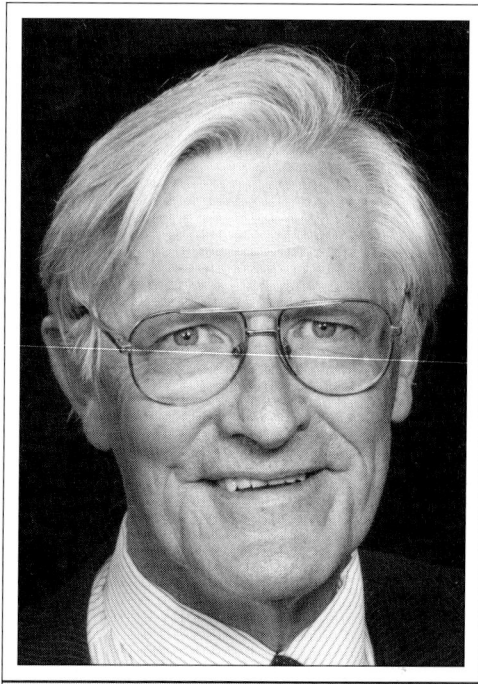
Plate 14. J G McLeod

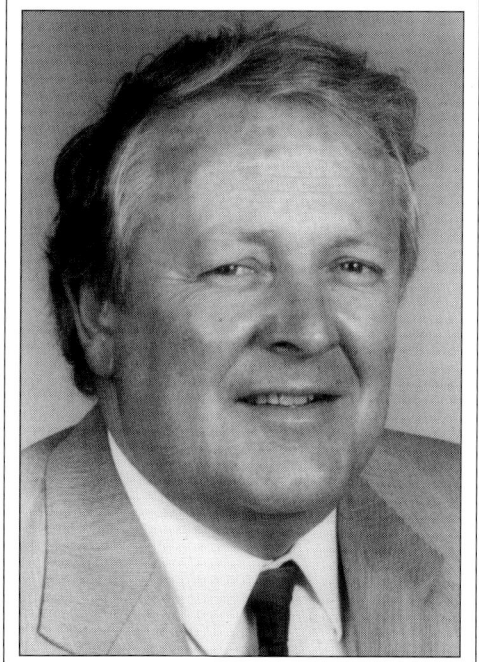
Plate 15. B S Gilligan

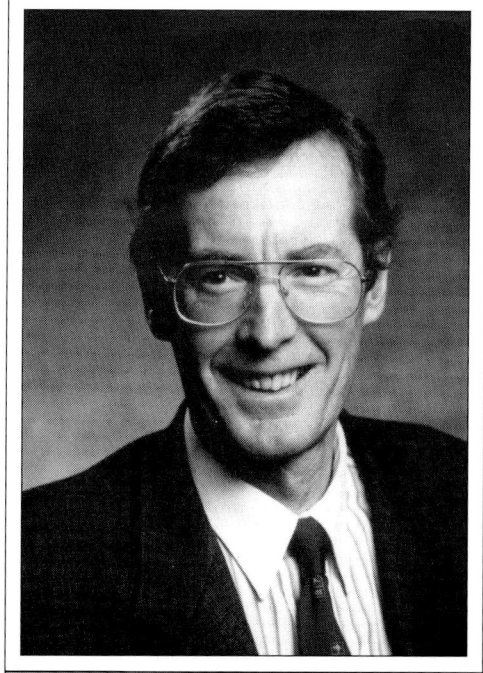
Plate 16. J King

Chapter 6 The Decades of Growth – the Australian Association of Neurologists

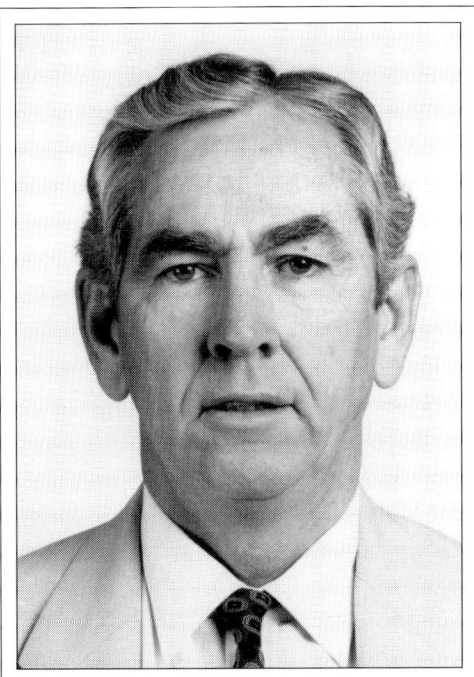

Plate 17. J P Rice

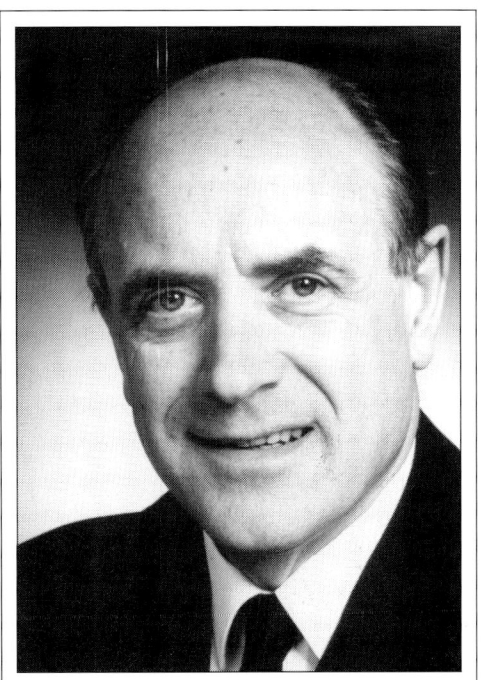

Plate 18. J G L Morris

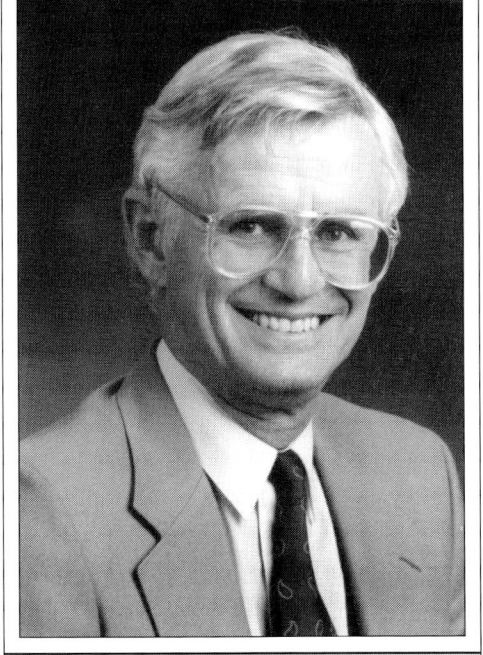

Plate 19. R Burns

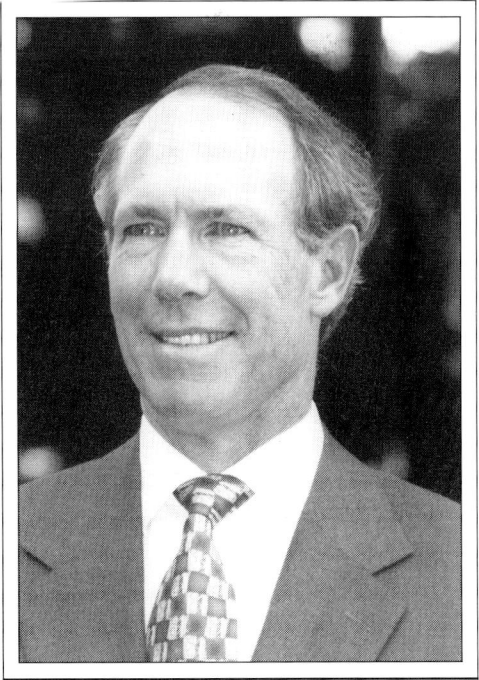

Plate 20. W M Carroll

The Association's Council adopted the practice of meeting just before each annual Ordinary General Meeting of the Association, and also meeting at one or two reasonably evenly spaced intervals during the intervening months. For a time in the early 1970s an Honorary Assistant Secretary attended Council Meetings and undertook the responsibility for compiling the Council's Minutes and those of the Ordinary General Meetings. After a few years the position was allowed to lapse.

The Secretariat

The first three Presidents of the Australian Association of Neurologists, whose combined term of office spanned some 20 years, lived and worked in Melbourne. Initially, the President and the Honorary Secretary provided the secretarial support for the Association from their own consultant practices, but in the latter part of Graeme Robertson's term of office, and throughout that of John Game, a part-time secretary was employed by the Association and worked in an office in the building of the Royal Australasian College of Surgeons in Spring Street, Melbourne. When the Presidency moved to Sydney in 1974, a part-time secretary was employed and based in the President's consulting rooms at the North Shore Medical Centre. Thereafter a pattern of shifting Presidents and shifting part-time secretariats every few years began, with its inevitable inefficiencies and discontinuities, and went on until quite recent times. Where possible, accommodation was found for the part-time secretary in the institution at which the President held his professional appointment. By the mid-1990s the Australian Association of Neurologists had grown too large, and its activities too complex, for such essentially makeshift arrangements to continue to be practicable. In 1997 it became possible for the Association to obtain space in the Royal Australasian College of Physicians building in Macquarie Street, Sydney as a permanent base for the secretariat. A continuing rather more senior part-time secretary was employed to work there, almost in the role of an executive officer. Additional part-time secretarial help was provided in the home city of the President and Honorary Secretary. Thus by the latter half of the 1990s the Association had achieved the situation in which it at last possessed a stable and continuing secretariat. There has not yet been time for all the anticipated dividends from this arrangement to become obvious.

Financial matters

The Australian Association of Neurologists began its financial existence in 1950 with an anonymous donation of £5.0.0 and a decision to set the annual subscription for each Ordinary and Associate Member at £1.1.0. Almost half a century later, it had accumulated assets of $285,652 and had an annual subscription of $320 for each Ordinary Member, $270 for each Provisional and Associate Member and $210 for each Affiliate-in-training. However, it should be appreciated that these latter subscription rates included the cost of receiving the six issues each year of the *Journal of Clinical Neuroscience* (whose cost was $ 208 per annum at the time of writing). No correction for the effects of inflation has been included in the above figures.

The Association's finances did not progress smoothly to their apparently satisfactory situation at the close of the 20th century. In the 1960s and early 1970s the financial state of the Association was sometimes rather precarious, mainly because of the cost of producing the annual volume which recorded the proceedings of its scientific meetings. The history of that publication and of its financing will be dealt with shortly. Once a mechanism was finally organised to relieve the Australian Association of Neurologists from having to provide full financial support for its publication, and when after 1973 a registration fee was charged for attendance at the Association's Annual Scientific Meetings, the Association's financial surplus began to grow, particularly as the Annual Scientific Meetings nearly always proved to yield a profit. During the period of high interest rates in Australia in the latter part of the 1980s, the Association's financial reserves were able to accumulate fairly rapidly. After that time the Association conducted its various operations so that they continued to produce a substantial profit each year. As well, at a time in the early 1980s when the annual subscription was raised, there was an unanticipated fall in the cost of producing the Association's publication over a few years, and this boosted the assets of the Association.

Details of the changes in the annual subscription rates, and in the value of the net assets of the Association, extracted from the Ordinary General Meeting Minutes and other Council documents, are shown in Figures 4 and 5 respectively, for the interest of those who wish to follow the annual trends. Because the timings of the Association's Annual Meeting (when the financial data were made available) varied from year to year in relation to the end of the Association's financial year, and also varied in relation to the dates at which subscriptions were due, the overall financial trends shown in Figure 5 provide a more valid indication of the Association's financial situation than the actual figure for each individual year. The changes with time in the cost of the *Journal of Clinical Neuroscience* and its predecessors *(Proceedings of the Australian Association of Neurologists* and *Clinical and Experimental Neurology)* per subscription-paying member, and the changes in the annual subscription for the Ordinary Members (the main category of member supporting the publication financially), are shown in Figure 6 for those years for which data are available. (Because the costs of the publication were recorded in the available records in different ways at different times, it seemed desirable to try to relate them to a common basis which could be calculated, the cost per subscription-paying member of the Association). Subsequent to 1996, the financial arrangements for the Association's annual publication have permitted the annual subscription to be adjusted so that the journal no longer imposes an unpredictable load on the finances of the Association from year to year.

Considered overall, the data suggest responsible and careful financial management of the Association in the hands of the various Honorary Treasurers, and also

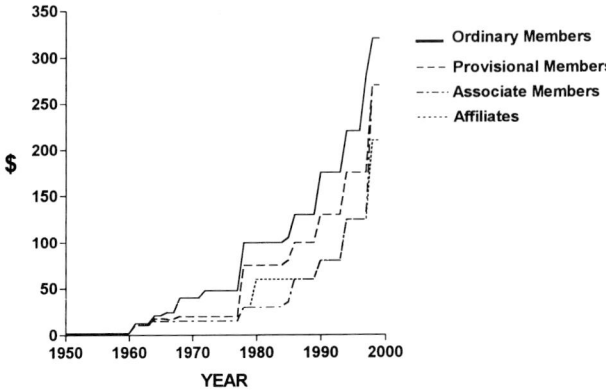

Figure 4. Annual subscriptions from the main classes of Member of the Association.

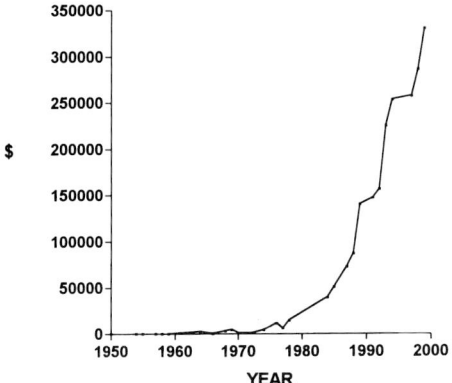

Figure 5. Growth in the assets of the Association.

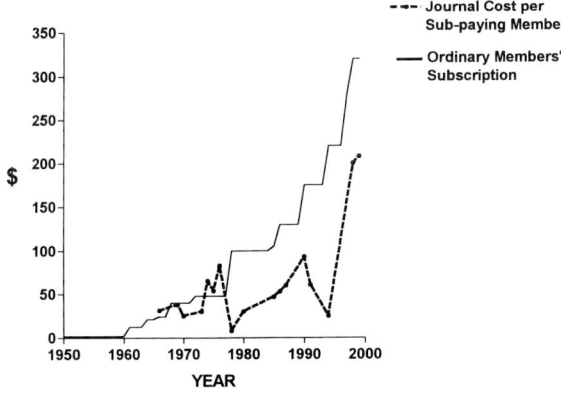

Figure 6. Changes in Ordinary Member subscriptions and in the cost of a volume of the Association's journals.

Chapter 6 The Decades of Growth – the Australian Association of Neurologists

relatively inexpensive day-to-day operation of the Association, once allowance is made for the effects of the costs of the Association's publications.

The Insigne of the Association

At the 1961 meeting of the Council of the Australian Association of Neurologists there was discussion concerning some form of insigne for the Association. At the next Annual General Meeting the idea was raised of an insigne comprising a picture of the head of John Hughlings Jackson ringed by a representation of the circle of Willis, but the matter was left in the hands of the President to progress it further. In the following year, Graeme Robertson returned to Council with the concept of using an illustration of a waratah (reproduced as the frontispiece of the present book) as the insigne. This illustration had been published in 1793, and was based on a specimen sent to London by John White, the first Surgeon-General to the newly founded colony at Sydney Cove. It could be regarded as an Australian parallel to the emblem (a rose, a thistle, a daffodil and a shamrock) of the National Hospital for Nervous Diseases at Queen Square in London, the institution to which Australian neurology had such a close relationship. Moreover, this particular illustration of the waratah had a historical association with some of the earliest medical activities in Australia.

Graeme Robertson's suggestion was accepted by the Council and the Annual General Meeting of the Association, and the insigne has been used by the Association since that time.

The E Graeme Robertson Book Collection

Near the end of his life, the second President of the Association, E Graeme Robertson, presented his collection of neurology books to the Australian Association of Neurologists. At the time of the bequest the Association possessed no property where the collection could be kept on a long-term basis. In 1974 Professor J H Tyrer offered to accommodate it in the Department of Medicine of the University of Queensland. There it remains at the time of writing. The collection comprises a considerable number of texts from the classical era of clinical neurology in the latter part of the 19th century, and some more recent works. It has been preserved intact in the Department of Medicine against the day when the Association will have a permanent home capable of housing the collection safely. It would probably be fair to say that the material in the collection would be of interest to neurologists, and is of moderate monetary value, but that it contains no really old or very rare and valuable works.

Scientific and educational activities

Scientific meetings

The Annual Scientific Meetings have been the main focus of the Australian Association of Neurologists' scientific activities. These meetings have been rotated around the Australian State capital cities and the national capital. Occasional meetings have been held overseas (Auckland, Singapore, Hong Kong) and in later years sometimes in easily accessible resort sites within Australia which possessed suitable conference facilities. Some of the earlier meetings were held in conjunction with those of other scientific bodies, e.g. the Royal Australasian College of Physicians and the Neurosurgical Society of Australasia, whilst the Association's meeting for 1967 was replaced by the Second Asian and Oceanian Congress of Neurology held in Melbourne. As the membership of the Australian Association of Neurologists grew, and increasing amounts of material for presentation at its meetings became available from within its own membership, the scientific meetings more and more have come to involve the Association only. As well, the meetings have become longer because special interest groups within the Association began to meet immediately before or after the meeting of the whole Association. The sites where the Annual Scientific Meetings have been held are listed in Appendix VI.

The scientific meetings began as one-day affairs, with a presentation scheduled each half hour. As time passed, and the numbers of papers on offer increased, spoken presentations were shortened to 20 minutes each (including five minutes for discussion), and in 1979 to 15 minutes each (the time again including five minutes for discussion). An increasing proportion of the scientific material on offer came to be presented in the form of posters, with the main thrust of the scientific content of these posters being delivered to the audience in a series of two-minute spoken presentations during the course of the meeting. Moreover, increasing proportions of the 15-minute presentations were given not to the meeting as a whole but in one or other of two concurrent sessions, in which papers on related tropics were grouped in the one session as far as possible. The necessity for such concurrent sessions was recognised in 1986. A little earlier, poster presentations had been introduced to permit more research to be reported to the meetings. Despite these devices for allowing a greater amount of scientific material to be accommodated within the programme of the meetings, the durations of the meetings had to be increased from one day to one and a half days in 1960, to two days in 1962, then to three days and finally, in 1997, to four days. Even so, as early as 1970, it sometimes proved necessary to reject papers that were offered simply because of lack of time to permit their presentation.

As time passed, the Annual Scientific Meetings ceased to involve predominantly reports of original observations and experimental studies on neurological topics. Sessions of a more didactic nature on recent progress in areas of basic or applied neuroscience were commissioned by those arranging the programme of the Annual Scientific Meetings. As well, from 1980, guest lecturers from overseas or from within Australia were invited to present formal lectures on topics relating to their areas of expertise. Once it was inaugurated in 1978, the E Graeme Robertson Memorial Lecture became a focal point of the Meeting programme.

The topics of the papers presented at the various Annual Scientific Meetings of the Association provide some indication of the types of case material that passed through the hands of Australian neurologists over the course of half a century, and of the scientific matters that proved of interest to them. A complete listing of the titles of the papers and posters presented at the Meetings would be too extensive to include in this book. However, the papers presented at the first 12 Annual Scientific Meetings, when the programme was much shorter than it later became, are listed in Appendix II. After the 12th Meeting it was possible for papers presented at the Annual Scientific Meetings of the Association to be published in the *Proceedings of the Australian Association of Neurologists,* and later in its successor *Clinical and Experimental Neurology*, and many such papers were. The contents of the various issues of those publications are set down in Appendix VII. They provide a record, though an incomplete one, of the material presented to Annual Scientific Meetings of the Association.

The Annual Scientific Meetings of the Association have served a number of purposes which collectively have advanced the practice of neurology in Australia. They have provided the mechanism and the stimulus for Australian neurologists once a year to discuss their problems, compare their experiences, express their views on various matters of concern to them and to plan together for the future. They have exposed Australian neurologists to educational opportunities relevant to their professional activities, made them aware of neurological research going on in the country and overseas at an early stage, and given them a forum at which they could describe and discuss their own original work and allow their younger colleagues an initiation into the techniques of presenting research material to an audience.

The E Graeme Robertson Memorial Lecture

In 1976, following the death of the second President of the Association, Edward Graeme Robertson, the Council of the Australian Association of Neurologists determined to fund an invited annual lecture in honour of his memory at each Annual Scientific Meeting of the Association. The first E Graeme Robertson Lecture was given in Hobart in 1978. There was a lecture given in each subsequent year with the exception of 1998 when circumstances prevented the lecturer from doing so. Many, but not all of the Lectures, have appeared in the pages of *Proceedings of the Australian Association of Neurologists* or those of the publications which have succeeded it. The names of the Graeme Robertson Lecturers, and the titles of their Lectures, are shown in Appendix VIII.

The Publications of the Australian Association of Neurologists

The journals

As already indicated (Chapter 4), within a few years of the foundation of the Australian Association of Neurologists, the Minutes of its Council and of its Ordinary General Meetings began to mention the possibility of preserving the contents of the presentations given at its Annual Scientific Meetings. The first venue considered for their publication (in 1954) was the Royal Australasian College of Physicians' journal, then the *Australasian Annals of Medicine*. Later (1960) having a stenographer record the presentations was mentioned. There was also some speculation about the possibility of founding a local neurology journal. Such ideas seem to have smouldered away for a few years. Then the decision was taken to publish the papers given at the Association's Scientific Meetings in the form of an annual volume to be called the *Proceedings of the Australian Association of Neurologists*, under the editorship of E Graeme Robertson. The first volume appeared a year later, in 1963. It comprised the papers from the 1962 Meeting, contained in a 74-page volume with a light grey cardboard cover with the title of the publication in red lettering (Plate 21). In the following year the cover took on the form it retained throughout the remaining 30 years of the publication's existence, white card (and after 1976 white hard-cover) featuring the Association's insigne, a waratah flower (in colour), with black lettering for the title and the other details.

Almost from the outset, the publication encountered difficulties. Potential authors sometimes proved reluctant to provide their manuscripts to the Editor, or provided them only after substantial delays. The editorial work, done in Graeme Robertson's private time, and the subsequent printing delays, often meant that the *Proceedings* from one meeting had not appeared by the time of the subsequent Annual Meeting. Such delays discouraged the publication of original work in the *Proceedings* and, though its contents were not copyrighted, editors of overseas journals were sometimes reluctant to accept work which had appeared in the *Proceedings*, or which was in press in it. Also, even though a paper had been accepted by the *Proceedings* earlier than by an overseas journal, if it first appeared in the public domain in a copyrighted overseas journal there were potential legal problems when its later publication in the *Proceedings* occurred. Although such matters always remained potential rather than actual problems, they tended to deter researchers from having their work appear in the *Proceedings* if they thought it might be accepted by an overseas journal with a higher profile and wider readership. Nevertheless, researchers were still prepared to present the material at the Association's Annual Scientific Meetings. Attempts were made to prevent presentation of such material at Annual Scientific Meetings unless it was guaranteed by the presenter that the material would be submitted to the *Proceedings*, and at one stage the Association's Council determined that this would become the Association's policy. Unfortunately, it was never practicable to implement the policy without denying the audience at Annual Scientific Meetings the opportunity to hear about the best

Chapter 6 The Decades of Growth – the Australian Association of Neurologists

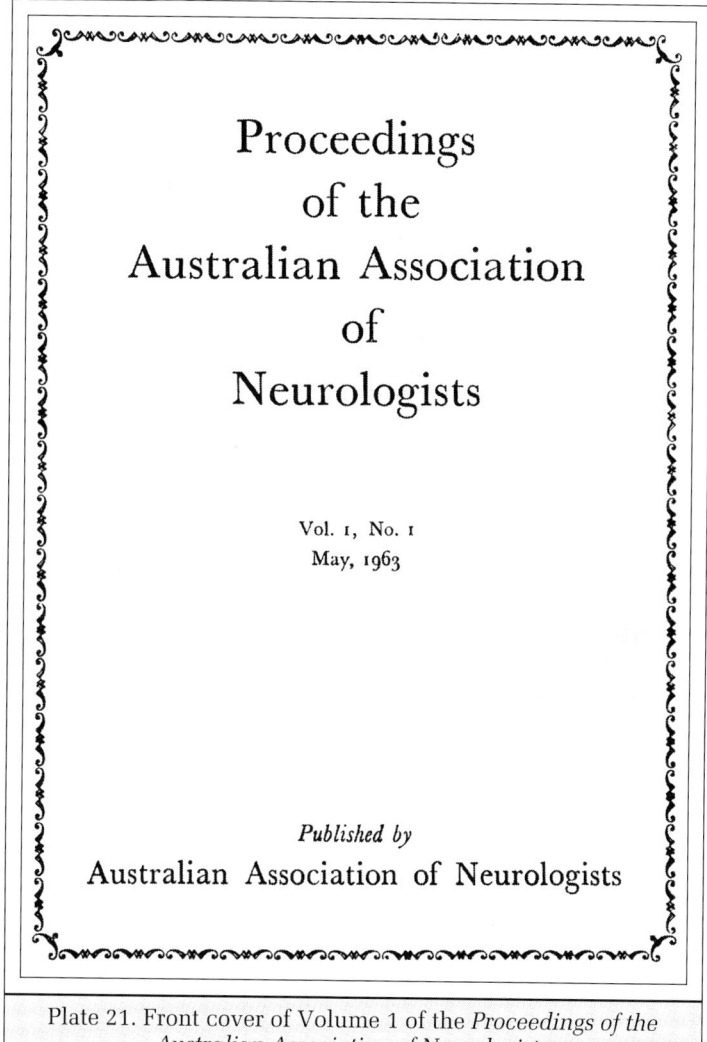

Plate 21. Front cover of Volume 1 of the *Proceedings of the Australian Association of Neurologists*

neurological research occurring in the country. Sadly, the difficulties in publishing such material militated against the success and wider dissemination of the *Proceedings*. In addition, the unavailability of the best Australian neurological research in its pages and the comparatively limited circulation of the publication denied the *Proceedings* the opportunity to publish the very work which might have allowed it to be more successful.

After almost a decade in the editorial role Graeme Robertson resigned from his office, to be replaced in 1974 by Professor John Tyrer, of Brisbane, with M J Eadie becoming Assistant Editor a year later.

In the mid-1970s the *Proceedings* faced problems resulting from several factors, viz. increasing annual printing costs, termination of the Commonwealth book bounty, a failure to find a cheaper source of printing, the impracticality of scaling back the length of individual publications too radically and thus reducing the size of each volume, and the possible reduction in the drug companies' contributions to the cost of the printing at a time of growing inflation. It then seemed that the *Proceedings* faced progressive financial strangulation. However, by 1977 the then President of the Association, George Selby, was able to inform the Ordinary General Meeting of the Association that Adis Press, of Sydney, had agreed to undertake responsibility for the publication of the *Proceedings*, and for its distribution. Adis were willing to promote the publication internationally. Copies for Australian Association of Neurologists' members were to be provided from their annual subscription to the Association. However, Adis Press considered that the title of *Proceedings of the Australian Association of Neurologists* was too limiting to encourage a wider readership. Therefore the publication's title was changed to that of *Clinical and Experimental Neurology*.

For several years the arrangement with Adis Press, and later with its successors Williams and Wilkins-Adis and MacLennan and Petty appeared to work well, though the anticipated expansion in circulation did not occur. The publication of each issue became slower as the publishers seemingly lost interest in the volume as their attempts to enhance its circulation faltered and failed. It became increasingly, indeed embarrassingly, apparent that the growing mass of academic neurological research in Australia was not being offered for publication in the volume.

John Tyrer resigned his editorship in 1984, Eadie taking on that role with C M Lander, later joined by M P Pender, as the Assistant Editors. The publication arrangement with MacLennan and Petty was terminated in 1990. After that time, the Australian Association of Neurologists reverted to its earlier role of publisher. The printing was carried out by the University of Queensland for the next two years. For the 1993 and 1994 volumes, the entire material was prepared by desk-top publishing within the Department of Medicine of the University of Queensland, with the final printing being done by Merino Lithographics in Brisbane. These changes considerably reduced costs for the Association, but nothing redressed the declining proportion of papers presented to Annual Scientific Meetings of the Association which was offered for publication in its journal. Some years earlier, in 1969, the Association's Council had authorised the Editor to accept papers dealing with neurological topics which had not been presented to Annual Scientific Meetings of the Association. This policy change led to the submission of some such papers, often from Asian countries, but publishing these involved an increased effort in organising refereeing and often considerable editorial correction. Unfortunately no papers of outstanding scientific merit became available as a result of the process. The issue of refereeing papers submitted to the journal had arisen at a much earlier stage, when the Australian National Health and Medical Research Council, the main source of medical research funding in the country, decreed that it would not take into account publications in non-refereed journals when determining the research track record of applicants for its grants. In relation to the available facilities, it would not have been logistically possible to send out for formal refereeing all the papers which would have been submitted to the journal in a single batch over a period of a few weeks in each year following the Annual Scientific Meeting of the Association. To have then engaged in further correspondence with authors about referees' criticisms, would have further delayed the already almost unacceptably slow production process of the journal. Rather than adopting such a practice, the discussion occurring after the presentation of papers at the Annual Scientific Meetings of the Association was taken as a form of refereeing. Formal refereeing by outside advisers was organised only for papers about which reservations were expressed at the time of their discussion, when doubts arose after the papers were subsequently read by the Editor, or when papers which had never been presented at Annual Scientific Meetings of the Association were on offer. In 1980 the National Health and Medical Research Council accepted that appearance of a paper in the Australian Association of Neurologists' journal was to be considered an instance of publication in a refereed journal.

At intervals over the years, at meetings of the Association, the possibility of an Australian neurological journal, not merely the publication of the contents of the Association's Scientific Meetings, continued to be mentioned. In 1987 and again in 1988, at the Ordinary General Meetings the matter was discussed at some length. By this time the shortcomings of *Clinical and Experimental Neurology* and its inability to meet the growing scientific aspirations of an increasingly academic and research-orientated body had become obvious. However, at that stage the majority of members present felt the time was not ripe, nor were the mechanisms available, for *Clinical and Experimental Neurology* to become a journal which appeared at regular intervals throughout the year.

In 1994 the situation changed. After making the Australian Association of Neurologists aware of its initiative, the Neurosurgical Society of Australasia launched the quarterly *Journal of Clinical Neuroscience*, with Professor Andrew Kaye of Melbourne as its Editor, and with its publisher the old Edinburgh firm of Churchill-Livingstone. The Australian Association of Neurologists was invited to make this new journal its official publication. Realising that *Clinical and Experimental Neurology* was withering away, the Association accepted the opportunity. It was decided that the existence of *Clinical and Experimental Neurology* would terminate after 31 years of production, with the appearance of the 1994 volume. Eadie was to become the Co-editor of the *Journal of Clinical Neuroscience*, and neurologists were to join its editorial board. The *Journal of Clinical Neuroscience* subsequently expanded in bulk, grew to six issues per year, and increased substantially in cost to subscribers. Unfortunately there has been no major increase in the number of papers from Australian neurologists which have been offered to it, though the journal has acquired a substantial queue of papers awaiting publication.

Financial aspects of the journals

The *Proceedings of the Australian Association of Neurologists* encountered financial problems from its beginning. Some of these have already been alluded to in relation to the financial affairs of the Australian Association of Neurologists. Some have been touched on immediately above in relation to the history of the Association's journals. The costs of printing each annual volume could not be anticipated, and at times came to imperil the solvency of the Association in the late 1960s and early 1970s. In Figure 6 the approximate cost of the annual volume per subscription-paying member of the Association is compared with the annual subscription applying at the time for Ordinary Members of the Association, the major category of subscription payers. In some of the early years of the *Proceedings'* existence, its cost per member exceeded that member's annual subscription to the Association. For several years in earlier times the Australian Association of Neurologists' finances were extricated from embarrassment only by virtue of grants to support publication of the *Proceedings* which were received from the three major Swiss drug companies of the time, and by the receipt of the book bounty which the Commonwealth Government of the day provided over a number of years to encourage the printing of books in Australia. As well, on at least one occasion, an injection of funds from the Van Cleef Foundation was needed to rescue the Association. However, receiving the book bounty precluded having the printing of the *Proceedings* done more cheaply, in an Asian country. In the late 1960s the cost of the *Proceedings* drove up the annual membership subscription. In the later 1970s, another financial crisis for the Association was impending before the arrangement with Adis Press referred to above came into operation. This relieved the situation for a time. Adis clearly overestimated their prospects of generating income from selling *Clinical and Experimental Neurology* outside the membership of the Australian Association of Neurologists. When this became apparent to their successor it resulted in rapidly mounting costs to the Association in the later 1980s. The Association then reduced its costs by reverting to the role of publisher and using a University-based printing mechanism, and later by making use of desk-top publishing and a commercial printing firm for the final stages of production. With the advent of the *Journal of Clinical Neuroscience* the Association finally reached a position in which it knew in advance the annual costs of the publication, and could adjust its annual subscription accordingly, making its whole financial operation more predictable.

Other Association publications

In 1994 John Morris, during his term as President of the Australian Association of Neurologists, brought out two small books under the aegis of the Association. One was *A Directory of Neurology in Australia*. It comprised a systematic listing of the various neurological units in institutions around the country, with details of their staffing, special interests and expertise and included an outline of their histories and philosophies. The second book, *Neurology in Australia,* comprised a collection of previously published and specially written accounts of events and persons significant in the development of Australian neurology. Overall, it provided a

Chapter 6 The Decades of Growth – the Australian Association of Neurologists

reasonably wide-ranging though not totally systematic brief account of the history of neurology in the country.

The significance of the Association's journals

As an outcome of a seemingly fortuitous though happy circumstance, in the face of mounting evidence of failure, *The Proceedings of the Australian Association of Neurologists* and its successor *Clinical and Experimental Neurology* came to arrive at the main final purpose for which they were devised. They were transmuted into an Australian-based neurological journal which had the potential to be commercially viable. Nonetheless, it can hardly be denied that the two earlier publications of the Australian Association of Neurologists fell short of achieving most of their more immediate intended purposes. Despite the editorial efforts, they never published the complete array of papers presented to any Annual Scientific Meeting of the Australian Association of Neurologists. They never became increasingly used by Australian neurologists as the venue for publication of their research. Rather, the reverse was the case. As Australian neurological research became increasingly competitive internationally, researchers saw to it that their work was published overseas and not locally. The Association's journal was forced into an inconsistent policy about the acceptance of papers from authors outside the Association's membership. As well, it always needed some financial subsidy to survive.

Yet the Association's two publications should not be considered total failures, even before their unexpected final and seemingly successful transformation. They were able to appear annually over a span of 31 years. Their very existence over this period proved a source of pride for Australian neurology. No other Australian medical specialist group of similar size, and relatively few neurological associations in overseas countries, were able to boast of possessing a publication which could be found on the shelves of medical libraries in many countries throughout the world. The publications yielded another dividend which could have been apparent only to those who had attended scientific meetings of the Australian Association of Neurologists before, and in the first few years after, the *Proceedings* began to appear. The discipline of having to prepare papers for presentation in a form suitable for publication, and the lessons to be learned from seeing the editorial corrections of submitted text, had a salutary effect on the standard of verbal presentation of material at the Association's Scientific Meetings. Over a few years the old discursive ways and evidences of lax thinking largely gave way to crisper, clearer, more direct and better reasoned and better delivered accounts. The generation that could learn the more rigorous and better structured ways of presentation prospered; that which could not ceased to offer material at the Scientific Meetings of the Association as the deficiencies in its presentations became more obvious. A standard of scientific presentation was achieved, and remained in force for over a quarter of a century, which has contributed to training more than a generation of Australian neurologists in the writing of scientific papers and in the public presentation of scientific material. It may be difficult to provide documentary evidence to support this assessment, but this training and discipline, as much as pioneering the way to a new national clinical neuroscience journal, appear to have been the great contributions that *The Proceedings of the Australian Association of Neurologists* and *Clinical and Experimental Neurology* have made to the development of the specialty of clinical neurology in Australia.

The training of Australian neurologists

At no stage of its existence did the Australian Association of Neurologists have direct responsibility either for the training of prospective neurologists in the country or for assessing their fitness to practise the specialty. However, members of the Association were at times involved in both of these activities in their individual capacities as consultants in various teaching hospitals throughout the country, and on occasions by virtue of the offices they held within the mechanisms of the Royal Australasian College of Physicians. This was the body which, throughout the latter half of the 20th century, granted the relevant specialist diploma which opened the door to recognition as a neurologist.

Nonetheless, the Australian Association of Neurologists was the acknowledged professional body which spoke for Australian neurology throughout the past half-century. Because of its carefully defined membership categories, and their qualifying criteria, the Australian Association of Neurologists was, in effect, though not *de jure*, a second body whose standard needed to be met before acceptance as a specialist neurologist was likely to be achieved in practice. This was a situation unlike that which applied for most of the other specialties of internal medicine where the relevant sub-specialty body's membership was neither so exclusive nor so tightly defined. The Australian Association of Neurologists had been positioned, almost certainly by the design of its founders, so that in time it could relatively easily become an examining body for assessing the matter of fitness to practise as a neurologist in Australia. The possibility of its taking on that role was broached within the confines of the Association as early as 1964, and continued to be raised on later occasions. This was particularly the case when, in the period around 1968 to 1970, the Royal Australasian College of Physicians revealed that it was in the process of altering its training programmes for all areas of internal medicine, converting them into a two-stage process. As explained in the previous chapter, the first stage of the training was to be in general internal medicine and to culminate in an examination. Success in this examination would open the way to two or three years of further apprenticeship-style training either in general medicine or in one of its sub-specialties. Following this, and subject to satisfactory reports being received from the training supervisors, Fellowship of the College was to be granted, allowing the consequent specialist registration to occur. There was some disagreement between the Australian Association of Neurologists and the Royal Australasian College of Physicians over certain of the details of the second stage of training. In these circumstances a degree of tension arose between those within the Association who took the broader College view of training, and those more concerned with the advancement of neurology *per se*. It was a partial recrudescence of

Chapter 6 The Decades of Growth – the Australian Association of Neurologists

what had gradually become the dwindling argument between those who expected the physician to be fully competent in all areas of medicine, and those who believed that the growing bulk of medical knowledge had made that no longer a reasonable expectation. It was at this time that the foundation of a College of Neurologists, with its potential for becoming an examining body, was mooted (Minutes of Council, 1976). In 1974, the Council had already sought legal advice about its becoming a diploma-granting body. However, over the subsequent few years the Royal Australasian College of Physicians gradually found itself increasingly in agreement with the Australian Association of Neurologists' views about the second stage of the College Fellowship. The issue of a separate College of Neurologists faded as the current pattern of Australian neurological training gained general acceptance in 1977 and then settled into place. Nonetheless, with the increasing numerical strength of the Australian Association of Neurologists as the years have passed, the increasing volume of neurological and basic neuroscience knowledge that must be mastered, and the tendency of neurology to become further separated from psychiatry, psychology, and areas such as speech pathology, it seems inevitable that the issue of a College of Neurologists will come to resurrect itself at some point in the future.

In 1977, the Australian Association of Neurologists negotiated the availability of a training position for one of its advanced trainees at the National Hospital, Queen Square, London and for another at the Mayo Clinic in the United States. From that time, these posts have continued to be occupied by Australian trainees. After 1989, a similar arrangement was entered into at Oxford, in the United Kingdom.

The Australian Neurological (Brain) Foundation

It could be argued that the story of the Australian Neurological Foundation is not a proper topic for discussion in relation to the affairs of the Australian Association of Neurologists. However, the Foundation was the brainchild of John Game and he became its first President. He conceived it, and he devoted years of his life to planning its organisation and its welfare, and continued to promote its purposes until his health by 1980 made that no longer possible. The Foundation had a long and painful gestation during John Game's years as President of the Australian Association of Neurologists. There was much negotiation with the neurosurgeons, with lawyers, and with the Taxation Department before the Foundation became a tax-exempt charity, a prerequisite to successful fundraising in Australia. The news of the granting of that tax exemption became available during a meeting of the Australian Association of Neurologists, and the restrained and dignified satisfaction with which John Game announced it to his colleagues on that occasion remains a pleasurable memory.

Sadly, the Foundation did not prosper as John Game had hoped. The main, though certainly not the sole original purpose of the Foundation in Game's mind, if not in the minds of the other main protagonists, was to obtain funds to set up one or more chairs of neurology in Australia. Game believed that this would do more than anything else to advance the cause of neurology in the country, and subsequent events suggested that he was right in his assessment. However, to obtain the tax exemption, it was necessary to make the Foundation's priorities those of patient care, education and research, so that the chairs had to accept a lowered publicly avowed precedence. When the Foundation was inaugurated, the late Henry Miller, that formidable and ebullient Northumbrian neurologist who had, by then, become Vice-Chancellor of the University of Newcastle-upon-Tyne, despite being in failing health, travelled the country attempting to make the Foundation's existence known. A selective appeal for support, rather than one directed to the wider community, was decided on, and met with some success. However, as time passed, the impetus died away and problems arose. The chief one centred on the argument that moneys raised within one State should be spent within that State and not be redistributed for national purposes. The issue came into the open in 1979. John Game had envisaged the Foundation as a national body which would have a national vision and not be dominated by more parochial concerns and influence. One can appreciate the force of the State argument, and in the end the Foundation had to be partly reconstituted to give it effect. Unfortunately, doing this added to the difficulties of the States which had less potential for fundraising. In general, in these States the Foundation, later renamed the Australian Brain Foundation to enhance its popular appeal, tended not to prosper, whereas it has been rather more successful in the more populous and wealthier States.

At one time, over a period of several years, the affairs of the Australian Neurological Foundation occupied some half of the contents of the Minutes of the Ordinary General Meetings of the Australian Association of Neurologists. However, after the Foundation was established that proportion declined and, whilst members of the Association of Neurologists may have continued to be members of the Foundation, the two bodies themselves reached a stage where they followed their own rather separate paths, though remaining in some degree of contact.

The story of the Australian Brain (Neurological) Foundation comprises a chapter in the history of the Australian Association of Neurologists. The Foundation was the product of a splendid vision. The initial high hopes which were held for it were not realised in full, but the Foundation continues to exist. The possibility remains that changing circumstances and new initiatives may give it opportunity to play something of the role that John Game envisaged for it a quarter of a century ago. Thus, at the time of writing, it appears likely to comprise the mechanism through which an Australian neurological Education and Research Foundation may be established.

Special interest groups within the Association

The Australian Association of Neurologists sprang from the membership of the Royal Australasian College of Physicians because of the perceived need for a venue and mechanism to cater for the peculiar interests of a sufficiently sized group of practitioners who worked solely, or chiefly, within the particular area of neurological medicine, and who still wished to retain links to the parent body. In like manner, as the Australian Association of Neurologists' membership grew, special interest groupings with that body developed which, at the time of writing, have remained within the purview of the Association. The first groupings to appear (in 1980) were those of the Child Neurologists, who had grown in number to some 21 persons by 1994, and the Neuropathologists, many of whom were Associate rather than Ordinary or Provisional Members of the Association of Neurologists. Both of these groupings tended to meet immediately before or after the Annual Scientific Meetings of the Association. A number of subsequently formed special interest groups have done likewise, e.g. the Movement Disorder group and the groupings of those interested in Neurological Rehabilitation and in Electroencephalography.

On the other hand, four special interest groupings, the Epilepsy Society of Australia, the Stroke Society (both originally based on the neurologists of the Austin Hospital in Melbourne), the Australian Headache Society (originally based on the Department of Neurology of the University of New South Wales) and the Neuro-ophthalmology group, commenced holding their meetings at separate times and at different sites from that where the Annual Association of Neurologists met in the same year. These various arrangements seem to have worked harmoniously enough, and the Epilepsy Society and Stroke Society Meetings, both held roughly six months from the time of the annual Australian Association of Neurologists' Meetings, in effect have provided a second opportunity for Australian neurologists to come together during each year.

Relationships with outside bodies

The Australian Medical Association

Over the past 40 years there have been ongoing interactions between the Australian Association of Neurologists and the Australian Medical Association. The main issue dealt with has been that of fees for the various professional activities provided by neurologists. At one stage (1973) the situation was reached at which the Australian Medical Association agreed to negotiate the listing of a fee for a neurological consultation which was 25 per cent greater than that which it recommended for a physician's consultation. However, the Australian Medical Association fairly rapidly reversed its position on the matter (in 1974), to the considerable disappointment of at least some Australian Association of Neurologists' members. There have also been interactions between the two bodies concerning the principles of specialist recognition, and about the changed basis of the composition of the representation of special interest groupings within the Australian Medical Association's structure.

The Royal Australasian College of Physicians

The major interaction between the Royal Australasian College of Physicians and the Australian Association of Neurologists has occurred in relation to neurological training, as discussed earlier in this chapter. Underlying the contacts and relationships between the two bodies, though to a lessening extent as the years have passed, has been the long-standing territorial tension between the claims of the self-acknowledged pluri-competent physician and those of the dedicated and focused specialised professional neurologist.

Government

A number of sections within the Australian Commonwealth Government have approached the Australian Association of Neurologists on different occasions to seek advice and comment on various matters. This has been particularly the case in relation to the variously named Department responsible for Health matters. There has also been ongoing interaction over the quantum of fees for certain professional services provided solely, or predominantly, by neurologists, including the appropriate costing for certain neurophysiological investigations. The matter remains unresolved after many years of negotiation. The issues concerning fees have often involved the Australian Medical Association as a third party, and on the whole usually have not led to a satisfactory outcome from the standpoint of the Australian Association of Neurologists, when any outcome at all has emerged. Nevertheless, the fact that the Commonwealth has chosen to consult, and to listen to the Australian Association of Neurologists on such matters is some recognition of the status in the community enjoyed by that Association.

By 1970 the Australian Association of Neurologists had found it desirable to set up a Drug Advice Committee to deal with the inquiries made by Government and other instrumentalities concerning the use of therapeutic drugs in neurological disorders. This Committee remained active over a number of years whilst its brief gradually broadened to take in a wider range of matters, e.g. the issue of vehicle driving and epilepsy. In time the Committee was re-designated the General Advisory Committee of the Association. In later years this Committee expanded its initial largely reactive role and began to initiate correspondence with Government bodies, in response to requests from Australian Association of Neurologists members, and sometimes from the Australian pharmaceutical industry.

International societies

The Australian Association of Neurologists has been affiliated with the World Federation for Neurology since the inception of the latter, and pays it a relatively nominal contribution for each Association member. The tangible dividend emanating from the linkage between the two bodies appears to have been relatively small. A reasonably similar situation has existed in relation to the International EEG Society.

Chapter 6 The Decades of Growth – the Australian Association of Neurologists

Other Australian professional societies

Throughout its existence, the Australian Association of Neurologists has maintained links with the Neurosurgical Society of Australasia and at least once, in earlier times, met in conjunction with that Society in Canberra. The existence of the *Journal of Clinical Neuroscience* depends on the linkage between the two societies. The journal would be likely to falter, or collapse, if either participating society withdrew.

The Australian and New Zealand Society of Neuropathologists, which began its existence as a club and became a society in 1980, was an offshoot of the Australian Association of Neurologists, as mentioned earlier. For several years, the abstracts of the Neuropathologists' Society were printed in *Clinical and Experimental Neurology*, and the Society usually met in conjunction with the Australian Association of Neurologists. However, some members of Neuropathologists' Society have not become members of the Australian Association of Neurologists.

There has been a long-standing relationship between the Society of EEG Technicians and the group of Australian Association of Neurologists members interested in this aspect of technology. The Australian Association of Neurologists has advised the EEG Technicians Society on a variety of matters of common interest, including aspects of technician training.

The Australian Council for Rehabilitation of the Disabled has also interacted with the Association of Neurologists over many years, though the relationship seems to have tended to be a rather distant one.

Social activities

From the time of the foundation of the Australian Association of Neurologists, it was the custom for its Members to attend a formal dinner on one evening during each Annual Meeting. In 1969 the decision was taken to invite Members' spouses to the dinner, and three years after that it became accepted that lounge suits rather than dinner jackets would be a suitable form of male attire for the occasion.

The Association also arranged for a necktie bearing its insigne to be produced in 1978. After only three such ties had been purchased by Members, the entire stock was inundated in a minor flood in the rooms of the then Honorary Treasurer. There was some delay before another batch of ties could be procured. About this time, through the generosity of a pharmaceutical firm, Members were provided with a set of cufflinks bearing the Association's insigne.

***

From small beginnings, over the space of 50 years, guided by wise foresight and a dedicated sense of purpose, and with prudent organisational and financial management, the Australian Association of Neurologists has grown into a very significant body which provides a well recognised public voice for Australian neurology.

Its view is a nationally based one, and parochialism has been almost non-existent within it. The Association has reached a stage where it appears to be stable and well established professionally and in the eyes of government and outside bodies. It is positioned by virtue of its size, cohesiveness, and Constitution to take on a more influential role and an enhanced titular status quite quickly, if that were seen as desirable at some stage in the future.

Chapter 7

Why and How?

When one looks back over what can be gleaned from the record of events, it would appear that clinical neurology has been practised in Australia for roughly a century, though its practice has not been acknowledged under this designation throughout all of that period. However, over at least the latter half of that time neurology has been fairly widely recognised as a specialty area within Australian medicine. Why did the recognisable specialty of neurology emerge in Australia when it did, and develop as it did? How, when clinical neurology began a good deal later in Australia than in Britain, did it manage to make up nearly all the leeway over a period of some 50 years?

The origin of Australian clinical neurology

British medicine has been the main source of Australian medicine. When neurology appeared in Northern Hemisphere countries as a distinct area of specialised medical practice more than a century ago, the Australian States were still British colonies which had been settled by several generations of immigrants, mainly of British stock. Prior to the latter part of the last century, when clinical neurology had already appeared in Britain, the Australian universities had not begun to produce their own medical graduates. Therefore Australians aspiring to be medical practitioners had to go overseas to be trained, and they nearly always went to Great Britain, mainly either to London or to Edinburgh. In these circumstances, it might reasonably have been expected that Australian medical practice would have followed the pattern of British medical practice, so that, after a few years delay, clinical neurology would have appeared in Australia. Because such a seemingly predictable development did not happen for many years, it seems likely that there may have been some circumstance applying in Australia in the latter part of the 19th century which deterred the emergence and subsequent development of the specialty of neurology. As was pointed out in Chapter 1, at the relevant time the demography of the Australian colonies was quite different from that of Great Britain, in that there was no single major centre of population in the country, a difference which remains today. As well, relative to Britain, Australian society at the time was probably rather less sophisticated and overall less affluent. At first sight these factors might seem a sufficient explanation for a considerable delay in clinical neurology developing in Australia, and no doubt they did contribute to that delay. However, a consideration of the factors which seemed to apply when clinical neurology emerged in Britain, suggests that additional matters may have been involved in the delayed appearance of neurology in Australia.

What factors were operating when clinical neurology developed as a recognised area of medical practice in Britain, and in France, around 1860 to 1870, the better part of a century before the specialty appeared in Australia? It could be argued that the circumstances which then seem to have applied in the Northern Hemisphere countries suggest that, for neurology to have emerged, there needed to exist an appropriate environment in which a person, or persons, of some original genius could produce something new, usually new knowledge, which could be seen to improve, immediately or in the foreseeable future, the welfare of patients with neurological illness. The appropriate environment for such an occurrence appeared to involve a sufficient number of patients with hitherto undiagnosed or unsatisfactorily treated neurological illnesses, and a sufficient level of background knowledge in the medical profession and the community to be able to appreciate the potential advantages accruing from continuing the activities which produced the new knowledge. It was not simply a matter of producing new knowledge which might benefit future patients with neurological illness. The knowledge had to be knowledge won from a mode of medical practice which involved managing neurological patients clinically, and which could be seen to do so.

Thus clinical neurology as an area of medical practice did not begin in London with Thomas Willis (1621–1675), the man who devised the word 'neurology'. He was a very great neuro-anatomical researcher with an extensive clinical practice in many areas of medicine, and wrote a number of books which brought new knowledge about the nervous system before a wide readership. Nor did it begin with Tissot (1728–1797) in Switzerland or with Romberg (1795–1873) in Germany, though their texts on neurology were widely read in their times. The new neurological knowledge that these three men conveyed was not for the most part derived from their own clinical practices. The situations were different at the newly founded National Hospital for Nervous Diseases in London and at the Salpêtrière in Paris, around 1860, when neurology did emerge. At both institutions there were substantial collections of neurological patients with inadequately understood and managed illnesses, and there were men such as Hughlings Jackson in London, and Charcot in Paris, who studied these illnesses, derived new knowledge from their study, and saw to it that this knowledge became more widely disseminated. In contrast, just a little later, in Edinburgh, that great expositor of clinical medicine Byrom Bramwell (1847–1931), who wrote a number of monographs on neurological topics, but did not commit himself predominantly or exclusively to neurology in personal clinical practice, certainly put neurological knowledge before a professional audience and readership. However, for the most part it was not new knowledge which could be seen to have emanated from his own mode of practice, and clinical neurology did not develop in the Scottish capital at the time.

Once neurology was underway in a particular city, persistence of the initiating set of circumstances was no longer so critical for maintaining the existence of the specialty – its own usefulness then provided a justification for its continuing. As well, once clinical neurology was known to have proved its worth at a number of different places, it may not have required men of such high level of genius for the specialty to have opened up elsewhere.

In Sydney, at the end of the 19th century George Rennie, with whose example Australian neurology might have begun, seems to have chosen not to practise exclusively or mainly in neurology. He also seems not to have derived new neurological knowledge from his mode of practice. On the other hand, Walter Campbell certainly produced new knowledge about the nervous system and, from 1905 onwards, demonstrated commitment to the exclusive clinical practice of the specialty in Sydney. However, Campbell lacked appointments to major teaching hospitals where he could display his expertise and his new knowledge was not derived so much from his clinical activities as from his laboratory studies. Perhaps for these reasons his example did not persuade other practitioners or the populace that neurology offered sufficient advantage to command a place in the local medical scene as a separate mode of practice. It was only in the fourth decade of the 20th century that, in Leonard Cox, Melbourne found a man with some investigative genius who held a teaching hospital and university appointment which gave him access to a collection of neurological patients whom he could study, and from whose study he could, and did, derive useful new knowledge which he made available to others. This happened at a time when in other countries there already was a growing measure of professional awareness of the usefulness of clinical neurology. The value of Cox's clinical activities, and those of Graeme Robertson soon afterwards, was realised locally. Thus out of their example clinical neurology in Australia commenced its years of self-sustaining growth.

The Australian catching-up process

Clinical neurology emerged in Australia as a medical specialty some two-thirds of a century after it first appeared in Britain. However, it would probably not be unfair to say that, after the passage of a further half-century, the standards and performance of Australian clinical neurology have become not dissimilar to those applying in contemporary Britain, if allowance is made for the difference in size of the populations and wealth of the two countries. It could be anticipated that if one country should begin to follow and imitate the methods and practices of another more advanced country, the gap between practices in the two would narrow with the passage of time. However, the gap would not be expected to disappear purely from adopting a follow-the-leader type of process, yet the gap appears to have become almost non-existent in relation to Australian clinical neurology *vis-à-vis* that of Britain. This suggests that Australian clinical neurology may have done rather more than emulate the pattern of British neurology. The additional factor may relate to the way in which academic neurology has been developed in the two countries. British neurology at its headquarters, the National Hospital for Nervous Diseases in London, remained virtually outside the British university system for a very long time. It was almost a full century from the founding of the Hospital before there was a professorial appointment in neurology within the institution. In contrast, if Australian clinical neurology is taken to have begun around 1940, it was only a little over a third of the century until there were several professorial appointments in neurology in the Australian university system, and there had been more junior academic appointments in the area more than a decade earlier than that. In recent times, it is probably its research, more than anything else, which enhances the stature and quality of practice in an area of medicine, and it is university chairs and other senior academic appointments which, more than anything else, facilitate research. It may therefore be the relatively more rapid development of academic neurology in Australia than in Britain which has enabled Australian clinical neurology by and large to catch up with the neurology of the country in which it originated.

Thus Australian clinical neurology, at least when viewed from within, appears to have arrived at a situation which might be regarded as a reasonably satisfactory one. If its founders were able to return briefly to this world to discover what had happened to their creation, they might not be too displeased with what had emanated from their efforts.

References

Abbie AA (1937) The anatomy of capsular vascular disease. Medical Journal of Australia 2:564–567.
Abbie AA (1941) The anatomy of the cerebellum. Medical Journal of Australia 1:159–163.
Abbie AA (1969) The original Australians. Wellington: Reed.
Abercrombie J (1828) Pathological and practical researches on diseases of the brain and the spinal cord. Edinburgh: Waugh & Innes.
Allen IM (1938) Results of the investigation of reflex epilepsy. Medical Journal of Australia 1:1052–1055.
Allen IM (1939) On compulsive grasping, the grasp reflex, tonic innervation and associated phenomena. Medical Journal of Australia 1:717–727.
Allen IM, Spencer FM (1935) Acute aseptic meningitis. Medical Journal of Australia 2:275–281.
Allsop JL (1954) Thallium poisoning. Australasian Annals of Medicine 3:144–160.
Allsop J (1994) A history of neurology in New South Wales. In: Morris J, ed. Neurology in Australia. Sydney: Australian Association of Neurologists: pp 35–45.
Anderson AG (1917) Some remarks on the occurrence of the 'Mysterious Disease' in Southern Queensland. Medical Journal of Australia 2:270–272.
Anderson C, English JC (1938) Streptococal meningitis treated with sulphanilamide. Medical Journal of Australia 2:287–288.
Anderson D (1933) John White: Surgeon-General to the first fleet. Medical Journal of Australia 1:183–187.
Anderson SG (1952) Murray Valley encephalitis: epidemiological aspects. Medical Journal of Australia 1:97–100.
Anderson SG, Donnelly M, Stevenson WJ, Caldwell NJ, Eagle M (1952) Murray Valley encephalitis: surveys of human and animal sera. Medical Journal of Australia 1:110–114.
Anderson SG, Price AVG, Nanadai-Koia, Slater K (1960) Murray Valley encephalitis in Papua and New Guinea. Medical Journal of Australia 2:410–413.
Anonymous (1917) Obituary: James Froude Flashman. Medical Journal of Australia 1:174–176.
Anonymous (1922) An historical account of the occurrence and causation of lead poisoning among Queensland children. Medical Journal of Australia 9:148–152.
Anonymous (1923) Obituary: George Edward Rennie. Medical Journal of Australia 2:211–213.
Anonymous (1924) Obituary. John Irvine Hunter. Medical Journal of Australia 2:669–671.
Anonymous (1926) Current comment. Sympathetic innervation and skeletal muscle tonus. Medical Journal of Australia 2:390–391.

Anonymous (1960) Queen Square and the National Hospital 1860–1960. London: Edward Arnold.

Baldwin AH, Heydon GM (1925) X disease in Townsville. Medical Journal of Australia 2:394–396.

Balls-Headley W (1896) Demonstration. Intercolonial Medical Journal of Australasia 1:380.

Bancroft J (1884) Queensland ticks and tick blindness. Australasian Medical Gazette 4:37, cited by Cleland JB (1912) *loc cit*.

Bancroft J (1892) Leprosy in Queensland. Australasian Medical Gazette 1:427–430.

Basten A, McLeod JG, Pollard JD, et al. (1980) Transfer factor in treatment of multiple sclerosis. Lancet ii:931–934.

Bell G, Latham O (1928) Tumour of the brain: spongioblastoma multiforme. Medical Journal of Australia 2:757–761.

Bentley BJ (1912) Some further points in the treatment of epilepsy with chloretone. Medical Journal of Australia 32:599–601.

Bentley J (1911) Epilepsy. Australasian Medical Gazette 30:121–126.

Bertrand S, Weiland S, Berkovic SF, Steinlein OK, Bertrand D (1998) Properties of neuronal nicotinic acetylcholine receptor mutants from humans suffering from autosomal dominant frontal lobe epilepsy. British Journal of Pharmacology 125:751–760.

Billings J, Robertson P (1955) Paraplegia following chest surgery. Australasian Annals of Medicine 4:141–144.

Black GHB (1934) Migraine. Medical Journal of Australia 2:37–46.

Blackburn CB, Latham O (1922) Pernicious anaemia with early spinal symptoms. Medical Journal of Australia 2:735–737.

Bochner F, Hooper WD, Tyrer JH, Eadie MJ (1972) Factors involved in an outbreak of phenytoin intoxication. Journal of the Neurological Sciences 16:481–487.

Bostock J (1926) Diabetic tabes so-called. Medical Journal of Australia 2:82–83.

Breinl A (1917) The mysterious disease. Medical Journal of Australia 1:454.

Breinl A (1918) Clinical, pathological and experimental observations on the 'mysterious disease', a clinically aberrant form of acute poliomyelitis. Medical Journal of Australia 5:209–213 & 229–234.

Breinl A, Young WJ (1914) The occurrence of lead poisoning amongst Queensland children. Annals of Tropical Medicine and Parasitology:575.

Brothers CRD (1964) Huntington's chorea in Victoria and Tasmania. Journal of the Neurological Sciences 1:405–420.

Brown-Sequard CE (1860) On the etiology, nature, and treatment of epilepsy, with a few remarks on several other affections of the nervous centres. In: Course of lectures on the physiology and pathology of the central nervous system. Philadelphia: Lippincott & Co: pp 178–186.

Buchanan AL (1929) Experiences with encephalography. Medical Journal of Australia 2:812–817.

Buchanan AR (1937) The Lange colloidal gold reaction as a routine test: a preliminary note on the results. Medical Journal of Australia 2:175–178.

Burkitt N (1944) Obituary. Norman Gilmore Royle. Medical Journal of Australia 1:570–571.

Burnell GH (1917) The Broken Hill epidemic. Medical Journal of Australia 2:157–163.

Burnell GH (1918) The Broken Hill epidemic. Medical Journal of Australia 1:278–280.

Burnell GH (1922) X disease. Medical Journal of Australia 1:126.

Burnet FM (1934) Louping ill virus as a possible cause of the X disease epidemics of 1917–1918. Medical Journal of Australia 1:679–681.

Burnet FM (1952a) Murray Valley encephalitis. American Journal of Public Health 42:1519–1521.

References

Burnet FM (1952b) Poliomyelitis and Murray Valley encephalitis: a comparison of two neurotropic virus diseases. Medical Journal of Australia 1:169–175.

Burns C (1963) Ivan Macdonald Allen. New Zealand Medical Journal 62:244–245.

Burns R, Thomas DW, Barron VJ (1974) Reversible encephalopathy possibly associated with bismuth subgallate ingestion. British Medical Journal 1:220–223.

Burrow JNC, Whelan PI, Kilburn CJ, Fisher DA, Currie BJ, Smith DW (1998) Australian encephalitis in the Northern Territory: clinical and epidemiological features, 1987–1996. Australian and New Zealand Journal of Medicine 28:590–596.

Burston RA (1988) Fry,Henry Kenneth. In: McDonald GL, ed. Roll of the Royal Australasian College of Physicians. v. 1. Sydney: Royal Australasian College of Physicians:pp 100–101.

Burt T, Blumbergs P, Currie B (1993) A dominant hereditary ataxia resembling Machado-Joseph disease in Arnhem Land, Australia. Neurology 43:1750–1752.

Burt T, Currie B, Kilburn C, et al. (1996) Machado-Joseph disease in east Arnhem Land, Australia: chromosome 14q32.1 expanded repeat confirmed in four families. Neurology 46:1118–1122.

Cade JF (1947) The anticonvulsant properties of creatinine. Medical Journal of Australia 2:621–623.

Calov WL (1940) Cerebro-spinal meningitis. Medical Journal of Australia 2:51–64.

Cameron J, Capra MF (1993) The basis of paradoxical disturbance of temperature perception in ciguatera poisoning. Journal of Toxicology and Clinical Toxicology 31:571–579.

Cameron J, Flowers AE, Capra MF (1991) Effects of ciguatoxin on nerve excitability in rats. Journal of the Neurological Sciences 101:87–92.

Campbell AW (1894a) Degenerations consequent on experimental lesions of the cerebellum. British Medical Journal 2:641–642.

Campbell AW (1894b) A contribution to the morbid anatomy and pathology of the neuro-nuscular changes in general paresis of the insane. Journal of Mental Science 40:177–195.

Campbell AW (1894c) On vacuolation of the nerve cell of the human cerebral cortex. Journal of Pathology and Bacteriology 2:380–393.

Campbell AW (1897) On the tracts of the spinal cord and their degenerations. Brain 20:488–535.

Campbell AW (1903) Communicated by Sherrington, CS. Histological studies on cerebral localisation. Proceedings of the Royal Society of London:488–492.

Campbell AW (1905) Histological studies on the localisation of cerebral function. Cambridge: Cambridge University Press.

Campbell AW (1910) The treatment of trigeminal neuralgia by injections of alcohol. Australasian Medical Gazette 29:66–75.

Campbell AW (1911) On the localisation of function in the cerebellum. Transactions of the Ninth Australasian Medical Congress, Sydney:847–852.

Campbell AW (1913) A case of syringomyelia. Australasian Medical Gazette 34:478–479.

Campbell AW (1916) Remarks on some neuroses and psychoses in war. Medical Journal of Australia 1:319–323.

Campbell AW (1919) A case for diagnosis (Thomsen's disease). Medical Journal of Australia 2:506–508.

Campbell AW (1924a) The evolution and functions of the labyrinth. Medical Journal of Australia Suppl:428–429.

Campbell AW (1924b) Infantile paralysis of cerebral origin. Medical Journal of Australia 1:512–515.

Campbell AW (1927a) The epilepsies of childhood. Medical Journal of Australia 1:774–775.

Campbell AW (1927b) Some modifications of nervous disease in childhood. Medical Journal of Australia 1:697–699.

Campbell AW (1928a) The sympathetic innervation of skeletal muscle. Medical Journal of Australia 1:258.

Campbell AW (1928b) The value of ocular signs in neurological diagnosis. Transactions of the Australasian Medical Congress 125–126.

Campbell AW (1930) Cerebro-spinal syphilis. Medical Journal of Australia 2:26–27.

Campbell AW (1931) Affections of peripheral nerves. Medical Journal of Australia 2:544–546.

Campbell AW (1933a) The nervous child. Medical Journal of Australia 2:535–538.

Campbell AW (1933b) The treatment of migraine. Medical Journal of Australia 1:36–37.

Campbell AW (1935) Dr John Hughlings Jackson. Medical Journal of Australia 2:344–347.

Campbell AW, Cleland JB, Bradley B (1918) A contribution to the experimental pathology of acute poliomyelitis (infantile paralysis). Medical Journal of Australia 5:123–128.

Campbell AW, Dowling N (1920) A case of nervous or hysterical fever. Medical Journal of Australia 1:171–172.

Cheek DB (1950) Pink disease: an investigation of its cause and treatment (preliminary report). Medical Journal of Australia 1:101–107.

Cheek DB, Hicks CS (1950) Pink disease or infantile acrodynia: its nature, prevention and cure. Medical Journal of Australia 1:107–121.

Chinner ME (1940) A clinical survey of nine cases of encephalomyelitis in association with measles. Medical Journal of Australia 2:526–529.

Clark FJ (1937) The treatment of trigeminal neuralgia. Medical Journal of Australia 2:784–785.

Clayton HJ (1923) Obituary. George Edward Rennie. Medical Journal of Australia 2:213–214.

Cleland JB (1912) Injuries and diseases of man in Australia attributable to animals (except insects). Australasian Medical Gazette 32:269–274; 295–299.

Cleland JB (1916) Some aspects of the aetiology and epidemiology of cerebro-spinal fever. Medical Journal of Australia 2:496–499 & 516–518.

Cleland JB (1917) Mysterious disease. Medical Journal of Australia 2:171–172.

Cleland JB (1923) Epidemic encephalitis. Medical Journal of Australia 2:594.

Cleland JB (1937) Small aneurysms at the base of the brain and subarachnoid haemorrhage. Medical Journal of Australia 1:141–142.

Cleland JB (1942) Injuries and diseases in Australia attributable to animals (insects excepted). Medical Journal of Australia 2:313–320.

Cleland JB, Campbell AW (1919) The nature of the recent Australian epidemics of acute encephalo-myelitis. Successful conveyance of the virus to sheep, a calf, and a horse. Medical Journal of Australia 1:232–236.

Cleland JB, Campbell AW (1920a) The epidemiology of acute encephalomyelitis ('X disease') in Australia. Proceedings of the Royal Society of Medicine 13:185–205.

Cleland JB, Campbell AW (1920b) An experimental investigation of an Australian epidemic of acute encephalomyelitis. Journal of Hygiene 18:272–316.

Clements FW (1940) Pink disease: a consideration of three aetiological possibilities. Medical Journal of Australia 2:430–432.

Clements FW (1960) The rise and decline of pink disease. Medical Journal of Australia 1:922–925.

Clendinnen FJ (1897) Skiagrams of the skull and intra-cranial blood-vessels. Intercolonial Medical Journal of Australasia 2:819.

Clubbe CPB (1925) Some aspects of infantile paralysis. Medical Journal of Australia 1:527–533.

Cohen A (1994) Beech, Ernest Robert. In: Wiseman JC, Mulhearn RJ, eds. Roll of the Royal Australasian College of Physicians. v. 2. Sydney: Royal Australasian College of Physicians: pp 14–16.

Collins AJ (1928) Epidemic encephalitis. Medical Journal of Australia 2:72–74.

References

Cook RD (1981) Multiple sclerosis: is the domestic cat involved? Medical Hypotheses 7:147–154.

Cook RD, Flower RL, Dutton NS (1986) Light and electron microscopical studies of the immunoperoxidase staining of multiple sclerosis plaques using antisera to a feline derived agent and to galactocerebroside. Neuropathology and Applied Neurobiology 12:63–79.

Corkill AB, Ennor AH (1937) Choline esterase in myasthenia gravis. Medical Journal of Australia 2:1121–1123.

Covernton JS, Draper MH (1947) A study of myotonia, with special reference to paramyotonia. Medical Journal of Australia 2:161–175.

Cox LB (1931) The origin of Sluder's or spheno-palatine neuralgia. Medical Journal of Australia 1:435–441.

Cox LB (1932a) Ganglioneuroma of the cerebrum, with an additional case. Medical Journal of Australia 1:347–351.

Cox LB (1932b) On the relation of Sluder's neuralgia to the trigeminal nerve, and other facial neuralgias. Medical Journal of Australia 1:292–298.

Cox LB (1933) The cytology of the glioma group: with special reference to inclusion of cells derived from the invaded tissue. American Journal of Pathology 9:839–898.

Cox LB (1934) Observations upon the nature, rate of growth, and operability of the intracranial tumours derived from 135 patients. Medical Journal of Australia 1:182–196.

Cox LB (1935) Tumour of the brain as met with in general practice. Medical Journal of Australia 1:425–541.

Cox LB (1937) Tumours of the base of the brain: their relation to pathological sleep and other changes in the conscious state. Medical Journal of Australia 1:742–752.

Cox LB (1938a) On the origin and treatment of syringomyelic cavities. Medical Journal of Australia 1:481–483.

Cox LB (1938b) The relation of myasthenia gravis and allied conditions to 'Prostigmin' therapy. Medical Journal of Australia 1:344–348.

Cox LB (1939a) Haemorrhage of the brain stem as a significant complication of intracranial tumours. Medical Journal of Australia 1:259–262.

Cox LB (1939b) Trauma and intracranial tumours. Medical Journal of Australia 1:256–259.

Cox LB (1949a) Medical sequelae of brain injury. Medical Journal of Australia 1:519–521.

Cox LB (1949b) The treatment of neurosyphilis. Medical Journal of Australia 1:449–451.

Cox LB, Fantl P, Fitzpatrick M (1949) The treatment of disseminated sclerosis by prolonged lowering of the blood prothrombin level. Medical Journal of Australia 1:577–579.

Cox LB, Tolhurst JC (1946) Human torulosis. Melbourne: Melbourne University Press.

Cox LB, Trumble HC (1939) Tumours and malformations of the blood vessels of the brain and spinal cord. Medical Journal of Australia 2:308–319.

Crago WH (1890) Notes on a case of ascending paralysis of Landry. Australasian Medical Gazette 10:19–21.

Crago WH (1923) Obituary: George Edward Rennie. Medical Journal of Australia 2:213.

Craig RG (1924) The treatment of spastic paralysis. Medical Journal of Australia 11:98.

Creed JM (1889) Leprosy: in its relation to the European population of Australia. Intercolonial Medical Congress of Australasia:499–503.

Critchley M (1990) The ventricle of memory. Personal recollections of some neurologists. New York: Raven Press.

Crowther WELH (1946) A case of so-called hydrophobia: a matter of diagnosis. Medical Journal of Australia 1:69–72.

Cullen W (1805 (originally 1789)) First lines of the practice of physick. v. 1 & 2. New York: Duyckinck, Swords, Falconer et al.

Current Comment (1927) Tick paralysis. Medical Journal of Australia 1:548–549.

Curtis JB, Miller D, Simpson D (1980) The neurosurgical society of Australasia: the first forty years. Australian and New Zealand Journal of Surgery 50:434–437.

Dawson WS (1928) The treatment of general paralysis by malaria. Medical Journal of Australia 1:10–13.

Dawson WS (1937) Cerebral arteriosclerosis: a review. Medical Journal of Australia 2:499–506.

Dawson WS (1938) Obituary. Alfred Walter Campbell. Medical Journal of Australia 1:183–185.

Dawson WS, Latham O (1931) A case of encephalomyelitis. Medical Journal of Australia 2:236–238.

Dawson WS, Latham O (1943) Pathological states in dementia praecox as revealed in a fatal case of picrotoxin medication. Medical Journal of Australia 1:245–248.

De Crespigny CT (1938) Cerebral vascular accidents and their treatment. Medical Journal of Australia 1:1077–1081.

De Crespigny CTC (1944) G E Rennie Memorial Lecture. Torula infection of the central nervous system. Medical Journal of Australia 2:605–615.

De Crespigny CTC, Hurst EW (1942) A demyelinating condition apparently localized in the brain stem. Medical Journal of Australia 1:408–410.

De Crespigny CTC, Woollard HH (1929) A case of Schilder's disease. Lancet ii:864.

Delasiauve LJF (1854) Traite de l'epilepsie. Paris.

Denny-Brown D, Robertson EG (1933a) On the physiology of micturition. Brain 56:149–190.

Denny-Brown D, Robertson EG (1933b) The state of the bladder and its sphincters in complete transverse lesions of the spinal cord and cauda equina. Brain 56:397–463.

Denny-Brown D, Robertson EG (1935) An investigation of the nervous control of defaecation. Brain 58:256–310.

Dew HR (1922) Tumours of the brain: their pathology and treatment. Medical Journal of Australia 1:515–521.

Dew HR (1936) Some aspects of intracranial surgery, with special reference to the meningiomata. Medical Journal of Australia 2:69–76.

Docaz C (1933) Pink disease (infantile acrodynia). (translated Wood, IJ) London: Martin Hopkinson.

Donnan GA, Bladin PF, Berkovic SF, Longley WA, Saling MM (1991) The stroke syndrome of striato-capsular infarction. Brain 114:57–70.

Donnan GA, McNeill JJ, Adena MA, Doyle AE, O'Malley HM, Neill GC (1989) Smoking as a risk factor for cerebral ischaemia. Lancet ii:643–647.

Donnan GA, O'Malley HM, Quang L, Hurley S, Bladin P (1993) The capsular warning syndrome: pathogenesis and clinical features. Neurology 43:957–962.

Douglas RA (1977) Dr Anton Breinl and the Australian Institute of Tropical Medicine. Medical Journal of Australia 1:713–716; 748–751; 784–790.

Downing JH (1919) Coma following influenza. Medical Journal of Australia 2:69.

Duhig JV (1922) Polio-encephalitis. Medical Journal of Australia 2:261–263.

Dunlop DB (1996) Obituary. Adrian Dawson. Medical Journal of Australia 164: 182.

Eadie MJ (1981) A W Campbell – Australia's first neurologist. Clinical and Experimental Neurology 17:27–35.

Eadie MJ ed. (1992) Drug therapy in neurology. Edinburgh: Churchill-Livingstone.

Eadie MJ (1994) Epileptic seizures in 1902 patients: a perspective from a consultant neurological practice (1961–1991). Epilepsy Research 17:55–79.

Eadie MJ, Sutherland JM, Doherty RL (1965) Encephalitis in the aetiology of Parkinsonism in Australia. Archives of Neurology 12:240–245.

References

Eadie MJ, Tyrer JH (1980) Neurological clinical pharmacology. Auckland: Adis Press.

Eadie MJ, Tyrer JH (1985) The biochemistry of migraine. Lancaster: MTP Press.

Eadie MJ, Tyrer JH (1989) Anticonvulsant therapy: pharmacological basis and practice. 3rd ed. Edinburgh: Churchill-Livingstone.

Eadie MJ, Vajda FJE eds (1999) Antiepileptic drugs: pharmacology and therapeutics. Berlin: Springer.

Eaton EM (1913) A case of tick-bite followed by wide-spread transitory muscular paralysis. Australasian Medical Gazette 33:391–394.

Eccles JC (1941) Changes in muscle produced by nerve degeneration. Medical Journal of Australia 1:573–575.

Editorial (1892) Leprosy in New South Wales. Australasian Medical Gazette 11:165–166.

Editorial (1927) Tick paralysis. Medical Journal of Australia 1:548–549.

Edwards AT, Latham O (1943) Alzheimer's disease. Medical Journal of Australia 1:251–253.

Edye BT (1926) The technique of cisternal puncture and its application in the treatment of general paralysis of the insane by arsenicalized serum. Medical Journal of Australia 1:272–273.

Elkin AP (1935) Primitive medicine men. Medical Journal of Australia 2:750–757.

Ellery RS (1926) On the treatment of general paralysis of the insane by malaria. Medical Journal of Australia 1:401–404.

Evans W (1925) Preanaemic combined degeneration of the cord. Medical Journal of Australia 2:508–509.

Evans W (1931) Pink disease or erythroedema polyneuritis. Medical Journal of Australia 2:86–87.

Fairley NH, Guest JV (1915) Cerebro-spinal fever: an analysis of fifty cases. Medical Journal of Australia 2:383–389.

Farquhar J, Gajdusek DC eds (1981) Kuru. Early letters and field notes from the collection of D Carleton Gajdusek. New York: Raven Press.

Ferguson EW (1924) Deaths from tick paralysis in human beings. Medical Journal of Australia 2:346–348.

Ferrier TM, Eadie MJ (1973) Clioquinol encephalopathy. Medical Journal of Australia 2:1008–1009.

Ferrier TM, Schwieger AC, Eadie MJ (1986) Delayed onset of partial epilepsy of temporal lobe origin following acute clioquinol encephalopathy. Journal of Neurology, Neurosurgery and Psychiatry 50:93–95.

Findlay JP (1933) Facial paralysis due to toxic inflammation of the geniculate ganglion. Medical Journal of Australia 1:251–253.

Flashman JF, Latham O (1915) A contribution to the study of the aetiology of disseminated sclerosis. Medical Journal of Australia 2:265–269.

Flecker H (1944) Sudden blindness after eating 'finger cherry' (Rhodomyrtus macrocarpa). Medical Journal of Australia 2:183–185.

Fleetwood TF (1889) A case of Thomsen's disease. Australian Medical Journal New Series 11:393–394.

Flynn J, Greenaway TM (1935) Diffuse 'encephalitis', presumably Schilder's disease. Medical Journal of Australia 2:120.

French EL (1952) Murray Valley encephalitis: isolation and characterization of the aetiological agent. Medical Journal of Australia 1:100–107.

Frith JA (1988) History of multiple sclerosis. An Australian perspective. Clinical and Experimental Neurology 25:7–16.

Frith JA, McLeod JG, Basten A, et al. (1986) Transfer factor as a therapy for multiple sclerosis: a follow-up study. Clinical and Experimental Neurology 22:149–154.

Fulton, JF (1879) On a case of chorea, treated by subcutaneous injection, in progressive doses, of curara. Australian Medical Journal New Series 1:273–278.

Fulton JF (1938) Obituaries: Alfred Walter Campbell MD ChM 1868–1937. Archives of Neurology and Psychiatry 40:566–568.

Gajdusek DC (1981) Introduction. In: Farquhar J, Gadjusek DC, eds Kuru. Early letters and field notes from the collection of D Carleton Gadjusek. New York: Raven Press: pp xv-xx.

Game J (1946) A case of periarteritis (polyarteritis) nodosa. Medical Journal of Australia 1:295–298.

Game J (1951) Cerebral tumour: early symptoms and methods of investigation. Medical Journal of Australia 1:367–373.

Game JA (1975) The Australian Association of Neurologists – a review of twenty-five years. Proceedings of the Australian Association of Neurologists 12:1–6.

Game J (1976) Obituaries. Edward Graeme Robertson. Proceedings of the Australian Association of Neurologists 13:1–3.

Gandevia B, Cobley J (1974) Mortality at Sydney Cove, 1788–1792. Australian and New Zealand Journal of Medicine 4:111–125.

Gibson JL (1896) Traumatic rupture of carotid into cavernous sinus – pulsating exophthalmos. Australasian Medical Gazette 5:147–149.

Gibson JL (1904) A plea for painted railings and painted walls of rooms as the source of lead poisoning amongst Queensland children. Australasian Medical Gazette 23:149.

Gibson JL (1905) Pulsating exophthalmos – post-mortem. Australasian Medical Gazette 24:107–108.

Gibson JL (1912) The importance of lumbar puncture in the plumbic ocular neuritis of children. Australasian Medical Gazette 31:25–27.

Gibson JL, Love W, Hardie D, Bancroft P, Turner AJ (1892) Notes on lead-poisoning as observed among children in Brisbane. Transactions of the Intercolonial Medical Congress of Australasia 3rd Session:76–83.

Gillespie NC, Lewis RJ, Pearn JH, et al. (1986) Ciguatera in Australia. Occurrence, clinical features, pathophysiology and management. Medical Journal of Australia 145:584–590.

Gillett BStP, Farmer F, Anderson M, Sadka M (1973) Obituary: Gerald Carew Moss. Medical Journal of Australia 59:44–45.

Gilligan BS (1996) John Aylward Game. Medical Journal of Australia 164:497.

Goulston DL (1930) The action of radiation from radium needles on nerves. Medical Journal of Australia 2:651–661.

Gowers WR (1888) A manual of diseases of the nervous system. 1st ed. v. 2. (vol. 1, 1986). London: Churchill.

Graham J (1893) Multiple neuritis among Chinamen in Sydney. Australasian Medical Gazette 12:357–360.

Gray DF (1948) Human botulism in Australia. Medical Journal of Australia 2:37–42.

Greenfield JG (1956) The spino-cerebellar degenerations. Oxford: Blackwell Scientific Publications.

Greenfield JG, Robertson EG (1933) Cystic oligodendrogliomas of the cerebral hemispheres and ventricular oligodendrogliomas. Brain 56:247–264.

Greenwood B (1967) The origins of sympathectomy. Medical History 11:165–169.

Griffiths (1922) Insular sclerosis. Medical Journal of Australia 2:658–659.

Guillain G (1959) J-M Charcot 1825–1893. His life – his work. London: Pitman.

References

Hagen PB, Noad KB, Latham O (1951) The syndrome of lamellar cerebellar degeneration associated with retinitis pigmentosa, hypertopias, and mental deficiency, with report of a case. Medical Journal of Australia 1:217–223.

Hall B, Noad KB, Latham O (1945) Familial cortical cerebellar atrophy: a contribution to the study of heredo-familial cerebellar disease in Australia. Medical Journal of Australia 1:101–108.

Ham BB (1905) The recent epidemic of infantile paralysis. Australasian Medical Gazette 24:193–199.

Hamilton DG (1940a) Tick paralysis: a dangerous disease in children. Medical Journal of Australia 1:759–765.

Hamilton DG (1940b) The treatment of meningitis due to the meningococcus, haemophilus influenzae and streptococcus. Medical Journal of Australia 2:342–346.

Hammond SR, de Wytt C, Maxwell IC, et al. (1987) The epidemiology of multiple sclerosis in Queensland, Australia. Journal of the Neurological Sciences 80:185–204.

Hammond SR, English DR, de Wytt C, et al. (1989) The contribution of mortality statistics to the study of multiple sclerosis in Australia. Journal of Neurology, Neurosurgery and Psychiatry 52:1–7.

Hammond SR, English D, de Wytt C, et al. (1988a) The clinical profile of MS in Australia: a comparison between medium- and high-frequency prevalence zones. Neurology 38:980–986.

Hammond SR, McLeod JG, Millingen KS, et al. (1988b) The epidemiology of multiple sclerosis in three Australian cities: Perth, Newcastle and Hobart. Brain 111:1–25.

Hammond WA (1871) A treatise on diseases of the nervous system. New York and London: Appleton & Co. and Trubner & Co.

Hare F (1903) Mechanism of the paroxysmal neuroses. Australasian Medical Gazette 22:283–291; 333–340; 387–394.

Hawkes CS (1903) The mechanism of trigeminal neuralgia. Australasian Medical Gazette 22:497–501.

Hawkes CS (1905) The treatment of epilepsy. Australasian Medical Gazette 24:644–650.

Haymaker W, Schiller F eds (1970) The founders of neurology. 2nd ed. Springfield: Thomas.

Head H, Campbell AW (1900) On the pathology of herpes zoster and its bearing on sensory localisation. Brain 24:353–523.

Hickey MF (1963) Obituary: Herbert John Wilkinson. Medical Journal of Australia 1:869.

Hiller K (1919) Encephalitis lethargica. Medical Journal of Australia 32:181.

Himmelhoch E, Latham O, McDonald CG (1947) Alzheimer's disease complicated by a terminal salmonella infection. Medical Journal of Australia 1:701–703.

Hogg CA, Latham O (1923) Encephalitis lethargica. Medical Journal of Australia 2:90–95.

Hogg GH (1902) On the medicine of the Tasmanian aboriginals. Transactions of the Sixth Session, Australasian Medical Congress, Hobart:176–177.

Hogg GH (1906) A case of myasthenia gravis in special relation to eye and throat conditions. Australasian Medical Gazette 25:184–186.

Hogg GH (1915) Leber's disease. Medical Journal of Australia 1:253.

Hogg GH (1928) Hereditary optic atrophy. Medical Journal of Australia 1:372–374.

Holmes G (1954) The National Hospital Queen Square. Edinburgh: E & S Livingstone.

Holmes GM (1904) On certain tremors in organic cerebral lesions. Brain 27:327–375.

Holmes GM (1956) The Croonian lectures on the clinical symptoms of cerebellar disease and their interpretation. In: Walshe FMR, ed. Selected papers of Sir Gordon Holmes. London: MacMillan & Co: pp 49–111.

Holmes à Court AW (1923) Discussion on encephalitis. Medical Journal of Australia Suppl:38.

Holmes à Court AW, Latham O (1935) Schilder's disease. Medical Journal of Australia 2:117–120.

Hood J (1902) Epidemic cerebro-spinal meningitis. Proceedings of the Sixth Session, Australasian Medical Congress:158–164.

Hooper R (1978) Graeme Robertson and the golden age of neurology. Clinical and Experimental Neurology 15:1–10.

Hopkins WF (1898) Case of gunshot wound of brain. Intercolonial Medical Journal of Australasia 3:486–489.

Howson F (1918) A case of muscular atrophy. Medical Journal of Australia 2:305.

Hughes JF (1940) Parkinsonism: an account of the disorder and its treatment, with special reference to high atropine dosage therapy. Medical Journal of Australia 2:174–176.

Hughes TD (1927) Arsenical neuritis treated by the intravenous injection of sodium thiosulphate. Medical Journal of Australia 1:543.

Hunter JI (1924a) The postural influence of the sympathetic innervation of voluntary muscle. Medical Journal of Australia 11:86–89.

Hunter JI (1924b) The significance of the double innervation of voluntary muscle illustrated by reference to the maintenance of the posture of the wing. Medical Journal of Australia 11:581–587.

Hunter JI (1924c) On the choice of procedure adopted in the operation of ramisection for spastic paralysis. Medical Journal of Australia 11:590–591.

Hunter JI, Latham O (1925) A contribution to the discussion of the histological problems involved in the conception of a somatic and sympathetic innervation of voluntary muscles. Medical Journal of Australia 1:27–36.

Hurley LE (1926) Disseminated sclerosis. Medical Journal of Australia 1:25.

Hurst EW (1941a) Acute haemorrhagic leucoencephalitis: a previously undefined entity. Medical Journal of Australia 2:1–6.

Hurst EW (1941b) G E Rennie Memorial Lecture. Demyelination: a clinicopathological and experimental study. Medical Journal of Australia 2:661–666.

Huxtable LR (1892a) Records of clinical cases. Case VI – paralysis agitans. Australasian Medical Gazette 11:211–213.

Huxtable LR (1892b) Records of clinical cases. Case VII – insular sclerosis. Australasian Medical Gazette 11:213–215.

Jackson ES (1924) Historical notes: a comparison of two annual lists, those of 1827 and 1832, from Brisbane Hospital records. Medical Journal of Australia 11:381–385.

Jackson ES (1926) Some early Australian doctors. Medical Journal of Australia 1:121–127.

Jackson JH (1870) A study of convulsions. Transactions of the St. Andrew's Medical Graduates Association 3:162–204.

Jamieson J (1873) On a case of chorea of unusual severity. Australian Medical Journal 18:47–48.

Jamieson J (1883) Diptheritic paralysis. Australian Medical Journal New Series 5:386–387.

Jamieson J (1886) Cases of multiple neuritis. Australian Medical Journal New Series 8:295–302.

Jamieson S (1894) Case of pseudo-hypertrophic paralysis. Australasian Medical Gazette 13:294–295.

Jamieson S (1895–6) Record of cases illustrating some of the effects of syphilis upon the central nervous system. Intercolonial Quarterly Journal of Medicine and Surgery 2:207–222.

Johnston WWS (1927) Disseminated sclerosis. Medical Journal of Australia 2:417.

Jones SE (1917) Huntington's chorea. Medical Journal of Australia 1:376–377.

Kelly M (1942) Headaches, traumatic and rheumatic: the cervical somatic lesion. Medical Journal of Australia 2:479–483.

Kennedy J (1944) Obituary. John Fullarton Mackeddie. Medical Journal of Australia 2:601–602.

Kenny G (1988) HJ Wilkinson – the travail of a pioneer with muscle. In: Pearn J, ed. Pioneer medicine in Australia. Brisbane: Amphion Press: pp 269–279.

References

Kneebone JleM, Cleland JB (1926) Acute encephalitis (X disease) at Broken Hill: probable successful transmission to a sheep. Australian Journal of Experimental Biology and Medical Science 3:119–127.

Lalor P, Haddow G (1920) Toxaemia in epilepsy. Medical Journal of Australia 1:251–260.

Lambie CG, Latham O, McDonald GL (1947) Olivo-ponto-cerebellar atrophy (Marie's ataxia). Medical Journal of Australia 2:626–632.

Lance JW ed. (1987) Mind, movement and migraine. Sydney: University of New South Wales.

Lance JW (1988) Robertson, Edward Graeme. In: McDonald GL, ed. Roll of the Royal Australasian College of Physicians. v. 1. Sydney: Royal Australasian College of Physicians: pp 247–248.

Lance JW, Goadsby PJ (1998) Mechanism and management of headache. 6th ed. Oxford: Butterworth-Heinemann.

Lance JW, McLeod JG (1981) A physiological approach to clinical neurology. London: Butterworth.

Larkins N (1959) Obituary. Eric Leo Susman. Medical Journal of Australia 2:339–340.

Latham LS (1922) Report of a case of encephalitis lethargica. Medical Journal of Australia 2:426.

Latham O (1926) Trophic glial states in spinal cord lesions. Medical Journal of Australia 1:507–510.

Latham O (1927) The pathology of two cases of sudden death. Medical Journal of Australia 1:121–123.

Latham O (1930) Some difficulties met with in the pathological diagnosis of encephalitis. Medical Journal of Australia 1:376–382.

Latham O (1931) Some thoughts on the term acute disseminated encephalomyelitis and its affinities. Medical Journal of Australia 2:677–681.

Latham O (1934) Some activities of a mental hospital laboratory during thirty years. Medical Journal of Australia 1:739–746; 767–776; 797–804.

Latham O (1938) The role of the small intracranial blood vessels in the pathology of brain conditions. Medical Journal of Australia 1:292–295.

Latham O (1939) Haematomyelia. Medical Journal of Australia 1:529–534.

Latham O (1941) Some notes on the pathology of the cerebellar system. Medical Journal of Australia 1:164–167.

Layton W, Sutherland JM (1975) Geochemistry and multiple sclerosis: a hypothesis. Medical Journal of Australia 1:73–77.

Lind WAT (1924) Epiloia. Medical Journal of Australia 2:290–294.

Lindon LCE (1936) Cerebral arteriography. Medical Journal of Australia 1:849–853.

Litchfield WF (1917) The mysterious disease. Medical Journal of Australia 1:384.

Litchfield WF, Latham O, Campbell AW (1917) A clinical and anatomical report of a case of Friedreich's disease. Medical Journal of Australia 1:135–140.

Littlejohn ES (1923) Pink disease – erythroedema. Medical Journal of Australia 1:689–692.

Lockwood L (1931) Post-vaccinal encephalomyelitis. Medical Journal of Australia 1:662–663.

Lowe RF (1940) Pneumococcal meningitis treated with sulphapyridine. Medical Journal of Australia 2:536–538.

Macdonald WL (1927) A case of chronic lenticular degeneration. Medical Journal of Australia 2:718.

Macewen W (1879) Tumour of the dura mater removed during life in a person affected with epilepsy. Glasgow Medical Journal 12:210.

Mackeddie JF (1926) Cisterna magna puncture. Medical Journal of Australia 2:447–449.

Mackeddie JF (1927) Localization of spinal tumours. Medical Journal of Australia 1:511.

Mackeddie JF (1929) Encephalography and the use of 'lipiodol'. Medical Journal of Australia 2:511.

Mackeddie JF (1931) Lipiodol; in neurological diagnosis. Medical Journal of Australia 2:221–227.

MacLaurin C (1917) Obituary. James Froude Flashman. Medical Journal of Australia 1:176.

MacLeod RA (1920) Congenital word blindness. Medical Journal of Australia 1:593–596.

Macnamara J (1929) The treatment of acute poliomyelitis by means of human immune serum. Medical Journal of Australia 2:838–850.

Macnamara J (1953) Elizabeth Kenny. Medical Journal of Australia 1:85.

Maddox K (1959) Obituary: Eric Leo Susman. Medical Journal of Australia 91:338–340.

Marten RH (1897) Notes on cases of post-herpetic neuralgia. Intercolonial Medical Journal of Australasia 2:195–196.

Mathewson THR (1921) A rare type of intra-cranial tumour. Medical Journal of Australia 2:400–402.

Mathewson THR (1922) Discussion following papers on epidemic encephalitis. Medical Journal of Australia 2:283.

Mathewson THR, Latham O (1917) Acute encephalitis of unknown origin. Medical Journal of Australia 2:352–356.

Maudsley HC (1906) Brachioplegia of cerebellar type, and rhythmical tremor, with an attempt to explain the symptoms and to localise the lesion. Intercolonial Medical Journal of Australasia 11:302–319.

Maudsley HF (1925) Disseminated sclerosis. Medical Journal of Australia 1:326.

Maudsley HF (1926) The sequelae of lethargic encephalitis. Medical Journal of Australia 1:696–703.

Maudsley HF (1927) Disseminated sclerosis. Medical Journal of Australia 1:836–837.

Maudsley HF (1928) Ocular signs in neurological diagnosis. Transactions of the Australasian Medical Congress 126–127.

Maund J (1856) Epilepsy produced by pressure on the brain. Australian Medical Journal 1:20–27.

McAdam RL (1895) Notes of a case of intractable epilepsy much relieved by borax. Australasian Medical Gazette 14:492–493.

McCall MG, Brereton TL, Dawson A, Millingen K, Sutherland JM, Acheson ED (1968) Frequency of multiple sclerosis in three Australian cities – Perth, Newcastle and Hobart. Journal of Neurology, Neurosurgery and Psychiatry 31:1–9.

McCall MG, Sutherland JM, Acheson ED (1969) The frequency of multiple sclerosis in Western Australia. Acta Neurologica Scandinavica 45:151–165.

McDonald JEF (1906) The treatment of cerebral haemorrhage. Australasian Medical Gazette 25:186–188.

McDonald SF (1933) Swift's or pink disease: recent work on pathology and treatment. Medical Journal of Australia 2:276–280.

McLean DM, Stevenson WJ (1954) Between Australian X disease and the virus of Murray Valley encephalitis. Medical Journal of Australia 1:636–638.

McLeod JG, Hammond SR, Hallpike JF (1994) Epidemiology of multiple sclerosis in Australia. With NSW and SA survey results. Medical Journal of Australia 160:117–122.

McWhae (1924) Headache. Medical Journal of Australia 2:78–81.

Miles JAR, Howes DW (1953) Observations on viral encephalitis in South Australia. Medical Journal of Australia 1:7–12.

Mills AE (1917) Obituary. James Froude Flashman. Medical Journal of Australia 1:176–177.

Mills AE (1919) Multiple peripheral neuritis due to toxaemia of pregnancy. Medical Journal of Australia 2:331–332.

References

Mills AE (1922) Encephalitis. Medical Journal of Australia 2:197–198.

Milroy WH, Hughes BL (1945) A case of pneumococcal meningitis successfully treated with penicillin. Medical Journal of Australia 2:434.

Minogue SJ (1926) The differential diagnosis of cerebral syphilis. Medical Journal of Australia 2:444–447.

Minogue SJ (1927) Progressive lenticular degeneration. Medical Journal of Australia 2:695–696.

Minogue SJ, Latham O (1945) Cerebellar degeneration with epilepsy. Medical Journal of Australia 1:430–433.

Molesworth EH (1926) The leprosy problem. Medical Journal of Australia 2:365–381.

Money A (1896) Epilepsies – cerebral paroxysms. Intercolonial Medical Journal of Australasia 1:578–581.

Monson RBP (1926) The surgical technique of pneumoventriculography with an illustrative case. Medical Journal of Australia 1:271–272.

Morgan F (1958) Obituary: Arthur Schuller. Medical Journal of Australia 2:241–242.

Morgan I (1920) A review of four cases of syphilis of the nervous system. Medical Journal of Australia 1:477–481.

Morlet C (1921) Hereditary optic atrophy as a possible menace to the community. Medical Journal of Australia 2:499–502.

Morris J (1994a) A directory of neurology in Australia. Brisbane: Australian Association of Neurologists.

Morris J (1994b) Neurology in Australia. Brisbane: Australian Association of Neurologists.

Morris JN (1908) Hereditary cerebellar ataxia. Intercolonial Medical Journal of Australasia 13:185–188.

Moss GC (1941) Meningococcal infections with special reference to meningococcal septicaemia. Medical Journal of Australia 1:548–552.

Moss GC (1949) Encephalitis and encephalomyelitis. Medical Journal of Australia 1:414–416.

Moss GC (1963) The mentality and personality of the Julio-Claudian emperors. Medical History 7:165–175.

Murphy E (1924) Amyotrophic lateral sclerosis. Medical Journal of Australia 1:10–11.

Newland H (1937) Obituary: Harry Swift. Medical Journal of Australia 2:976.

Newman AK (1875) On insular sclerosis of the brain and spinal cord. Australian Medical Journal 20:369–374.

Nicholson GA, Yeung L, Corbett A (1998) Efficient neurophysiologic selection of X-linked Charcot-Marie-Tooth families: ten novel mutations. Neurology 51:1412–1416.

Noad KB (1933) Simulation of vascular disease of the geniculo-calcarine pathway by cerebral tumour. Medical Journal of Australia 2:400–404.

Noad KB (1943) Head injuries. Medical Journal of Australia 2:141–144.

Noad KB (1944) Uncinate epilepsy: the subjective symptoms of an attack. Medical Journal of Australia 2:641.

Noad K (1975) Obituary: Oliver Latham. Medical Journal of Australia 2:492.

Noad KB, Haymaker W (1953) Neurological features of tsutsugamushi fever, with special reference to deafness. Brain 76:113–131.

Noble R (1926) The value of the ventriculogram in the localization of cerebral tumours. Medical Journal of Australia 1:268–271.

Nowland HH, Hunter JI, Latham O (1924) Supra-pituitary tumour with Frohlich's syndrome. Medical Journal of Australia 2:194–196.

Nye LJJ (1933) Chronic nephritis and lead poisoning. Sydney: Angus & Robertson.

Officer DM (1903) Case of disseminated sclerosis in a child. Intercolonial Medical Journal of Australasia 8:347–349.

O'Hara HM (1893) A case of trigeminal neuralgia of five years' duration – curetting of Gasserian ganglion from cavum Meckelii. Australian Medical Journal New Series 15:513–517.

Ouvrier RA, Nicholson GA (1995) Advances in the genetics of hereditary hypertrophic neuropathy in childhood. Brain Development 17 (Suppl):31–38.

Parker LR (1938) Obituary. Alfred Walter Campbell. Medical Journal of Australia 1:181–183.

Parker N (1958) Observations on Huntington's chorea based on a Queensland survey. Medical Journal of Australia 1:351–359.

Parker N (1985) Hereditary whispering dysphonia. Journal of Neurology, Neurosurgery and Psychiatry 48:218–224.

Parry D (1892) A case of hydatid of the brain. Australasian Medical Gazette 11:315.

Paton RT (1894) On beri beri in New South Wales. Australasian Medical Gazette 13:363–365.

Patrick R (1985) Fraud or medical genius. In: Horsewhip the doctor. St Lucia: University of Queensland Press: pp 194–204.

Penfold WJ, Butler HM, Wood IJ (1932) The aetiology of erythroedema (Swift's disease, pink disease, erythroedema polyneuritis, juvenile acrodynia, trophodermatoneurose), with special reference to blood culture. Medical Journal of Australia 2:131–136.

Phillips G (1931) On the apparent diminution in skeletal muscle tonus following removal of the lumbar sympathetic trunk. Medical Journal of Australia 1:628–632.

Phillips G (1937) Protein in the cerebro-spinal fluid: clinical significance and quantitative determination. Medical Journal of Australia 2:179–181.

Phillips G (1939) Recent work in the study of epilepsy. Medical Journal of Australia 1:922–924.

Phillips G (1951) Obituary. Geoffery Trahair. Medical Journal of Australia 1:100–101.

Pockley E (1915) Leber's disease (hereditary optic atrophy). Medical Journal of Australia 1:189–191.

Pockley FA (1891) Notes on a case of ophthalmoplegia acuta and double optic neuritis. Australasian Medical Gazette 10:273–275.

Pridmore SA (1990) The large Huntington's disease family of Tasmania. Medical Journal of Australia 153:593–595.

Prior GPU (1937) Syphilis and neuro-syphilis treated by electropyrexia. Medical Journal of Australia 1:895–910.

Prior GUP, Jones SE (1916) Calcium and epilepsy: a preliminary report. Medical Journal of Australia 1:199–203.

Read SJ, Pettigrew L, Schimmel L, et al. (1998) White matter medullary infarcts: acute subcortical infarction in the centrum ovale. Cerebrovascular Disease 8:289–295.

Reeves E (1861) Clinical illustrations of acute softening of the corpus striata. Australian Medical Journal 6:155–167.

Reid WL (1940) The use of histamine in the treatment of neuro-vascular headache. Medical Journal of Australia 2:307–310.

Reid WL (1948) Studies on the tremor-rigidity syndrome: 1. Surgical treatment of human subjects. Medical Journal of Australia 2:481–492.

Rennie GE (1895) Death after head injuries. Australasian Medical Gazette 14:374–378.

Rennie GE (1897) Some recent work on the cerebellum and its connections. Australasian Medical Gazette 16:575–578.

Rennie GE (1902) Three cases of meralgia paraesthetica. Australasian Medical Gazette 21:446–448.

References

Rennie GE (1903) The physiology of voluntary movements. Australasian Medical Gazette 22:135–141.

Rennie GE (1905a) Epilepsy: is it incurable? Proceedings of the Seventh Session, Australasian Medical Congress:48–53.

Rennie GE (1905b) Some points in the treatment of chronic nerve disease. Australasian Medical Gazette 24:359–363.

Rennie GE (1915) The influence of occupation on the localization of syphilitic nervous disease. Medical Journal of Australia 1:375–377.

Rennie GE (1919) Exophthalmic goitre combined with myasthenia gravis. Medical Journal of Australia 2:416–417.

Rennie GE (1921) The symptomatology of complete transverse lesions of the spinal cord. Medical Journal of Australia 1:185–189.

Reye RDK, Morgan G, Baral J (1963) Encephalopathy and fatty degeneration of the viscera. A disease entity in childhood. Lancet ii:749–752.

Reynolds JR (1861) Epilepsy: its symptoms, treatment, and relation to other chronic convulsive diseases. London: Churchill.

Rischbieth RH (1994) Neurology in South Australia. In: Morris J, ed. Neurology in Australia. Sydney: Australian Association of Neurologists: pp 90–93.

Robertson EG (1935) A clinical study of micturition. Medical Journal of Australia 2:890–895.

Robertson EG (1936) Intracranial aneurysms. Medical Journal of Australia 2:381–389.

Robertson EG (1937) Epilepsy as a symptom of organic lesions of the brain. Medical Journal of Australia 2:331–341.

Robertson EG (1938) Spinal arachnoiditis. Medical Journal of Australia 1:1043–1047.

Robertson EG (1940) An examination of the olfactory bulbs in fatal cases of poliomyelitis during the Victorian epidemic of 1937–1938. Medical Journal of Australia 1:156–162.

Robertson EG (1941) Encephalography. Melbourne: Macmillan.

Robertson EG (1946a) Further studies in encephalography. Melbourne: Macmillan.

Robertson EG (1946b) Toxoplasmic encephalomyelitis, with the report of two cases. Medical Journal of Australia 2:449–452.

Robertson EG (1947) Some physical aspects of encephalography. Brain 70:1–16.

Robertson EG (1949a) Developmental defects of the cisterna magna and dura mater. Journal of Neurology, Neurosurgery and Psychiatry 12:39–51.

Robertson EG (1949b) Cerebral lesions due to intracranial aneurysms. Brain 72:150–185.

Robertson EG (1952) Murray Valley encephalitis: pathological aspects. Medical Journal of Australia 1:107–110.

Robertson EG (1954) Photogenic epilepsy: self-precipitated attacks. Brain 77:232–251.

Robertson EG (1955) James Parkinson and his essay on the shaking palsy. Royal Melbourne Hospital Clinical Reports 25:1–14.

Robertson EG (1957) Pneumoencephalography. 1st ed. Oxford: Blackwell.

Robertson EG (1959) A perspective of epilepsy. Postgraduate Medicine 25:31–44.

Robertson EG (1967) Pneumoencephalography. 2nd ed. Springfield: Charles C Thomas.

Robertson EG (1968) John White, Surgeon-General to the colony. Proceedings of the Australian Association of Neurologists 5:1–18.

Robertson EG (1974) Investigation of intracranial tumours by pneumoencephalography. In: Vinken PJ, Bruyn GW, eds. Handbook of clinical neurology. v. 16. Amsterdam: North Holland: pp 530–621.

Robertson EG (1984) Decorative cast iron in Australia. Melbourne: Currey O'Neil.

Robertson EG, McLorinan H (1952) Murray Valley encephalitis: clinical aspects. Medical Journal of Australia 1:103–107.

Robertson J (1860) Report on a case where a large tumour was discovered in the brain at the post-mortem examination. Australian Medical Journal 5:37–42.

Robertson J (1881) Notes on two cases of hemiplegia. Australian Medical Journal New Series 3:296–310.

Robinson HE (1939) Successful treatment of pneumococcal meningitis with 'Soluseptasine' and 'M&B693'. Medical Journal of Australia 1:433–434.

Rocaz C (1933) Pink disease (infantile acrodyia). London: Hopkinson.(translated Wood,IJ)

Romberg MH (1853) A manual of the nervous diseases of man. London: New Sydenham Society. Translated Sieveking, EH.

Ross-Lee L, Heazlewood V, Tyrer JH, Eadie MJ (1982) Aspirin treatment of migraine attacks: plasma drug level data. Cephalalgia 2:9–14.

Royle ND (1924a) A new operative procedure in the treatment of spastic paralysis and its experimental basis. Medical Journal of Australia 11:77–86.

Royle ND (1924b) The operation of sympathetic ramisection. Medical Journal of Australia 11:587–590.

Royle ND (1927) The treatment of congenital spastic paraplegia by sympathetic ramisection. Medical Journal of Australia 1:632–642.

Royle ND (1928) The sympathetic innervation of skeletal muscle. Medical Journal of Australia 2:257–258.

Royle ND (1930) The treatment of blindness associated with retinitis pigmentosa: a preliminary note. Medical Journal of Australia 2:364–365.

Royle ND (1932a) The function of the sympathetic nervous system. Medical Journal of Australia 1:550–553.

Royle ND (1932b) The treatment of blindness associated with retinitis pigmentosa. Medical Journal of Australia 1:111–116.

Royle ND (1933) The surgical treatment of disseminated sclerosis. Medical Journal of Australia 1:586–588.

Royle ND (1935) A new treatment for anterior poliomyelitis and its experimental basis. Medical Journal of Australia 1:486–488.

Royle ND (1937) The surgical treatment of spastic paralysis. Medical Journal of Australia 1:979–982.

Rudall JT (1859) Case of cysticercus in the brain, with remarks. Australian Medical Journal 4:161–166.

Russell KF, Bradley KC (1977) Obituary: Leonard Bell Cox. Medical Journal of Australia 1:37–38.

Ryan G (1993) Professor Emeritus Sir Sydney Sunderland. Medical Journal of Australia 159:828–829.

Sadka M (1988) Moss, Gerald Carew. In: McDonald GL, ed. Roll of the Royal Australasian College of Physicians. v. 1. Sydney: Royal Australasian College of Physicians: pp 217–218.

Sawers WC, Thomson E (1935) Torulosis, with a report of a case of meningitis due to torula histolytica. Medical Journal of Australia 2:581–593.

Schwieger AC (1994) Cox, Leonard Bell. In: Wiseman JC, Mulhearn RJ, eds. Roll of the Royal Australasian College of Physicians. v. 2. Sydney: Royal Australasian College of Physicians: pp 67–69.

Selby G (1956) Parietal lobe syndromes. Australasian Annals of Medicine 5:89–100.

Selby G (1972) Subacute myelo-optic neuropathy in Australia. Lancet i:123–125.

Selby G (1974) Obituary: Brian Turner. Proceedings of the Australian Association of Neurologists 11:248.

Selby G (1983) Migraine and its variants. Sydney: Adis.

Selby G (1988) Susman, Eric Leo. In: McDonald GL, ed. Roll of the Royal Australasian College of Physicians. v. 1. Sydney: Royal Australasian College of Physicians: pp 284–285.

Selby G, Lance JW (1960) Observations on 500 cases of migraine and allied vascular headache. Journal of Neurology, Neurosurgery and Psychiatry 23:23–32.

Sewell SV (1915) The function of maturition. Medical Journal of Australia 1:231–233.

Sewell SV (1920) Discussion. Medical Journal of Australia 2:42–43.

Sewell SV (1926) Disseminated sclerosis. Medical Journal of Australia 2:161.

Sewell SV (1937) Listerian oration. Medical Journal of Australia 2:1019–1027.

Shallard B, Latham O (1945) A case of acute haemorrhagic leucoencephalitis. Medical Journal of Australia 1:145–148.

Shields A (1889) Leprosy in Australia. Australian Medical Journal New Series 11:274–282.

Simpson DA, Jamieson KG, Morson SM (1974) The foundations of neurosurgery in Australia and New Zealand. Australian and New Zealand Journal of Surgery 44:215–227.

Sippe C (1938) Migraine from the allergic viewpoint: results of treatment in 105 cases. Medical Journal of Australia 1:893–895.

Sippe C, Bostock J (1932) Some observations on bromide therapy and intoxication. Medical Journal of Australia 1:85–90.

Smith ET (1920) A case of encephalitis lethargica. Medical Journal of Australia 1:553–554.

Smith P (1873) On the treatment of epilepsy by large doses of bromide of potassium. Australian Medical Journal 18:258–267.

Smith W (1871) On paralysis with apparent hypertrophy of the muscles. Australian Medical Journal 16:161–171.

Southby R (1949) Pink disease, with a clinical approach to possible aetiology. Medical Journal of Australia 2:801–807.

Spark EJS (1897) Notes on three cases of Friedreich's ataxy. Australasian Medical Gazette 16:408–409.

Springthorpe JW (1886) Notes on twenty-one cases of epilepsy. Australian Medical Journal New Series 8:101–112.

Springthorpe JW (1887) Treatment of epilepsy by removal of peripheral irritants. Australian Medical Journal New Series 9:177–180.

Springthorpe JW (1888) Notes on fifty cases of epilepsy. Australian Medical Journal New Series 10:3–6.

Stawell RH (1915) Huntington's chorea. Medical Journal of Australia 1:245.

Stawell RR (1895) Two cases of Friedreich's disease. Australian Medical Journal New Series 17:452–460.

Stawell RR (1919) Encephalitis lethargica. Medical Journal of Australia 2:97.

Stawell RR (1920) Encephalitis lethargica. Medical Journal of Australia 2:387.

Stawell RR (1923) Epidemic encephalitis. Medical Journal of Australia 2:594–595.

Stewart-Wynne E, Jamrozik K, Ward G (1987) The Perth community stroke study: attack rates for stroke and TIA in Western Australia. Clinical and Experimental Neurology 24:39–44.

Stoller A (1966) Obituary: Jacob Mackiewicz. Medical Journal of Australia 2:1120.

Stoller A, Emmerson R (1969) General paresis in Victoria, Australia: historical study. Medical Journal of Australia 2:607–611.

Sunderland S (1978) Nerves and nerve injuries. 2nd ed. Edinburgh: Churchill-Livingstone.

Sunderland S (1991) Nerve injuries and their repair: a critical appraisal. Edinburgh: Churchill-Livingstone.

Sunderland S (1994) The Cox-Trumble contribution to Australian neurology. In: Morris J, ed. Neurology in Australia. Sydney: Australian Association of Neurologists: pp 99–111.

Susman E (1949) The treatment of neurosyphilis. Medical Journal of Australia 2:829–831.

Susman E, Maddox K (1940) Guillain-Barré syndrome. Medical Journal of Australia 1:158–162.

Sutherland JM (1981) Fundamentals of neurology. New York: Adis Press.

Sutherland JM (1989) A far-off sunlit place. Brisbane: Ampion Press.

Sutherland JM, Eadie MJ (1980) The epilepsies. Modern diagnosis and treatment. 3rd ed. Edinburgh: Churchill-Livingstone.

Sutherland JM, Tyrer JH, Eadie MJ, Casey JH, Kurland LT (1966) The prevalence of multiple sclerosis in Queensland, Australia. Acta Neurologica Scandinavica 42 (Suppl 19):57–67.

Swift H (1914) Erythroedema. Transactions of the Australasian Medical Congress 10th Session:547–552.

Swift H (1917) A case of progressive lenticular degeneration. Medical Journal of Australia 2:310.

Swift H (1923) Erythroedema. Medical Journal of Australia 2:159–160.

Swift H, Bull LB (1917) Notes on a case of systemic blastomycosis – Blastomycotic cerebrospinal meningitis. Medical Journal of Australia 2:265.

Syme GA (1895) Case of tumour of the dura mater, pressing on the brain, successfully removed by operation. Australian Medical Journal New Series 17:60–67.

Taylor RJ (1938) Muscular atrophies and dystrophies in childhood. Medical Journal of Australia 2:889–892.

Thompson JA (1898) On the history and prevalence of lepra in Australia. Intercolonial Medical Journal of Australasia 3:65–77.

Thomson JRM (1898) Notes on two cases of peripheral neuritis following febrile diseases. Intercolonial Medical Journal of Australasia 3:539–545.

Tiegs OW, Coates AE (1928) The sympathetic innervation of skeletal muscle. Medical Journal of Australia 1:140–143.

Tissot SA (1840) Traite des nerves et de leurs maladies. Reprint of 1st (1778) edition. Paris.

Trahair G (1950) Some modern trends in electroencephalography. Medical Journal of Australia 1:146–148.

Trahair G, Garven AK (1948) Electroencephalography: the localization of cerebral lesions. Medical Journal of Australia 1:458–461.

Trumpy DE (1922) Epidemic encephalitis. Medical Journal of Australia 2:282.

Turner AJ (1897) Lead-poisoning among Queensland children. Australasian Medical Gazette 16:475–479.

Turner AJ (1908) Lead-poisoning in childhood. Transactions of the Australasian Medical Congress 8th Session:3–9.

Turner EK (1946) Purulent meningitis in infancy and childhood: a twelve months' survey of the results of treatment with penicillin. Medical Journal of Australia 1:14–18.

Tyrer JH (1993) History of the Brisbane Hospital. A pilgrim's progress. Brisbane: Boolarong Publications.

Tyrer JH, Sutherland JM (1961) The primary spino-cerebellar atrophies and their associated defects, with a study of the foot deformity. Brain 84:289–300.

Tyrer JH, Sutherland JM, Eadie MJ (1981) Exercises in neurological diagnosis. 3rd ed. Edinburgh: Churchill-Livingstone.

Verco JC (1912) Paramyoclonus multiplex epilepticus of Unverricht. Australasian Medical Gazette 31:77–80.

References

Vickers W (1921) The treatment of acute anterior poliomyelitis. Medical Journal of Australia 1:396–397.

Vinken PJ, Bruyn GW eds (1975) Handbook of clinical neurology. v. 21. Amsterdam: North Holland Publishing Co.

Von Bonin G (1970) Walter Campbell (1868–1937). In: Haymaker W, Schiller F, eds. The founders of neurology. 2nd ed. Springfield: Thomas: pp 102–104.

Wallace DC (1972) Huntington's chorea in Queensland. A not uncommon disease. Medical Journal of Australia 1:299–307.

Wallace JAL, Latham O (1914) A case of sudden dementia from massive cerebral glioma of unusual nature. Medical Journal of Australia 2:516–519.

Walshe FMR, Robertson EG (1933) Observations upon the form and nature of the 'grasping' movements and tonic innervation" seen in certain cases of lesion of the frontal lobe. Brain 56:40–70.

Watson JF (1911) The history of the Sydney Hospital from 1811 to 1911. Sydney: Government Printer.

Whitcomb WP (1862) Case III – epilepsy treated by trepanning – death. Australian Medical Journal 7:41–42.

White AER (1949) Obituary: Sidney Valentine Sewell. Medical Journal of Australia 1:666–669.

Wilkinson HJ (1927) The Argyll-Robertson pupil: a contribution towards its understanding. Medical Journal of Australia 1:267–272.

Wilkinson HJ (1929) The innervation of striated muscle. Medical Journal of Australia 2:768–793.

Wilkinson JF (1920) Encephalitis lethargica. Medical Journal of Australia 2:205–206.

Williams (1881) Intracranial aneurism. Australian Medical Journal New Series 3:310.

Williams H, Macdonald WB, Callow V (1951) Pink disease: its relation to adrenal function and the value of salt and desoxy corticosterone in treatment. Medical Journal of Australia 1:363–365.

Williams S (1937) Sydenham's chorea: its course and relationship to rheumatic fever. Medical Journal of Australia 2:590–593.

Willis T (1683) De anima brutorum. (Two discourses concerning the soul of brutes). London: Dring, Harper and Leigh. (Translated by Pordage, S)

Willis T (1684) Pathology of the brain and nervous stock: on convulsive diseases. In: Pordage S, ed. The remaining medical works of that famous and renowned physician Dr Thomas Willis of Christ Church in Oxford, and Sidley Professor of Natural Philosophy in that Famous University. London: Dring, Harper, Leigh & Martyn: pp 1–89.

Wilson SAK (1918) Epidemic encephalitis. Lancet 2:91.

Wilson SAK (1928) Modern problems in neurology. London: Edward Arnold.

Wolfenden WH (1994) Noad, Sir Kenneth Beeson. In: Wiseman JC, Mulhearn RJ, eds. Roll of the Royal Australasian College of Physicians. v. 2. Sydney: Royal Australasian College of Physicians: pp 241–244.

Wolff HG (1963) Headache and other head pain. 2nd ed. New York: Oxford University Press.

Wood AJ (1921) Erythroedema or pink disease. Medical Journal of Australia 1:145.

You R, McNeill JJ, O'Malley HM, Davis SM, Donnan GA (1995) Risk factors for lacunar infarction syndromes. Neurology 45:1483–1487.

Young JA, Sefton AJ, Webb N eds (1984) Centenary book of the University of Sydney Faculty of Medicine. Sydney: Sydney University Press.

Youngman NV (1942) Some aspects of epilepsy. Medical Journal of Australia 1:433–438.

Youngman NV (1945) Can epilepsy be cured? The results of treatment. Medical Journal of Australia 2:332–335.

Appendix I

Minutes of the Inaugural Meeting of the Australian Association of Neurologists

MINUTES OF THE INAUGURAL BUSINESS MEETING OF THE ORIGINATING MEMBERS, HELD IN THE ANATOMY DEPARTMENT OF THE UNIVERSITY OF MELBOURNE AT 10AM, ON WEDNESDAY, 25th OCTOBER, 1950

PRESENT: Dr. Leonard B. Cox, M.D., F.R.A.C.P., M.R.C.P. (Edin.) of Melbourne, Dr. K.B. Noad M.B., Ch.M. (Syd.), F.R.A.C.P., M.R.C.P. (London), of Sydney, Dr. E. Graeme Robertson, M.D., F.R.A.C.P., F.R.C.P., of Melbourne, Dr. E. Susman; M.B., Ch.M. (Syd.), F.R.A.C.P., M.R.C.P. (London), of Sydney, Dr. J.J. Billings, M.D., M.R.A..C.P., M.R.C.P. (London), of Melbourne.

By unanimous agreement of those present as originating members, Professor S. Sunderland, D.Sc., M.D., B.S., F.R.A.C.P. of Melbourne and Dr. J. A. Game, M.D. of Melbourne were admitted as originating members and joined the meeting.

APOLOGIES: Apologies were received from Dr. Gerald Moss, M.B., B.S., M.R.C.P., (London) of Perth.

The meeting was opened by Dr. Cox, who suggested that the order of business should be the election of officers and consideration of a constitution.

ELECTION OF OFFICE BEARERS:

Thereupon Dr. Graeme Robertson proposed, and Dr. K. Noad seconded that Dr. Leonard B. Cox be elected President of the Association. This was agreed unanimously and Dr. Cox formally accepted his appointment. He thanked those present for the trust they had placed in him by electing him as their first President, and gave his assurance that he would help in any way he could to make the Association a success.

Dr. Cox then suggested from the Chair that the posts of Honorary Secretary and Honorary Treasurer be combined for the present, and called for nominations. Having been proposed by Dr. Graeme Robertson and seconded by Dr. K. Noad, Dr. John Game was appointed.

DRAFT CONSTITUTION:

The President then submitted for the consideration of the meeting a draft constitution which he had prepared. He suggested that the essential provisions should be considered and decided by the meeting. The draft would then be circulated for the detailed consideration of members before submission to a legal firm. Finally, the permanent copies of the Constitution would be signed by the Originating Members and the Association registered.

The Chairman then called for discussion of the separate clauses of the draft constitution.

Clause 1 – Name. "The Australian Association of Neurologists."

Dr. E. Susman asked the President whether the alternative of "The Association of Australian Neurologists" should be considered. Dr. Graeme Robertson mentioned the possibility of members who may not be Australians, and the former title was then unanimously adopted.

The remaining clauses of the draft, clauses II to XVIII, were accepted without discussion.

Dr. Graeme Robertson then moved that it be recorded in the proceedings of the Association that the Originating Members greatly appreciated Dr. Cox's work in forming the Association and preparing the Constitution. This was seconded by Dr. Noad and unanimously approved.

APPOINTMENT OF COUNCIL:

The President said an Ad Hoc Council had been formed by Dr. Cox, Dr. Robertson, Dr. Noad and Dr. Susman.

Professor Sunderland moved that the ad hoc council, including the elected Secretary and Treasurer, become the first Council. Dr. Billings seconded this.

Dr. Graeme Robertson proposed an amendment that Dr. Game be added to the Council as an elected member, apart from his ex-officio membership as Hon. Secretary and Treasurer, thus conferring the right to vote in Council.

Professor Sunderland and Dr. Billings wished their motion to be re-submitted accordingly.

This was adopted by the meeting.

DINNERS:

The President proposed that the cost of social functions should be shared by participating members. This Çculd ensure an equitable distribution of costs when the Association met in any State with a small membership.

FINANCE:

Dr. Cox announced an anonymous gift of £5.

Dr. Graeme Robertson proposed that initially the subscription be £1.1.-. per member per annum. Dr. Susman seconded this and proposed that the Associate Members' fees be also £1.1.-.

Dr. Robertson agreed to incorporate this in the motion, which was adopted by the meeting.

MEMBERSHIP:

Dr. Susman asked the President whether the terms of membership of the Association as defined in the draft constitution might be considered too exclusive of General Physicians who had some interest in neurology.

The President expressed the view that in order to attain the objects of the Association the existing provisions of the draft constitution allowed sufficient discretion in the appointment of members. He hoped, however, that the Scientific Meetings of the Association would be open to all who may be interested, and that guests would be invited to give papers and take part in the scientific discussions of the Association.

Dr. Robertson endorsed these views and added that he thought a high standard of membership should obtain.

It was agreed that the existing provisions of the draft constitution allowed sufficient discretion in these matters.

In the absence of any further business the President declared the meeting closed at about 10.55 a.m.

Confirmed this 10th day of April, 1951.

Leonard B Cox

President.

Appendix II

Programmes of the Early Scientific Meetings of the Australian Association of Neurologists

(the original spellings are reproduced)

INAUGURAL SCIENTIFIC MEETING OF THE ASSOCIATION HELD IN THE ANATOMY SCHOOL, UNIVERSITY OF MELBOURNE, on 25th OCTOBER, 1950.

The following Papers were presented: –

The capacity of muscles to function efficiently following re-innervation after prolonged denervation	Professor S. Sunderland
The deformation of nerves	Dr. K. Bradley
Psychogenic impotence	Dr. E. Susman
Brief attacks of muscular weakness of endocrine origin	Dr. E. Graeme Robertson
Cavitation of the brain-stem and basal ganglia, (Syringo-encephalia)	Dr. Leonard B. Cox
(1) The differential filling of arterio-venous malformations by arteriography of the internal carotid of the same and opposite sides, and of the external carotid	Dr. John A. Game & Dr. H. Luke
(2) The blood supply of the brain after carotid ligation demonstrated by angiography	Dr. John A. Game & Dr. H. Luke

SCIENTIFIC MEETING OF THE ASSOCIATION HELD IN THE MAITLAND LECTURE THEATRE OF SYDNEY HOSPITAL on TUESDAY 10th APRIL, 1951.

The following papers were presented: –

Peripheral Neuritis and Bronchial Carcinoma	Mr. Gilbert Phillips
Hallevorden-Spatz Disease and its Relation to Wilson's Disease	Dr. Leonard B. Cox
Lesions of Nerves in Typhus and their Pathology	Dr. K .B. Noad
What a Cerebellar Section might reveal	Dr. Oliver Latham
Some unusual Sub-dural Haematomas	Dr. John A. Game
Examination of Twins Joined at the Vertex	Dr. E. Graeme Robertson

SCIENTIFIC MEETING OF THE ASSOCIATION, HELD AT THE ANATOMY SCHOO(L), UNIVERSITY OF MELBOURNE, ON MONDAY, 16th MARCH, 1953.

The following papers were presented: –

A Short Review of the Work of a New Neurological Diagnostic Centre in Sydney	Dr. E. Susman
Case Reports –	
(1) Leprosy	
(2) Uni-lateral Proptosis	Dr. John Billings
Report of the First Thousand Electroencephalograms at the Alfred Hospital	Dr. John A. Game
The Heart in Friedreich's Ataxia: Short Case	Dr. K. Noad
Injury in the Congenitally Diseased Spinal Cord	Dr. Leonard B. Cox
The Parietal Lobe	Dr. McDonald Critchley
Self Induced Photic Epilepsy	Dr. E. Graeme Robertson

SCIENTIFIC MEETING OF THE ASSOCIATION HELD AT THE SYDNEY GENERAL HOSPITAL, SYDNEY ON THE 12th OCTOBER, 1954.

The following papers were presented: –

Migraine – A Clinical Study of 250 cases	Dr. G. Selby
The Clinical Importance of the Brain Stem and Thalamic Reticular Formation	Dr. L. Rail
A Clinical Survey of Optic Atrophy	Dr. J. Billings
Permanent Paralysis in Myasthenia	Dr. K. Noad
Myasthenia Gravis and Pulmonary Lesions	Dr. L. Cox
A Case of Thyrotoxicosis, Exophthalmic Opthalmoplegia and Myasthenia Gravis	Dr. J. Game
The Use of Encephalography in Suprasellar Tumours	Dr. E. Graeme Robertson

SCIENTIFIC MEETING OF THE ASSOCIATION HELD AT THE ANATOMY SCHOOL UNIVERSITY OF MELBOURNE, ON SATURDAY, 15th OCTOBER, 1955.

The following papers were presented: –

An unusual case of Spinal Cord Disease	Dr. J. Game & Dr. Ross Anderson
Carcinomatous Neuropathy	Dr. J.J. Billings
Internal Carotid Thrombosis	Dr. George Selby & Dr. Brian Turner
Cystic pineal glands, and long supra-pineal recess	Dr. E. Graeme Robertson
Infection of Tumours of the Pituitary Region	Dr. Leonard B. Cox
Some aspects of Status Epilepticus	Dr. Leonard Rail

SCIENTIFIC MEETING OF THE ASSOCIATION HELD AT THE SYDNEY GENERAL HOSPITAL, SYDNEY ON THE 17th OCTOBER 1957.

The following papers were presented: –

Speech Development and Hemispherectomy	Dr. L.S. Basser
A Group of Cases of Cerebral Embolism	Dr. John Billings
Ulnar Symptoms in Cortical Lesions	Dr. John Gordon
A film Depicting some well-known Neurologists	Dr. E. Graeme Robertson
Trigeminal Nerve Lesions	Sir Geoffrey Jefferson

Appendix II Programmes of the early Scientific Meetings

SCIENTIFIC MEETING OF THE ASSOCIATION HELD IN THE MAITLAND LECTURE HALL, SYDNEY HOSPITAL, on WEDNESDAY 4th JUNE and FRIDAY 6th JUNE, 1958.

A Symposium on the subject of the management of Cerebro-Vascular Disease included the following papers: –

Experiences with Long-Term Anticoagulant Therapy in C.V.D.	Dr. G. Selby
Two Cases of Internal Carotid Artery Syndrome	Dr. J.J. Billings
Basilar Artery Syndrome	Dr. W. Burke
Treatment of Recurrent Attacks Suggestive of Localised Cerebral Ischaemia by Cervical Sympathectomy	Dr. Graeme Robertson
Some Aspects of Collateral Cerebral Circulation	Dr. John A. Game

Friday 6th June, 1958.
The following papers were presented: –

Familial Polyneuritis with Four Generations of Pes Cavus	Dr. J.W. Lance
Sensory Neuropathy	Dr. L.S. Basser
Necrotic Myelitis	Dr. J.L. Allsop & Dr. Brian Turner
Episodic Behaviour Disorders in Childhood	Dr. E. Davis
A Case of Kinnier Wilson's Disease	Dr. John A. Game
Severe Torula Meningitis	Dr. G. Selby

SCIENTIFIC MEETING OF THE ASSOCIATION HELD IN THE MEDICAL SCHOOL, FROME ROAD, ADELAIDE on TUESDAY 26th MAY, 1959.

The following papers were presented: –

Failure of Initial Investigations to Disclose Cerebral Tumour, later proven	Dr. George Selby
The Radiological Demonstration of the Full Length of the Carotid and Vertebral Arteries	Dr. H.A. Luke
Steroid Therapy of Encephalomyelitis. (Cancelled due to illness)	Dr. W. Burke
Neurological Manifestations of Methyl Bromide Poisoning	Dr. P.J. Landy
Cerebellar Atrophy Associated with Alcoholism	Dr. Brian Turner
Sub-Acute Inclusion Encephalitis	Dr. J.V. Gordon
Late Infantile Metachromic Leuco-encephalopathy.	Dr. Leon Basser & Dr. Brian Turner
A Case of Megalencephaly with Hyaline Pan-Neuropathy	Dr. R. McD. Anderson
Some Atypical Manifestations Of Acoustic Nerve Tumour	Dr. Anthony Fisher
Upward Deviation of the Eyes	Dr. Arthur Schweiger

SCIENTIFIC PROGRAMME FOR THE PLENARY SESSION OF THE ROYAL AUSTRALASIAN COLLEGE OF PHYSICIANS' MEETING held in the ACADEMY CONFERENCE CHAMBER, CANBERRA on SATURDAY 17th OCTOBER 1959.

CEREBRO-VASCULAR DISEASE

Introduction	Dr. L.B. Cox
Pathology	Dr. R. McD. Anderson
Difficulties in Diagnosis	Dr. K.B. Noad
Cerebral Ischaemic Attacks	Dr. John Billings
Management	Dr. W. Burke
Concluding Remarks	Dr. E. Graeme Robertson

THE FLOWERING OF A WARATAH

SCIENTIFIC MEETING OF THE ASSOCIATION HELD AT THE WOOD-JONES LECTURE THEATRE, ANATOMY SCHOOL, UNIVERSITY OF MELBOURNE on 24th MAY 1960

Anticonvulsants in the treatment of facial pain	Dr. R.H.S. Rischbeith
The Neurophysiology of Kuru	Dr. L.R. Rail
On Cerebellar Localisation Using Positive Contrast	Dr. A. Fisher
Olivo-ponto Cerebellar Degeneration with Extrapyramidal Involvement	Dr. B. Turner
Familial Myoclonic Epilepsy and its Association with Cerebellar Disorder	Dr. J.W. Lance & Dr. K.B. Noad
Some Observations on Parkinsonism. (Thoughts and Questions About the Pathological Anatomy and Physiology of Certain Aspects of the Various Forms of Parkinsonism)	Dr. G. Selby
The Symptomatology of Multiple Sclerosis Based on the Review of 555 Patients	Dr. J.M. Sutherland
Experimental Encephalomyelilis	Dr. R. Anderson & Dr. G. Szego
Recent experiences in the investigation and treatment of Temporal Lobe Epilepsy, particularly in relation to Surgery	Dr. Eric Davis

AUSTRALIAN ASSOCIATION OF NEUROLOGISTS
SCIENTIFIC PROGRAMME

Thursday 31st. May 1962

Dystonic Seizures: Striatal or Extra-pyramidal Epilepsy	Dr. J. Lance
Some Aspects of Disseminated Sclerosis in Queensland	Dr. P. Landy
Progressive Multifocal Leukoencephalopathy – A Clinical and Pathological Study	Dr. M. Sadka
Acute Toxic Encephalopathy	Dr. R. Anderson
The Present Status of Immunization Against Poliomyelitis	Dr. J. Billings
The Stiff Man Syndrome	Dr J. Allsop
Temporal Lobe Epilepsy: A Critical Review of Some Thirty Cases Submitted to Temporal Lobectomy	Dr E. Davis
Visual Mechanisms and the Electro-encephalogram	Dr. Ross Davis
Film – The Neurological Examination of the Newborn	

Friday 1st June 1962

The Falling Attacks of Myoclonus	Dr J. Lance
The Supra-pineal Arachnoid Body	Dr G.C. T. Kenny
Some Recent Laboratory Aids to Neurological Diagnosis	Dr. B. Turner
Clinical Features of Obstruction of the Proximal Part of the Major Extracranial Arteries	Dr. G. Selby
By-passing Vertebral Artery Occlusion by Extracranial Anastomotic Channels	Dr. J.A. Game
Observations on the Prognostic Signs Following Relief of Spinal Cord Compression	Dr. A. Fisher
Deep Sensibility	Prof. A. McIntyre
Psychomimetics and Synaptic Transmission	Dr. D. Curtis
The Problems of Subdural Gas After Pneumoencephalography	Dr. E. Graeme Robertson
Film – The Neurological Examination of the One-year Old	

Appendix II Programmes of the early Scientific Meetings

PLENARY SESSION WITH THE ROYAL AUSTRALASIAN COLLEGE OF PHYSICIANS held at the UNION THEATRE, UNIVERSITY OF SYDNEY on THURSDAY 6th JUNE 1963.

Evaluation of Investigation of the Nervous System Introduction	Dr. E. Graeme Robertson
Evaluation of Pneumoencephalography	Dr. E. Graeme Robertson
The Scope and Limitations of E.E.G. Examinations in Clinical Diagnosis	Dr. Leonard Rail
The Value of Angiography in the Investigation of Cerebral Disease	Dr. George Selby
Motor and Sensory Nerve Conduction Studies as Applied to the Hand	Dr. Peter Ebeling
Laboratory Investigations of Mental Retardation	Dr. Brian Turner

SCIENTIFIC MEETING HELD IN THE MAITLAND THEATRE SYDNEY HOSPITAL on SATURDAY 8th JUNE, 1963

Discussion of the Reasons for Doing Lumbar Puncture	Dr. John A. Game
Activation of the E.E.G.	Dr. George Preswick
Positron Scanning in the Diagnosis of Intracranial Lesions	Dr. Paul Farrar
An Evaluation of the Echogram in Neurological Diagnosis (By Invitation)	Mr. Robin Lowe
Cortical Biopsy in Childhood	Dr. Peter Ebeling & Dr. Ross Anderson
Total Cerebral Angiography, *and* Anterior Mediastinography in the Demonstration of the Thymus	Dr. W.S.C. Hare (By Invitation)
Experience with Cortical Biopsy	Dr. Mervyn Eadie
The Hyperkalaemic Type of Periodic Paralysis	Dr. John Allsop
Necrosis of the Brain in Newborn Babies (By Invitation)	Dr. H.F. Bettinger
Serotonin and the Nervous System: A Review	Dr. J.W. Lance
Experimental Demyelination	Dr. George Szego
Experiences with Myasthenia Gravis	Dr. Arthur Schweiger
Reading Epilepsy	Dr. John V. Gordon
Study of Vascular Malformation of the Brain	Dr. Anthony Fisher

(Each paper was 20 minutes long and was followed by 10 minutes' discussion)

Appendix III

The Original Constitution of the Australian Association of Neurologists

CONSTITUTION
of
THE AUSTRALIAN ASSOCIATION OF NEUROLOGISTS

NAME

1 The name of the Association shall be "The Australian Association of Neurologists".

OBJECTS

2 The objects of the Association are –

    (a)   to bring together physician Neurologists and scientific workers in the field of the nervous system and its diseases for their mutual benefit and for the better understanding of the nervous system and its diseases.

    (b)   to hold scientific meetings in which all matters pertaining to the nervous system and its diseases may be discussed.

    (c)   to provide special facilities for members of the Association.

    (d)   to assist as may from time to time be considered advisable in the publication of matter pertaining to the nervous system and its diseases.

    (e)   generally to utilise the funds and credit of the Association in any manner which in the opinion of the Council is conducive or incidental to the encouragement of the study or appreciation of the nervous system and its diseases.

ASSOCIATION PROPERTY

3 (a)   the property of the Association shall be vested in three trustees who shall be appointed and may be removed by the Council. The Council shall also have the right to fill any vacancy occurring by resignation, death, unwillingness to act or other reasons. The following powers shall be deemed to be vested in the trustees, and may be exercised by them, subject to the direction of the Council, as hereinafter mentioned: –

	(i)	To invest money and adopt such measures as may appear to them necessary in the interests of the Association, subject to the approval of the Council.
	(ii)	To purchase or otherwise acquire any land or property of any tenure which the Council may deem desirable for, or partly for, the purposes of the Association, at such price, on such terms and upon such conditions as the Council shall think fit, and to use the Association's moneys and funds for such purposes and to hold such property on behalf of the Association and the members thereof.
	(iii)	To sell and procure the selling of any property of the Association, real or personal, for such consideration, on such terms and upon such conditions as the Council shall think fit.
	(iv)	To let any part or parts of such last-mentioned property which the Council may think is or are not required for the purposes of the Association at such rent, for such term and upon such conditions as the Council shall think fit.
	(v)	To borrow and arrange for borrowing, either with or without giving security, such sum or sums of money as the Association shall be of the opinion may be required by it upon such terms and at such rate or rates of interest as the Council shall think proper, and for such purpose to give (if thought fit by the Council) such security or securities over any property, real or personal, held by or on behalf of the Association as the Council shall think fit, and adopt such other measures as may appear to them necessary in the interest of the Association, subject to the approval of the Council. All securities shall be taken and investments made in the names of the trustees the property the subject matter of the trust to be nevertheless subject to the disposition of the Council.
	(vi)	The powers aforesaid shall only be exercised by the Trustees in accordance with the directions of the Council and the authority in writing of a majority of those assembled at a duly constituted meeting of the Council and signed by the President of the day, and attested by the Honorary Secretary, shall be binding upon and a justification to the trustees as to any purchase, sale, investment, or disposal as aforesaid, or any exercise of such powers or any of them.
(b)	(i)	The income and property of the Association whencesoever derived shall be applied solely towards the promotion of the objects of the Society and no portion thereof shall be paid or transferred directly or indirectly by way of dividend bonus or otherwise howsoever by way of profit to the persons who at any time are or have been members of the Association or to any of them or to any person claiming through any of them. Provided that nothing herein shall prevent the payment in good faith of remuneration to any officers or servants of the Association or to any member thereof or other person in return for services actually rendered to the Association or for goods supplied in the ordinary way of business nor prevent the payment of interest on money borrowed or the payment of rent for premises let to the Association. If the Association is dissolved and there remains after the satisfaction of its liabilities any property whatsoever the same shall not be paid to or distributed among the members of the Association but shall be given or transferred to some body whose aims are conducive to the appreciation or study of the nervous system and its diseases selected by the Council and having objects which prohibit the distribution of its or their income amongst its or their members.

Appendix III Constitution of the Australian Association of Neurologists

MEMBERSHIP

4. THE members of the Association shall be –
   (a) The signatories to this Constitution and any other persons who in addition to such signatories are hereinafter named as members of the Council.
   (b) Every person who may be admitted by the Council to membership of the Association as hereinafter provided.
5. Members shall be divided into the following classes, namely –
   Ordinary Members.
   Associate Members.
   Honorary Members.
   Provisional Members.
6. Candidates for membership shall be nominated by any ordinary member.
7. All nominations for membership shall be placed before the Council which may elect the applicant for membership or refrain from so doing. An applicant shall not become a member of the Association unless and until elected, and the decision of the Council on nomination for membership and as to the class of membership for which the applicant is eligible shall be conclusive.
8. In judging which applicants for ordinary or associate membership shall be elected the Council shall take into consideration its knowledge of the qualifications of the applicant in the practice of neurology, his general medical and other scientific qualifications and his contribution to the knowledge of the nervous system and its diseases.
9. The Council may elect any person to honorary membership.
10. The Council may elect as provisional members those who practice neurology and who do not hold senior neurological appointments at approved hospitals although this will not of necessity preclude them from ordinary membership, and who in the opinion of the Council may not adhere to the practice of neurology, or who for other reasons should not in the opinion of the Council be appointed as ordinary members. It shall be the practice of the Council to appoint a provisional member for a period of three years after which his appointment shall be reconsidered in the light of his known professional skill and such other qualities as may seem relevant to the Council.

TERMINATION OF MEMBERSHIP

11. Membership may be terminated –
    (a) by written resignation
    (b) by death
    (c) by resolution of the Council pursuant to Rule 4 for non-payment of subscription.
    (d) by resolution of the Council pursuant to Rule 11.
12. The Council may by resolution suspend the membership of any member for such period as the Council thinks fit or may expel any member for any conduct which in the opinion of the Council is detrimental to the interests of the Association PROVIDED ALWAYS that no resolution for suspension or expulsion shall be passed unless the Council has given the member concerned an opportunity of showing cause against his proposed suspension or expulsion.

FEES AND CONTRIBUTIONS

13. The annual subscription shall be such sums respectively as are from time to time fixed by the Council of the Association but shall not be less than –

	(a)	for Ordinary Members	$1.1.0 per annum
	(b)	for Associate Members	$1.1.0 per annum
	(c)	for Provisional Members	$1.1.0 per annum

14 The annual subscription shall be paid in advance in the month of October in each year and shall be for the fiscal year 1st October to 30th September.

15 If any subscription is not paid within three calendar months after notification of election or after 31st October in any year membership may at any time thereafter be terminated by resolution of the Council.

16 The members shall be expected to assist the Association by their honorary work especially in technical and professional spheres.

17 Contributions or donations may be accepted from members to supplement their annual subscriptions which are to be regarded as minima.

VOTES OF MEMBERS

18 Each Ordinary Member shall have one vote.

19 Votes may be given either personally or by proxy or by Attorney.

20 The instrument appointing a proxy shall be in writing under the hand of the appointer or of his Attorney duly authorised in writing. No person shall be appointed a proxy who is not an ordinary member of the Association.

21 The instrument appointing a proxy and the Power of Attorney (if any) under which it is signed, or a notarially certified copy thereof, shall be deposited at the office not less than forty-eight hours before the person named in such instrument purports to vote in respect thereof but no instrument appointing a proxy shall be valid after the expiration of twelve months from the date of its execution.

22 A vote given in accordance with the terms of an instrument of proxy shall be valid notwithstanding the previous death of the principal, or revocation of the proxy, provided no intimation in writing of the death or revocation shall have been received at the office or by the Chairman of the meeting before the vote is given.

23 Every instrument of proxy, whether for a specified meeting or otherwise shall as nearly as circumstances will admit, be in the form or to the effect following –

"I   of
being an ordinary member of the Australian Association of Neurologists hereby appoint   of   or failing him   of
as my proxy to vote for me and on my behalf at the (ordinary or extraordinary as the case may be) general meeting of the Association to be held on the
    day of   and at any adjournment thereof.
As witness my hand this   day of   195 ."

or in such other form as the Council may from time to time prescribe or accept. Any instrument of proxy deposited at the office in which the name of the appointee is not filled in shall be deemed to be given in favour of the Chairman of the Meeting to which it relates.

PRIVILEGES OF MEMBERS

24 The members shall be entitled to admission to all meetings and functions held by the Association.

Appendix III Constitution of the Australian Association of Neurologists

25   The members shall be entitled to other privileges such as will be determined by the Council from time to time.

GENERAL MEETING

26   A general meeting shall be held once in each year commencing in the year 1951 unless in the Judgment of the Council such is not practicable.

27   The annual general meeting shall be called the Ordinary General Meeting. All other general meetings shall be called Extraordinary General Meetings.

28   The Ordinary General Meetings shall where considered practicable by the Council be held at the time of a scientific session of the Association.

29   The Council may whenever it thinks fit convene an Extraordinary General Meeting and shall convene an Extraordinary General Meeting on the requisition of at least ten per centum of the ordinary members.

30   Twenty-eight days' notice at the least specifying the place day and hour of any general meeting and in the case of special business the general nature of such business shall be given to members but the accidental omission to give notice to any member shall not invalidate the proceedings at such meeting.

PROCEEDINGS AT GENERAL MEETINGS

31   The business of an Ordinary General Meeting shall be –

     (a)   to receive and consider the report of the Council.

     (b)   to receive and consider the statement of accounts and the Auditor's report.

     (c)   to elect officers and other members of the Council.

     (d)   to transact any other business which ought under the Constitution or the Rules to be transacted at an ordinary General Meeting.

All other business transacted at an ordinary General Meeting and all business transacted at an Extraordinary General Meeting shall be special business.

32   No member shall be at liberty to introduce any special business unless he has given not less than twenty-one days' previous notice in writing to the Council or unless he has the approval of the Council.

33   The quorum for a general meeting shall be thirty per cent. of the ordinary members of the Association present in person or by proxy.

34   The president shall be entitled to take the chair at every general meeting or if at any general meeting he shall not be present within fifteen minutes after the time appointed for the holding such meeting or is unwilling to act the Council may choose a chairman and in default of their doing so the ordinary members present shall choose one of the Councillors to be Chairman and if no Councillor present be willing to take the chair shall choose some one of their number to be Chairman.

35   Every question submitted to a meeting shall be decided, in the first instance, by a show of hands, and in the case of an equality of votes the chairman shall, both on a show of hands and on a poll, have a casting vote in addition to the vote or votes to which he may be entitled as a member.

36   At any General Meeting, unless a poll is demanded by the Chairman or by at least five ordinary members present at the meeting, a declaration by the Chairman that a resolution has been carried, or carried by a particular majority, or lost, or not carried by a particular majority and an entry to that effect in the book of proceedings of the Association, shall be conclusive evidence of the fact without proof of the number or proportion of the votes recorded in favour of or against such resolution.

37 If a poll is demanded as aforesaid, it shall be taken in such manner and at such time and place as the chairman of the meeting directs and either at once, or after an interval or adjournment, and the result of the poll shall be deemed to be the resolution of the meeting at which the poll was demanded. The demand of a poll may be withdrawn. In case of any dispute as to the admission or rejection of a vote, the chairman shall determine the same, and such determination made in good faith shall be final and conclusive.

38 Associate members, Honorary members and Provisional members shall be entitled to notice of general meetings and to attend and speak thereat but shall not be entitled to vote.

POSTAL BALLOT

39 Whenever the Council thinks fit it may submit any question to the vote of all ordinary members by means of a postal ballot in such form and returnable in such manner as the Council decides. A resolution approved by a majority or specific majority of such members voting by such ballot shall have the same force and effect as such a resolution would have if carried by such majority or specific majority at a duly constituted general meeting competent to pass such resolution.

COUNCIL AND MANAGEMENT

40 The affairs of the Association shall be managed by a Council which may exercise all powers and do all things which are not by the constitution or Rules of the Association required to be exercised or done by a general meeting.

41 The Council shall consist of the President, Honorary Treasurer, Honorary Secretary and three other ordinary members. The offices of Honorary Treasurer and Honorary Secretary may be held by one person in which case there shall be four other ordinary members. No Associate or Honorary member or Provisional member may be a member of the Council.

42 The Council shall define the duties of the President, Honorary Treasurer and Honorary Secretary, who shall in all respects be subject to the control of the council.

43 The first Council shall be

    Dr. Leonard Bell Cox (President).

    Dr. John Aylward Game (Honorary Treasurer and Secretary).

    Dr. Kenneth Beeson Noad.

    Dr. Edward Graeme Robertson.

    Dr. Eric Leo Susman.

and they shall hold office until the Ordinary General Meeting to be held in the year 1952.

44 The election of officers and other members of the Council shall take place in the following manner: –

(a) Any two ordinary members shall be at liberty to nominate an ordinary member as a candidate for office or otherwise to serve on the Council. The name of each member so nominated shall be sent in writing to the Honorary Secretary twenty-one days at least before the annual general meeting, accompanied by a letter from the candidate consenting to serve if elected.

(b) Notices of the names of the nominated members shall be sent to the members fourteen days at least before the ordinary general meeting. Balloting lists shall be prepared containing the names of the candidates only and each ordinary member present at the annual general meeting shall be entitled to vote for any number of such candidates not exceeding the number of vacancies. In case there shall not be a sufficient number of candidates nominated the Council shall fill up the remaining vacancies. If two or more obtain an equal number of votes, the Council shall select by lot from such candidates the candidate or candidates who are to be members of the Council.

45 At the Ordinary General Meeting in 1952 and thereafter at every succeeding ordinary general meeting one-half of the Councillors or if their number is not a multiple of two then the number nearest to, but not exceeding one half shall retire from office and shall be eligible for re-election. The Councillors or Councillor to retire in every year shall be determined as follows: –

  (a) At the ordinary general meeting in 1952 by lot.

  (b) And thereafter at every succeeding ordinary general meeting the Councillors or Councillor to retire shall be those who have been longest in office and for this purpose the length of time a Councillor has been in office shall be computed from his last election. In the event of it being necessary to decide as between two or more Councillors who were elected on the same day which of them should retire the question shall (in default of agreement between them) be determined by lot.

46 Any casual vacancy on the Council shall be filled up by the Council, and any member so chosen shall retire at the following annual meeting, but shall be eligible as a candidate for election on the Council at such annual meeting. The service of any member on the Council chosen to fill a casual vacancy shall not be reckoned in calculating the seniority of such member if subsequently elected to serve on the Council.

47 The Council may from time to time make, alter and repeal bye laws for the furtherance of the objects of the Association and generally for the good conduct of the affairs of the Association. Such bye laws shall, providing they are not inconsistent with the rules of the Association for the time being, be binding on all members and be construed as part of the rules of the Association until they are rescinded or varied by the Association in general meeting.

48 The Council may meet together for the despatch of business adjourn and otherwise regulate its meetings and proceedings as it thinks fit and may from time to time determine the quorum necessary for the transaction of business. Until otherwise determined three Councillors shall be a quorum.

49 A member of the Council may at any time and the Honorary Secretary upon the request of a member of the Council shall convene a meeting of the Council.

50 The President shall be entitled to take the chair at every meeting of the Council or if at any such meeting he shall not be present within fifteen minutes after the time appointed for holding such meeting or is unwilling to act the Council may choose a Chairman from one of its members.

51 Questions arising at any meeting of the Council shall be decided by a majority of votes. In case of an equality of votes the Chairman of the Meeting of the Council shall have a second or casting vote.

EXECUTIVE COMMITTEE

52 The Council shall have the power at any time to appoint an Executive Committee consisting of Honorary Treasurer and Honorary Secretary and any member or members of the Association.

53 The Executive Committee shall appoint one of its members to be Chairman.

54 The Executive Committee shall subject to any directions from time to time given by the Council exercise all the powers of the Council.

55 The proceedings of the Executive Committee shall be in accordance with the proceedings of the Council and the number of members to be a quorum shall be determined by the Council.

SPECIAL COMMITTEES

56 The Council may from time to time appoint and delegate any of its powers to special committees upon and subject to such conditions as the Council thinks proper in relation to such matters as the Council determines.

57 Any person whether a member of the Association or not shall be eligible for appointment to a special committee.

58 Cheques and other negotiable instruments shall be drawn made signed and endorsed in such manner as the Council or Executive Committee from time to time directs.

ALTERATION OF CONSTITUTION

59 The Council may from time to time alter or amend this Constitution by a resolution passed by a majority of not less than two-thirds of the ordinary members of the Council present and voting at the meeting at which such resolution is proposed, but no such resolution shall be proposed at any meeting of the Council unless not less than twenty-eight days' notice of such resolution has been given to each member of the Council.

NOTICES

60 Any notice to members may be given by advertisement published in an authorised Medical Journal circulating in Australia or by posting the same by prepaid letter addressed to members at their respective addresses appearing in the Association's records.

Appendix IV

Amendments to the Constitution Made in 1961

AMENDMENTS TO CONSTITUTION
1961
Articles 4 – 10A altered to read –

4   THE members of the Association shall be –

    (a)   The signatories to this Constitution and any other persons (male or female) who in addition to such signatories are hereinafter named as members of the Council.

    (b)   Every person (male or female) who may be admitted by the Council to membership of the Association as hereinafter provided.

        For the purposes of interpretation in this Constitution the masculine shall include the feminine.

5   MEMBERS shall be divided into the following classes, namely –

    Ordinary Members
    Associate Members
    Honorary Members
    Provisional Members

6   CANDIDATES for membership shall be nominated by any two members, one as proposer and one as seconder. The proposer and seconder shall request a member of Council to act as sponsor. The sponsor shall present the nomination for membership at the Council Meeting at which it is considered. The proposer or seconder shall act as guarantor to the sponsor for the identity of the candidate and for the substantiation of the candidate's qualifications for membership as hereinafter prescribed. The proposer and seconder shall provide the sponsor with the candidate's curriculum vitae, including his present occupation and appointments and the relative amount of time devoted to the various occupations and appointments.

    The sponsor shall submit the application together with qualifications and curriculum vitae and guarantee to the Honorary Secretary twenty-eight days at least before the next Council Meeting so as to enable inclusion of the nomination in the agenda for the Council Meeting and circulation of details of the candidate to other Council members if so desired. The proposer and seconder may if they wish suggest the suitable category of membership for the candidate.

7   Council may elect the applicant for membership, or refrain from so doing. An applicant shall not become a member of the Association unless and until elected, and the decision of the Council on Nomination for membership and as to the class of membership for which the applicant is eligible shall be conclusive.

8   AFTER the Nineteenth day of May 1961 the Council may elect to Ordinary Membership any candidate who

(a) (i) Is either a graduate of a Faculty of Medicine already existing in one of the Universities in Australia in the year 1960 or in a Faculty of Medicine established after that date in any University in Australia and which in the opinion of the Council establishes a standard of the Faculties of Medicine in those Universities already established in Australia.

    (ii) Who holds the Degree of Doctor of Medicine in one of the abovementioned Universities and/or is a Fellow or Member of the Royal College of Physicians of London or of the Royal Australasian College of Physicians or any other British Royal College of Physicians approved by the Council.

    (iii) Who has been engaged preferably as a house physician in a period of training of at least one year in the clinical practice of neurology including clinical responsibility for in-patients in either a special hospital or institute for the treatment of patients suffering from disease of the nervous system or in a clinic or department for the treatment of such patients in a hospital recognised by one of the abovementioned Universities as a teaching hospital of the University:

and

    (iv) Who has been occupied in the practice of clinical neurology as a primary occupation for a period of at least three years and has the purpose and intention to continue that occupation as a career.

OR

(b) Is a graduate of any Faculty in any one of the Universities mentioned in (a) who in the opinion of Council has achieved eminence and distinction as a result of his scientific contributions to the knowledge of the nervous system and its diseases and who is engaged predominantly in the scientific study of the nervous system.

Notwithstanding the possession of these qualifications by any candidate the Council shall retain the option of accepting or rejecting the candidate for membership.

9   THE Council may elect to Associate Membership any candidate who is a graduate of the Faculty of Medicine in any of the Universities mentioned in Article 8 and who is not engaged in clinical practice as a primary occupation but who in the course of his work is especially engaged with problems relating to the nervous system and who in the opinion of the Council is by virtue of his proficiency, scientific qualification, or contributions to knowledge, worthy of Associate Membership and is likely to make valuable contributions to the objects of the Association.

10   THE Council may elect to provisional membership any candidate who is a graduate of any of the Universities mentioned in Article 8 (a) (i), (ii) and (iii) of this Constitution but who has not yet attained the other qualifications of Article 8.

It shall be the practice of the Council to appoint a provisional member for a period of three years after which his appointment shall be reconsidered by the Council who may retain the member in the category of provisional membership for a further period or appoint him to the category of Ordinary Membership providing he has fulfilled all the requirements of Article 8 or terminate his provisional membership on the grounds that the member has not or is not likely to adhere to the practice of clinical neurology as a primary occupation or for other reasons is considered unsuitable by the Council.

[At this time Articles 43, 44, 45 and 46 were also modified, but these deal only with the organisation of the composition of future Councils, specifying the pattern of retirement and replacement of Council members.]

Appendix V

Memberships of the Council of the Australian Association of Neurologists

AUSTRALIAN ASSOCIATION OF NEUROLOGISTS COUNCIL MEMBERS

1950 – 1957

President:	Dr. Leonard B. Cox
Treasurer & Secretary:	Dr. John A. Game
Members:	Dr. K.B. Noad, Dr. E.G. Robertson, Dr. E. Susman

1957 – 1959

President:	Dr. E. Graeme Robertson
Secretary:	Dr. John A. Game
Treasurer:	Dr. J.J. Billings
Members:	Dr. Leonard B. Cox, Dr. K.B. Noad, Dr. E. Susman

1959 – 1961

President:	Dr. E. Graeme Robertson
Secretary:	Dr. John A. Game
Treasurer:	Dr. J.J. Billings
Members:	Dr. Leonard B. Cox, Dr. Leonard R. Rail, Dr. George Selby

1961 – 1963

President:	Dr. E. Graeme Robertson
Secretary:	Dr. John A. Game
Treasurer:	Dr. J.J. Billings
Members:	Dr. Leonard R. Rail, Dr. George Selby, Dr Gerald C. Moss

1963 – 1965

President:	Dr. E. Graeme Robertson
Secretary:	Dr. John A. Game
Treasurer:	Dr. W.J.G. Burke
Members:	Dr. Leonard R. Rail, Dr. George Selby, Dr Gerald C. Moss

1965 – 1967

President: Dr. John A. Game
Secretary: Dr. P. Ebeling
Treasurer: Dr. W.J.G. Burke
Members: Dr. Leonard R. Rail, Dr. George Selby, Dr Gerald C. Moss

1967 – 1968

President: Dr. John A. Game
Secretary: –
Treasurer: Dr. W.J.G. Burke
Members: Dr. Leonard R. Rail, Dr. George Selby, Dr Gerald C. Moss

1968 – 1969

President: Dr. John A. Game
Secretary: –
Treasurer: Dr. W.J.G. Burke
Members: Dr. George Selby, Dr Gerald C. Moss, Dr. John L. Allsop

1969 –

President: Dr. John A. Game
Secretary: Dr. J. Barrie Morley
Treasurer: Dr. W.J.G. Burke
Members: Dr. George Selby, Dr Gerald C. Moss, Dr. John L. Allsop

1969 – 1970

President: Dr. John A. Game
Secretary: Dr. J. Barrie Morley
Treasurer: Dr. W.J.G. Burke
Members: Dr Gerald C. Moss, Dr. John L. Allsop, Dr. John M. Sutherland

1970 – 1971

President: Dr. John A. Game
Secretary: Dr. J. Barrie Morley
Treasurer: Dr. W.J.G. Burke
Members: Dr. John L. Allsop, Dr. John M. Sutherland, Dr. Arthur C. Schwieger

1971 – 1972

President: Dr. John A. Game
Secretary: Dr. J. Barrie Morley
Treasurer: Dr. John L. Allsop
Members: Dr. John M. Sutherland, Dr. Arthur C. Schwieger, Dr. George Selby

Appendix V Memberships of the Council of the Australian Association of Neurologists

1972 – 1973

President:	Dr. John A. Game
Secretary:	Dr. J. Barrie Morley
Treasurer:	Dr. John L. Allsop
Members:	Dr. John M. Sutherland, Dr. Arthur C. Schwieger, Dr George Selby, Professor Byron A. Kakulas

1973 – 1974

President:	Dr. John A. Game
Secretary:	Dr. J. Barrie Morley
Treasurer:	Associate Prof. J.W. Lance
Members:	Dr. John M. Sutherland, Dr. Arthur C. Schwieger, Dr. George Selby, Professor Byron A. Kakulas

1974 – 1975

President:	Dr. George Selby
Secretary:	Dr. Peter M. Williamson
Treasurer:	Dr. John V. Gordon
Members:	Dr. Mervyn J. Eadie, Professor Byron A. Kakulas, Associate Professor J.W. Lance, Professor James G. McLeod

1975 – 1977

President:	Dr. George Selby
Secretary:	Dr. Peter M. Williamson
Treasurer:	Dr. John V. Gordon
Members:	Professor David R. Curtis, Dr. Mervyn J. Eadie, Professor J.W. Lance, Professor James G. McLeod

1977 – 1978

President:	Dr. George Selby
Secretary:	Dr. Peter M. Williamson
Treasurer:	Dr. Bernard S. Gilligan
Members:	Professor David R. Curtis, Dr. Mervyn J. Eadie, Professor J.W. Lance, Professor James G. McLeod

1978 – 1980

President:	Professor J.W. Lance
Secretary:	Dr. M. Anthony
Treasurer:	Dr. B.S. Gilligan
Members:	Professor D R. Curtis, Professor M.J. Eadie, Professor J.G. McLeod, Dr J.P. Rice
In Attendance:	Dr. D. Burke (Hon. Assistant Sec.)

1980 – 1981

President:	Professor J.W. Lance
Secretary:	Dr. M. Anthony
Treasurer:	Dr. B.S. Gilligan
Members:	Professor D.R. Curtis, Dr. A.G. Fisher, Dr. J.P. Rice, Dr. J.C. Walsh
In Attendance:	Dr. D. Burke (Hon. Assistant Sec.)

1981 – 1983

President:	Professor J.G. McLeod
Secretary:	Dr. M. Anthony
Treasurer:	Dr. B.S. Gilligan
Members:	Dr. D.B. Appleton, Dr. A.G. Fisher, Dr. J.P. Rice, Dr. J.C. Walsh
In Attendance:	Dr. G.M. Halmagyi

1983 – 1984

President:	Professor J.G. McLeod
Secretary:	Dr. M. Anthony
Treasurer:	Dr. J.O. King
Members:	Dr. D.B. Appleton, Dr. A.G. Fisher, Dr. J.P. Rice, Dr. J.C. Walsh
In Attendance:	Dr. G.M. Halmagyi

1984 – 1987

President:	Dr. B..S. Gilligan
Secretary:	Dr. R.J. Stark
Treasurer:	Dr. J.O. King
Members:	Dr. D.B. Appleton, Assoc. Professor D. Burke, Dr. A.G. Fisher, Dr. R. Rischbieth

1987 – 1990

President:	Dr. J.P. Rice
Secretary:	Dr. C. Kneebone
Treasurer:	Dr. J. King
Members:	Professor D. Burke, Professor F. Mastaglia (from May 1988), Dr. R. Rischbieth

1990 – 1992

President:	Dr. J. King
Secretary:	Dr. Christine Kilpatrick
Treasurer:	Dr. Geoff Donnan
Members:	Dr. Christopher Kneebone, Professor F. Mastaglia, Dr. John Morris

1992 – 1993

President:	Dr. J. King
Secretary:	Dr. Christine Kilpatrick
Treasurer:	Dr. Geoff Donnan
Members:	A/Prof. Richard Burns, Dr. William Carroll, Dr. Stephen Davis, Dr. John Morris

1993 – 1996

President:	A/Prof. John Morris
Secretary:	Dr. Ivan Lorentz
Treasurer:	Dr. Barry Cant
Members:	A/Prof. Richard Burns, Dr. William Carroll, A/Prof. Stephen Davis, Dr. R. Joffe

Appendix V Memberships of the Council of the Australian Association of Neurologists

1996 – 1998

President:	A/Prof. Richard Burns
Secretary:	A/Prof. John Willoughby
Treasurer:	Dr. Barry Cant (till 1997); Dr. Richard Stark
Members:	Professor Edward Byrne, Dr. William Carroll, Professor Michael Pender, Dr. Catherine Storey

1998 – 1999

President:	Dr. William Carroll
Secretary:	Dr. Allan Kermode
Treasurer:	Dr. Richard Stark
Members:	Professor Geoff Donnan, Professor Malcolm Horne, A/Prof. Christine Kilpatrick, Dr. Catherine Storey

Appendix VI

Dates and Venues of the Annual Scientific Meetings of the Australian Association of Neurologists

Date	City	Venue
25 October 1950	Melbourne	Anatomy Dept, University of Melbourne
10 April 1951	Sydney	Sydney Hospital
16 March 1953	Melbourne	Anatomy Dept, University of Melbourne
12 October 1954	Sydney	Sydney Hospital
15 October 1955	Melbourne	Anatomy Dept, University of Melbourne
18 October 1957	Sydney	Sydney Hospital
4 & 6 June 1958	Sydney	Sydney Hospital
26 May 1959	Adelaide	Medical School
17 October 1959	Canberra	Academy of Sciences
24 May 1960	Melbourne	Anatomy Dept, University of Melbourne
31 May & 1 June 1962	Canberra	John Curtin School of Medical Research
6 & 8 June 1963	Sydney	University of Sydney & Sydney Hospital
27–28 October 1964	Canberra	John Curtin School of Medical Research
11 May 1965	Melbourne	Royal Australasian College of Surgeons Building
16–17 May 1966	Adelaide	University of Adelaide
27–28 May 1968	Sydney	University of Sydney
26–27 May 1969	Brisbane	Physiology Building, University of Queensland
14–15 May 1970	Canberra	Australian National University
26 November 1971	Perth	University of Western Australia
10–11 May 1972	Canberra	John Curtin School of Medical Research
24–25 May 1973	Adelaide	Hotel Australia
1–3 May 1974	Canberra	John Curtin School of Medical Research
16–18 April 1975	Sydney	Sydney Hospital
19–21 February 1976	Auckland	University of Auckland

23–25 March 1977	Melbourne	Royal Australasian College of Surgeons Building
16–18 May 1978	Hobart	University of Tasmania
16 May 1979	Brisbane	University of Queensland
23 May 1980	Canberra	Canberra Rex Hotel
26 May 1981	Adelaide	Gateway Inn
22 April 1982	Sydney	Sebel Town House
3 May 1983	Perth	University of Western Australia
8 May 1984	Melbourne	Hilton Hotel
14 May 1985	Singapore	Meriden Hotel
5 May 1986	Hobart	Wrest Point Hotel
28 April 1987	Broadbeach, Qld	Conrad International Hotel
11 May 1988	Sydney	Menzies Hotel
2 May 1989	Adelaide	Adelaide Convention Centre
1 May 1990	Fremantle	Fremantle Hospital
7 May 1991	Hong Kong	Sheraton Hotel
2 June 1992	Melbourne	World Congress Centre
6 July 1993	Cairns	International Hotel
24 May 1994	Canberra	Hyatt Hotel
25 May 1995	Auckland	Sheraton Hotel
23 May 1996	Broome	Cable Beach Resort
1 May 1997	Sydney	Hilton Hotel
21 May 1998	Brisbane	Sheraton Hotel
25 May 1999	Hobart	Wrest Point Hotel

Appendix VII

Contents of the Journals Published by the Australian Association of Neurologists (1963–1994)

An * following the names of an author, or a number of authors, indicated that they were not members of the Australian Association of Neurologists.

PROCEEDINGS of the AUSTRALIAN ASSOCIATION of NEUROLOGISTS

Volume 1 – 1963

CONTENTS

Immunization against poliomyelitis in Australia	J Billings
By-passing vertebral artery occlusion by extracranial anastomotic channels	J A Game
Progressive multifocal leuko-encephalopathy	G Selby
The stiff man syndrome	J L Allsop
Some aspects of disseminated sclerosis in Queensland	P J Landy
A review of the features and treatment of temporal lobe epilepsy, with special reference to surgery	E Davis
Observations on the prognostic signs following relief of spinal cord compression	A Fisher
Acute encephalopathy in childhood	R McD Anderson
Deep sensibility	A K McIntyre
Cytogenic studies in mental retardation	B Turner
Psychomimetics – a neuropharmacological study	D R Curtis
Dystonic seizures: striatal or extrapyramidal epilepsy	J W Lance
The falling attacks of myoclonus	J W Lance
Visual mechanisms and the electroencephalogram	R Davis
Further observations of the suprapineal arachnoid body	G C T Kenny
The problem of subdural gas after pneumoencephalography	E G Robertson

THE FLOWERING OF A WARATAH

Volume 2 – 1964

CONTENTS

The insigne of the Australian Association of Neurologists	
A comparative evaluation of pneumoencephalography in the diagnosis of cerebral neoplasms with and without increased intracranial pressure	E Graeme Robertson
The scope and limitations of the electro-encephalograph	L Rail
The value of angiography in the investigation of cerebral disease	G Selby
Laboratory investigation of mental retardation	B Turner
Discussion of the reasons for doing lumbar puncture	J A Game
The place of positron-scanning in the diagnosis of intracranial tumours	P A Farrer
Activation of the electroencephalogram	G Preswick
Cortical biopsy in childhood	P Ebeling & R McD Anderson
Experience with cortical biopsy	M Eadie
Total cerebral arteriography	W S C Hare
Anterior mediastinography in the demonstration of the thymus	W S C Hare
Some experiences with cerebral vascular malformation	A Fisher
Hyperkalemic periodic paralysis	J Allsop
Some experiences with myasthenia gravis	A Schwieger
Reading epilepsy	J V Gordon
Serotonin and the nervous system: a review	J W Lance
Cerebral necrosis in newborn babies	H F Bettinger*
Experimental demyelination	G Szego
A contribution to the study of the extrapyramidal system: cerebello-rubral pathway in the cat	R Davis

Volume 3 – 1965

CONTENTS

The nature of dystonia	D Denny-Brown
Inhibitory systems in the cerebellar cortex	J C Eccles, R Llinás & K Sasaki
The nature of the representation of the visual fields in the lateral geniculate nucleus	P O Bishop
Tactile sensory pathways from the face	I Darian-Smith
Agenesis of the corpus callosum-physio-pathological and clinical aspects	M A Jeeves*
An auditory feed-back system, involving the organ of hearing	Jürgen Fex*
The neuromuscular junction with special reference to myasthenia gravis	J I Hubbard
The myasthenic syndromes and their reactions	G Preswick
Perception of vibration	A K McIntyre
The mechanism of reflex irradiation	J W Lance
The effects of barbiturate anaesthesia and a muscle relaxant on an extrapyramidal centre: red nucleus	R Davis
Trigeminal neuralgia – a therapeutic trial of Tegretol	W J G Burke & G Selby
Are anticoagulants of value in disease of the extracranial and intracranial arteries?	P J Landy
Observations upon a predominantly sensory hereditary neuropathy	D C Wallace*
Subacute spongiform encephalopathy	R H Rischbieth
Cerebellar degeneration associated with chronic alcoholism	B Turner & J Allsop

Dietary deficiency and experimental allergic encephalomyelitis   G Szego
The innervation of the Mammalian pineal body   G C T Kenny
Aneurysms of superficial cerebral arteries   R McD Anderson
On chiasmal arachnoiditis with reference to the pneumographic diagnosis   A Fisher
The value of pneumoencephalography in pediatrics   E G Robertson

Volume 4 – 1966

CONTENTS

Posttraumatic epilepsy   A Earl Walker*

Symposium on Muscle

Some historical and clinical notes   J A Game
Duchenne-type dystrophy: selective aspects of diagnosis
and management   G Preswick
McArdle's disease: three cases in an
Australian family   J F Hammelt, P Bale, L S Basser & F C Neale
Autoimmune aspects of myasthenia gravis   S Whittingham & I R Mackay*
Type and incidence of lesions found in a human necropsy
survey of skeletal muscle   B A Kakulas & F L Mastaglia
The reflex effects of muscle vibration   J W Lance
Fine control of human muscular movement   D J Dewhurst*

Theme: Neurology and General Medicine

The association between diffuse sclerosis and Addison's disease   M J Eadie
Hypoglycaemia resulting from insulin secreting tumours
of the pancreas   J M Sutherland, J H Tyrer & M J Eadie
The neurological manifestations of subacute bacterial endocarditis   J L Allsop

Free Papers

Studies in migraine   J W Lance
The early diagnosis of acoustic neurilemmoma   W H Wolfenden
Ultrasound in neurological diagnosis   E Davis
Four cases of subacute necrotizing encephalomyelopathy in childhood
(Leigh's syndrome)   R McD Anderson
Some aspects of the neuron-neuroglia relationship   C P Wendell-Smith
The origin of brain macrophages in the rat   R McD Anderson, S Arumugam & G B Ryan
Some aspects of the development of knowledge of the pineal body   G C T Kenny
Immunological studies in experimental allergic encephalomyelitis
and in multiple sclerosis with special reference to pathogenesis and diagnosis   G Lamoureux*
Virus-like particles in proximity to myelin in a case of progressive
multifocal leukoencephalopathy   J M Papadimitriou, B A Kakulas & M Sadka

Volume 5 – 1968

CONTENTS

Part one

Preface

Symposium I

*The application of recent neurophysiology and neurochemistry
to clinical neurology*

THE FLOWERING OF A WARATAH

Presidential address: John White, Surgeon-General to the colony	E Graeme Robertson
The neuronal mechanism of the cerebellar efferent system	M Ito*
Cerebellar control of alpha motoneurone function	J G McLeod & I P Van Der Meulen
Projection of muscle afferents to the human thalamus	H Narabayashi, A Goto & K Kubota*
Diagnostic value of steady potential recording in man	K Sano, H Miyake & Y Mayanagi*
Picture of cerebral palsy by clinical neurophysiology	H Narabayashi & M Nagahata*
Studies on the mechanisms of spasticity and rigidity following spinal lesions and ischaemia	B Fujimori, M Shimamura, M Kato, T Yamauchi, M Aoki & J Tanji*
Central effect of the secondary endings of muscle stretch receptors in man	R F Mark*
Suppression of the H reflex by peripheral vibration	J W Lance, P D Neilson & C A Tassinari
Spinal pathways for impulses from mechanoreceptors of the hind-limb	A K McIntyre
The relation of the permeability of the vasa nervorum to degeneration and regeneration in peripheral nerves	R Mellick & J B Cavanagh
The neuropathy of Friedreich's ataxia	G Preswick
Lactic acid dehydrogenase (LDH) and creatine phosphokinase (CPK) isozymes in muscle from neuromuscular diseases	S Katsuki, M Nagamine, T Ishirnatsu, M Okumura & I Goto*
Normal and abnormal human muscle in tissue culture	B A Kakulas, J M Papadimitriou, I O Knight & F L Mastaglia
Ultrastructure of skeletal muscle in muscular dystrophy, the carrier state and other human myopathies	J M Papadimitriou & B A Kakulas
Dopamine and dopamine metabolites in Parkinson's disease	A Barbeau*
Recent advances in neuropharmacology of neurological interest	D R Curtis
Studies in serotonin metabolism in migraine	M Anthony, H Hinterberger & J W Lance
Extractum belladonnae as an adjuvant to Luminal in the therapy of epilepsy with a possible explanation in neurophysiological and neurochemical terms	P-G Sic*
Certain problems of enzyme quantitation in brain histochemistry	J H Tyrer, M J Eadie & J R Kukums
Citric acid cycle dehydrogenases and hexose monophosphate dehydrogenases in macroglia	M J Blunt

Symposium II
Mental effects and disorders of behaviour in children

Mental defects and disorders of behaviour in children	Y Fukuyama, I Matsui & M Higurashi*
The contribution of constitutional chromosomal abnormalities to mental deficiency	A G Baikie, O M Garson & S M Weste*
The pseudo-Hurler syndrome	B Turner
Phenylketonuria	D B Pitt*
Clinical and neuropathological observations in phenylketonuria	B A Kakulas, G I L Hamilton & F L Mastaglia
Temporal lobe epilepsy in childhood	R B Aird & D L Crowther*
Intellectual impairment and behaviour disorder in 500 epileptic patients	Tsu-pei Hung*

Intelligence in cerebral palsy	P E Bharucha, S Patel, E P Bharucha & P K. Mulla-Firoze*
Congenital minor anomalies in mentally retarded children	M Arima, K Komiya, K Ono & K Hisada*
Neurological abnormalities in primary hyperammonaemia	I J Hopkins, J F Connelly, B Hocking & T G Maddison
The neuropathology of the 17–18 trisomy syndrome	B A Kakulas, H R Trowell, G I Cullity, K Al Hockey & P L Masters
Prevention of Wilson's disease in asymptomatic patients	M Arima, K Komiya, A Fujisawa & K Matsuoka*
Electron microscopic findings in subacute sclerosing leucoencephalitis	J M Papadimitriou, S S Gubbay, J S Lekias & B A Kakulas

Part two
Symposium III
Neurological cause of blindness

Modes of reaction to central blindness	M Critchley
Metamorphosia of macular origin	D M O'Day
Neural mechanisms concerned in the development of amblyopia ex anopsia	J D Pettigrew, T Nikara & P O Bishop
Cranial arteritis	W H Smith & J Billings
The sella turcica in space-taking lesions	K Thumnoon, U Chaikittisilp & J Edmeads*
The evaluation of presellar expanding lesions causing blindness	A Fisher
Optic neuritis	W J Burke
The diagnosis of visual failure in clinical practice	J J Billings
Benign amaurosis fugax of uncertain cause	M J Eadie
Difficulties in pneumographic demonstration of suprasellar lesions	E G Robertson

Symposium IV
Clinical and physiological lessons from stereotactic procedures

Clinical evaluation of thalamic surgery in cerebral palsy	H Narabayashi*
Clinical and physiological data obtained in stereotaxic surgery of the hypothalamus	K Sano, M Ogashiwa & H Sekino*
Stereotaxic amygdalotomy	V Balasubramaniam & B Ramanurthi*
Successful operations in Parkinson's disease: observations on pathological findings	M C Smith*
The adverse effect of akinesia on the success of stereotactic surgery in Parkinson's disease	R S Schwab*
Cerebral atrophy in parkinsonism	G Selby
Cryosurgical thalamotomy	R G Robinson
Analysis of cogwheel rigidity	H Narabayashi*
Stereotaxic capsulotomy for epilepsy	S Kalyanaraman & B Ramanurthi*
A study of the fibre connections in the human substantia nigra	S Masuda*

Symposium V
Neurological diseases of regional interest

Kuru	R W Hornabrook

The central nervous system in kuru	R McD Anderson
A transmission model for kuru	J D Mathews*
Recent studies of amyotrophic lateral sclerosis and Parkinsonism-dementia on Guam	J A Brody & K Chen*
Motor neuron disease in the Kii peninsula, Japan	Y Yase, N Matsumoto, F Yoshimasu, Y Handa & T Kumamoto*
Clinical features of demyelinating disease in Japan	Y Kuroiwa*
Multiple sclerosis in Australia	M McCall, T Le Gay Brereton, A Dawson, K S Millingen, J M Sutherland, J H Tyrer, M J Eadie & E D Acheson
Acute necrotizing inclusion encephalitis in Taiwan	W-S Lin*
Cerebral paragonimiasis	J Y Shim & C S Park*
Neurological sequelae of anti-rabic inoculation	A Vejjajiva*
Neurological diseases in Korea	H K Lee & C S Park*
Neurological pattern in Singapore	A L Gwee*
A clinical study of cerebrovascular diseases in Djakarta	L Toen-Kiong & M Mardjono*
Carbon monoxide poisoning in Korea	M W Kim & C S Park*
Absorption studies in neurological disorders	B D Pimparker, E P Bharucha & V P Mondlkar*

Symposium VI

Malignancy and the nervous system

Peripheral neuropathy and carcinoma	R A Henson & H Urich*
Aspects of chronic polyneuropathy associated with myeloma	J B Morley & A C Schwieger
Some comments on surgical and non-surgical adjuncts to the treatment of intracranial tumours	E B Boldrey*
Brain perfusion for tumour—the effect of nitrogen mustard on brain adenosine triphosphate	B Woodhall & A P Sanders*
A malignancy involving the cranial nerves with a possible geographic distribution	M Mardono, S Supeno & S Markham*
Myelopathy following radiotherapy of nasopharyngeal carcinoma	T Hung*
Clinical study on metastatic meningeal carcinomatosis	K Takeuchi & Y Yahagi*
Neurologic manifestations in metastatic choriocarcinoma	T E Tupasi, E A de Veyra Jr, M C Perez & M R Agustines*
Central nervous system infiltration in acute childhood leukaemia	J A Corrie, J H Colebatch, M S Rice & H Ekert*

Part three

Free Papers

Further observations on Tourette's syndrome	K B Corbin, J R Feild, N P Goldstein & D W Klass*
Neurological diagnosis of ruptured cervical discs	R M Stuck*
Specific neural stimulation for inhibition of pain	W H Sweet*
The post-traumatic syndrome in closed head injuries accident neurosis	P J Landy
Cerebrospinal pressure mechanisms and their clinical applications	R Gye & J Pennybacker*
Preliminary experience with ^{99m}Tc cerebral scanning	J B Morley

Appendix VII Contents of the Journals

Displacement of the superior cerebellar artery in the diagnosis of the cerebello-pontine angle tumour	M Sato, K Yoda & M Tsuru*
Electroencephalography of cerebral paragonimiasis	C S Park*
Complications of tuberculous meningitis	C Suwanwela*
Computer analysis of cortical evoked potentials – application to agnostic syndrome study	Y Kuroiwa, M Kato & H Umezaki*
Staining tissues of central nervous system with lac dye	R Wanissorn*
Regional inhibition of brain monoamine oxidase measured by microscopic photometry	M J Eadie, J H Tyrer & J R Kukums
Treatment of congenital atlanto-axial disclocation	G Sinh & S K Pandya*
Haematomyelia during pregnancy: pathogenic discussion	B Q Huong, L D Hue & N Q Khanh (with the cooperation of N L Vien, N H Can, Lichtenberger & D H Anh)*
The function of the perineurium and its relation to the flow phenomenon within the endoneurial spaces	R Mellick & J B Cavanagh
Cranial polyneuritis – a distinct clinical entity	G S Ratnavale
Femoral neuropathy with abdominal pain	M Kase & E Hiyamuta*
The natural history of human muscle diseases studied by means of serial biopsy	F L Mastaglia & B A Kakulas
The detection of female carriers of pseudohypertrophic muscular dystrophy	B A Kakulas, J O Knight, S S Gubbay & F L Mastaglia
Muscle lesions associated with bony injuries	N C Anastas & B A Kakulas
Nervous system involvement in progressive muscular dystrophy	K Nakao, S Kito, T Muro, M Tomonaga & T Mozai*
The myocardinal lesions in the Rottnest quokka with nutritional myopathy	B A Kakulas, C G Owen, J M Papadimitriou & D T Durack
Retrobulbar neuritis in the state of South Australia	R H C Rischbieth
Febrile convulsions: a clinical and encephalographic study	M P Bhagat, N M Katie & A D Desai*
Hereditary kinaesthetic reflex epilepsy	Y Fukuyama & R Okada*
Application of electro-encephalographic monitoring and intra-carotid therapy in reiterative focal motor seizures	P F Bladin
A particular form of muscular inhibition in epilepsy: the related epileptic silent period (R.E.S.P.)	C A Tassinari, H Regis & H Gastaut*
Gliomas and epilepsy	J B Morley
Spinal vascular malformations and their treatment	R N Chatterlee & R N Roy*
An angiographic analysis of the cheiro-oral syndrome	G W Bruyn & J C Gathier*
Vascular changes in tuberculous meningitis – an arteriographic study in 33 patients	N H Wadia & B S Singhal*
Vascular disease with cerebral effects in young identical twins	J D Bergin
The effect of serotonin on cranial vessels and its significance in migraine	J W Lance & M Anthony
Migraine and methysergide – an appraisal	G W Bruyn & J C Gathier*
Application of the averaged photopalpebral reflex in clinical neurology	K Inanaga*

Volume 6 – 1969

CONTENTS

Admiral Lord Nelson's neurological illnesses	W Gooddy*
Introduction to the problems of dementia	W Gooddy*
Dementia in the adult due to occult hydrocephalus	K Lethlean & R Gye
Progressive dementia in childhood due to cerebral lipidosis	B S Gilligan
On meningioma presenting with dementia	A Fisher
Post-traumatic dementia	N Parker*
The major and minor hemispheres of the human brain	W Gooddy*
Outside time and inside time	W Gooddy*
Classification and treatment of myoclonus	J W Lance
Electro-physiological observations in a patient with segmental myoclonus	M J Eadie
Paroxysmal choreo-athetosis	C A Tassinari & R D Fine
Facial myokymia	J I Balla
Post-vaccinial sensory polyneuropathy with myoclonus	I T Lorentz & J G McLeod
The natural history of Duchenne muscular dystrophy – an ultrastructural study	J M Papadimitriou, F L Mastaglia & B A Kakulas
Regeneration in Duchenne muscular dystrophy – a histological electron-microscopic and histochemical study	F J Mastaglia, J M Papadimitriou & B A Kakulas
Restricted forms of muscular dystrophy: a study of 11 cases	F J Mastaglia, J M Papadimitriou & B A Kakulas
A correlative clinico-pathological study of spinal cord injury	B A Kakulas & G M Bedbrook
The blood vessel permeability of peripheral nerve during primary demyelination and the effect of A.C.T.H. therapy on the permeability and on the functional disability	R Mellick
A case of cerebral cysticercosis	J B Morley & K Langlord
The additional role of the scan in the diagnosis of cerebral tumours	J B Morley & R G Sephton
Experimental allergic encephalomyelitis, experimental allergic neuritis and multiple sclerosis: an electromyographic study	T A McPherson, Z S Kiss, G Robson, R L G Kirsner & D J Dewhurst*

Volume 7 – 1970

CONTENTS

Dr. Brown-Séquard in space and time	W Gooddy*
Aspects of diphenylhydantoin metabolism	M J Eadie, J H Tyrer & W D Hooper
Investigation of an outbreak of anticonvulsant intoxication	J H Tyrer, M J Eadie & J M Sutherland
Movement induced epilepsy: three case reports and comparison with a case of hemiballismus	J B Morley
Use of the ketogenic diet in epilepsy in childhood	I J Hopkins & B C Lynch
A comparative trial of serotonin antagonists in the management of migraine	J W Lance & M Anthony
A clinical trial of an antiserotonin drug, bc–105, in the prophylaxis of migraine	G Selby

Monoamine oxidase inhibitors in the control of migraine	M Anthony & J W Lance
A critical review of the treatment of migrainous neuralgia	P Mann, J M Sutherland & M J Eadie
Central synaptic transmitters	D R Curtis
The effect of germine diacetate on neuro-muscular transmission	S F Jones, J Brennan & J G McLeod
Optic neuritis and its relationship to disseminated sclerosis	P J Landy & G D Ohlrich
Cryptococcal meningitis	J L Allsop, J G McLeod & R S Gye
Alcoholic neuropathy	J C Walsh & J G McLeod
The carrier problem in progressive muscular dystrophy	J O Knight & B A Kakulas
Electrophysiological and sural nerve biopsy studies in patients with Friedreich's ataxia and Charcot-Marie-Tooth disease	J G McLeod
The mechanism of the suppression of the monosynaptic reflex by vibration	J D Gillies, J W Lance & C A Tassinari
A neurological appraisal of autistic children: results of a Western Australian survey	S S Gubbay, M Lobascher & P Kingerlee
Differing cerebral scan characteristics of different pathological lesions	J B Morley, R G Sephton, L W Steven, J T Andrews & S N Cornell
The necropsy demonstration of cerebral aneurysms by intra-arterial injection	R Rodda

Volume 8 – 1971

CONTENTS

Memory	A K McIntyre
Kuru and Creutzfeld-Jakob disease: clinical and aetiological aspects	M Alpers & L Rail
Lymphocytic studies in kuru patients	M J Simons, M G Fitzgerald & M P Alpers
Myasthenia gravis and horror autotoxicus	E Davis
Non-progressive sensory neuropathy	R E Vlietstra & M Pollock*
Histochemical and biochemical studies in pseudohyperparathyroidism	M Pollock & J G Sneyd*
Further observations on an outbreak of diphenylhydantoin intoxication	J H Tyrer, M J Eadie & W D Hooper
Whole blood histamine and plasma serotonin in cluster headache	M Anthony & J W Lance
The influence of hormonal change upon migraine in women	B W Somerville
Abnormal prothrombin times in cerebrovascular disease	J B Morley, M Korman & W G Parkin
Oxidative enzyme activity in single neurones in relation to selective vulnerability to ischaemia	M J Eadie, J H Tyrer & J R Kukums
Clinical and pathological aspects of central nervous system involvement in the haemolytic uraemic syndrome	J C Rooney, R McD Anderson & I J Hopkins
The use of immunosuppressive agents in peripheral nerve homograft surgery: an experimental study	J R Pollard, J G McLeod & R S Gye

In vitro destruction of human foetal muscle cultures by peripheral blood lymphocytes from patients with polymyositis and lupus erythematosus — B A Kakulas, G H Shute & J S Lekias

Thrombosis of the internal carotid artery after closed head injury — F L Mastaglia, S Savas, B A Kakulas & J S Lekias

The vascular lesions associated with cerebellar infarcts — R Rodda

Neuropathy associated with lymphoma — J C Walsh

Ultrastructural changes in the peripheral nerves in experimental dying-back polyneuropathies — J W Prineas

Onion bulb formations in chronic polyneuropathies — J G McLeod, J W Prineas & J C Walsh

An objective assessment of a gamma aminobutyric acid derivative in the control of spasticity — D Burke, J D Gillies & J W Lance

An electromyographic analysis of the clasp-knife phenomenon — D Burke, J D Gillies & J W Lance

The supraspinal control of the tonic vibration reflex — J D Gillies, D Burke & J W Lance

Different cerebral scan characteristics of different cerebral pathologies: double isotope scanning — J B Morley & R G Sephton

Volume 9 – 1973

CONTENTS

Polymyositis: new light on pathogenesis and treatment — J N Walton*

The nature of syringomyelia disease or syndrome? — P Hudgson & J B Foster

Chronic neuropathies of infancy and childhood — J G McLeod & J W Prineas

Infantile polymyoclonia — J I Manson

Subacute myelo-optico-neuropathy (SMON) – neurotoxicity of clioquinols — G Selby

Facial thermography in cerebral vascular insufficiency and migraine — J W Lance, M Anthony & B Somerville

A-mode echoencephalography (experience with 1300 midline echos) — J T Holland & G Kossoff

Familial amyotrophic lateral sclerosis — W H Wolfenden, A F Calvert, E Hirst, W Evans & J G McLeod

Tuberose sclerosis in childhood — J I Manson

Hyperkalaemic periodic paralysis associated with Addison's disease — A C Schwieger

Periodic megaphagia and hypersomnia – an example of the Kleine-Levin syndrome in an adolescent girl — B S Gilligan

Cerebrovascular 'moyamoya' disease — D J O'Sullivan

Limb kinetic apraxia (including case report) — J Vernea

Dysaesthesia-dyskinesia: a syndrome of painful legs and moving toes — J W Lance & C Andrews

Spinal cord cyst – case report — V E Edwards & G Merry

A case of cauda equina tumour presenting with stupor and papilloedema — W J Burke

Geomedical aspects of neurological cryptococcosis — J M Sutherland & V E Edwards

Pathological reflexes in presenile dementia – preliminary report — J Vernea

Subacute spongiform encephalopathy – a clinical and pathological study with attention to liver involvement — P M Williamson, W H Payne, G Selby & E Davis

The treatment of self-induced photic epilepsy	L R Rail
Spasmodic torticollis	E Davis
Results of surgical treatment of the carpal tunnel syndrome	B Mendelson & J Balla
Studies on cerebral circulation in man indicating presence of neurogenic control	J L Corbett & B H Eidelman
Bicuculline, GABA and central inhibition	D R Curtis
Reconsideration of the role of serotonin in subarachnoid haemorrhage	K M A Welch, K Hashi & J S Meyer*
The explanation of the 1968 Australian outbreak of diphenylhydantoin intoxication	F Bochner, W Hooper, J Tyrer & M Eadie
Clinical implications of certain aspects of diphenylhydantoin metabolism	F Bochner, W Hooper, J Tyrer & M Eadie
Incidence of hypertensive intracerebral haemorrhage in Thailand: an autopsy study of sixty-seven cases	P Tangchai*
Astrocytoma in Thailand: a study of 119 cases	S Shuangshoti & R Panyathanya*
Acromegaly: assessment and selection for treatment	L Lazarus*
Radiology of the pituitary	J Bull*
Pneumographic demonstration of suprasellar tumours	E G Robertson
Cervical spondylotic myelopathy: the use of one-radiography to select certain cases for surgery	K Bleasel, T J Connelley & N G Dan*
Timing of surgery for leaking cerebral aneurysms: clinical, radiological and radio-isotopic considerations	T A R Dinning*
Computer-assisted radioisotope studies with the scintillation camera in cerebrovascular disease	R J O'Reilly, P M Ronai & R E M Cooper*

Volume 10 – 1973

CONTENTS

Central nervous system dysfunction with open heart operations	I M Williarns
Carotid sinus syncope	J L Allsop
Pathologic changes in the greater splanchnic nerve of subjects with diabetic peripheral neuropathy	C Y Huang & J C Walsh
A standardized test battery for the assessment of clumsy children	S S Gubbay
Ocular motor apraxia in childhood	J I Manson
Familial spastic paraplegia	R H Rischbieth
Progressive supranuclear palsy (the Steele – Richardson – Olszewski syndrome): clinical and electrophysiological observations in eleven cases	F L Mastaglia, K Grainger, F Kee, M Sadka & R Lefroy
Huntington's chorea – the rigid form (Westphal variant) treated with L-dopa: a case report	P A Low & J L Allsop
Central pontine myelinolysis	M G Darke & B A Kakulas
Diphenylhydantoin dosage	M J Eadie, J H Tyrer & W D Hooper
Clonazepam – a clinical study of its effectiveness as an anticonvulsant	V E Edwards & M J Eadie
Clonazepam in the treatment of epilepsy	C Y Huang, J G McLeod, D Sampson & W J Hensley

An experimental animal model for the effect of ketogenic diet on epilepsy	D B Appleton & D C De Vivo
The pathogenesis of trigeminal neuralgia	G Selby
Plasma free fatty acid changes in migraine	M Anthony
A serial section study for Charcot-Bouchard aneurysms in hind-brain	G Caravella, P F Jacobsen & B A Kakulas
The effect of humoral agents on the cranial circulation of the monkey	P J Spira, K M A Welch & J W Lance
A radioimmunoassay for creatine kinase	G A Nicholson & W J O'Sullivan
Experimental autonomic neuropathy	E J Post & J G McLeod
Electromyographic studies of the orbicularis oculi reflex	J Vernea & T Horvath
Activity of motor neurones during isometric contraction	H Kranz & R von der Heydt
Unit analysis of the F wave	J L Veale & N D Hewson
Segmental reflex changes in acute and chronic spinal cats	J Hancock, L Knowles & D Gillies

Obituary – Gerald Moss

Volume 11 – 1974

CONTENTS

Subarachnoid haemorrhage in children	D B Appleton, P J Smith & W J S Earwaker
Long segment stenotic lesions of cervical arteries in cerebrovascular disease	P F Bladin
Cardio-vascular responses to prolonged head-up tilting in tetraplegic man	J L Corbett
Cardio-vascular responses to infused noradrenaline in tetraplegic man	J L Corbett
Cortical blindness with anosognosia subsequent simultaneous agnosia and persistent gross recent memory defect	J B Morley & F N Cox
Neuro-ophthalmic deterioration after burns	Isla M Williams
Headaches occurring during sexual intercourse	J W Lance
Landry-Guillain-Barré syndrome: a clinical and electrophysiological follow-up study	J C Walsh, J G McLeod, J W Prineas & J D Pollard
Colchicine and the peripheral nerve	R Mellick, R Kirkby, A Tait Smith & G Ratnavale
Demyelination in the central nervous system of the cat studied by single fibre isolation	G D Ohlrich & W I McDonald
Sensory function of the median nerve: preliminary studies using micro electrode techniques in man	D Burke, N F Shuse & A K Lethlean
Hypothesis: a biological model of schizophrenia	V I Karlov
The Aicardi syndrome	G Wise & R Ouvrier
Pituitary fossa demineralization in normal subjects	L A Cala, J Black & D W K Collins
Neurophysiologlcal mechanism of acupuncture analgesia	J G McLeod
Subacute sclerosing panencephalitis: a study of 25 patients	P G Procopis
Giant axonal neuropathy – a third case	R A Ouvrier, J Prineas, J C Walsh, R D K Reye & J G McLeod
Genetic counselling in neuromuscular diseases in Western Australia	P V Hurse & B A Kakulas
A new myopathy with type II muscle fibre hypoplasia	Y Matsuoka, S S Gubbay & B A Kakulas

A neurophysiological analysis of paramyotonia congenita	D Burke, N F Skuse & A K Lethlean
Neurological features in Freon freakout	J R Moon & P F Bladin
Chuckling and glugging seizures at night – Sylvian spike epilepsy	P F Bladin & G Papworth
Selective vulnerability of the hippocampus to hypoxia; cytophotometric studies of enzyme activity in single neurones	J E Penny, J R Kukums, J H Tyrer & M J Eadie
Palatal myoclonus and associated movements	F L Mastaglia, K M R Grainger & B A Kakulas
Preliminary observations on the clinical pharmacology of carbamazepine ('Tegretol')	W D Hooper, D K Dubetz, M J Eadie & J H Tyrer
Side effects of clonazepam therapy	V E Edwards
Progressive myoclonic epilepsy. The response to sodium di-n-propylacetate	E B Tomlinson
Visual hallucinations as a symptom of right parieto-occipital lesions	J W Lance, B Cooper & J Misbach
Hypercalcaemia and epilepsy	I T Lorentz
Partial status epilepticus with speech arrest	J J Vernea
Epilepsy and the frontal lobe	P F Bladin & J Woodward
Social problems confronting a person with epilepsy in modern society	V E Edwards
Temporal lobectomy for epilepsy – a follow-up	E Davis
Obituary – Brian Turner	

Volume 12 – 1975

CONTENTS

The Australian Association of Neurologists – a review of twenty-five years	J Game
Geniculate hemianopias: incongruous visual defects from partial involvement of the lateral geniculate nucleus	W F Hoyt*
Certain neuro-ophthalmological aspects of multiple sclerosis	J M Sutherland
A family with Charcot-Marie-Tooth disease and Leber's optic atrophy	J G McLeod, P A Low & J A Morgan
Superior oblique myokymia	K M R Grainger & S S Gubbay
The low intracranial pressure syndrome	J J Billings, E J Gilford & J K Henderson
Mechanism in cerebral lesions in trauma to high cervical portion of the vertebral artery – rotation injury	P F Bladin & J Merory
Amine turnover in migraine	M Anthony & H Hinterberger
The headaches of phaeocytochroma	J W Lance & H Hinterberger
Sodium valproate in the management of intractable epilepsy: comparison with clonazepam	J W Lance & M Anthony
Fluctuations of plasma phenytoin levels on single dose and twice daily dose regimes	F J E Vadja, J Merory & P F Bladin
Fibre function and perception during cutaneous nerve block	R A Mackenzie, D Burke, N F Skuse & A K Lethlean
Muscular dystrophy in young girls	B A Kakulas, P E Cullity & P Maguire

Autonomic disturbances produced by lung cancer: a report of two unusual cases	J C Walsh, P A Low & J L Allsop
Enteric coated levo-dopa in clinical practice	E P Hicks & M W O'Halloran
Frontal agraphia (including a case report)	J J Vernea & J Merory
The surgical management of extracranial cerebrovascular occlusive disease: a review of 200 consecutive surgical cases	D A Horton, R Fine & R G Hicks
Reversible cortiocospinal abnormality in the alcoholic	C Y Huang, G A Broe & P G Procopis
Interactions between anticonvulsants	C M Lander, M J Eadie & J H Tyrer
Remyelination after transient compression of the spinal cord	B M Harrison, R F Gledhill & W I McDonald
The bioavailability of carbamazepine	L M Cotter, G Smith, W D Hooper, J H Tyrer and M J Eadie
Tay Sachs disease in a child and management of a subsequent pregnancy	D B Appleton, T J Gaffney, H McGeary & N J Nicolaides
The action of thalidomide on the peripheral nervous system of the embryo	J McCredie
Ocular complications of varicella	P G Procopis
Congenital deficiency of horizontal gaze	P G Procopis
The autonomic nervous system in alcoholic and diabetic neuropathy	P A Low, J C Walsh, C Y Huang & J G McLeod
A case of spontaneously resolving 'papilloedema'	G Selby & G C Hipwell
Neuromyelitis optica following infectious mononucleosis	P M Williamson
Periodic alternating nystagmus	L de Silva, B P Cooper & J G McLeod
Opsoclonus with myoclonus	J T Holland
The ocular myasthenia syndrome	W G Burke
Familial cerebellar ataxia with sex-linked recessive inheritance	P J Spira & J W Lance
Microembolism and the visual system. Part II	I M Williams, N C R Merrillees & P M Robinson
The value of the brain scan and cerebral arteriogram in the Sturge-Weber syndrome	B McCaughan, R A Ouvrier, K de Silva & A McLaughin
The chiasmal enigma	B Hughes*
Obituary – Dr Oliver Latham	

Volume 13 – 1976

CONTENTS

Obituaries

    E Graeme Robertson

    Henry Miller

    Bryan Cooper

Pattern visual evoked potentials in the diagnosis of multiple sclerosis and other disorders	A L Hume & B R Cant
Evoked potential studies in neurological disorders	F L Mastaglia, J L Black & D W K Collins
Computerized axial tomography for intracranial diagnosis	L A Cala
Hereditary hypertrophic neuropathy in the trembler mouse: electrophysiological studies	P A Low & J G McLeod

Computerized axial tomography findings in a group of patients with migrainous headaches	L A Cala & F L Mastaglia
Neurophysiological aspects of peripheral neuropathies	R A MacKenzie, N F Skuse & A K Lethlean
Three cases of post traumatic vascular headache treated by surgery	J T Holland
The influence of previous stereotactic thalamotomy on l-DOPA therapy in Parkinson's disease	G Selby
A unique case of derangement of vitamin B 12 metabolism	M Anthony & A C McLeay
Epilepsy and driving	K S Millingen
Some aspects of tuberculous meningitis in Surabaya	B Chandra*
An animal model for the study of drugs in the central nervous system	G J G Parry
The effects of phenobarbitone dose on plasma phenobarbitone levels in epileptic patients	M J Eadie, C M Lander, W D Hooper & J H Tyrer
On the visual disturbances associated with massive basal aneurysms	A Fisher & R L Cooper
Progressive facial herniatrophy (Parry-Romberg syndrome)	R H C Rischbieth
Electrophysiological and pathological studies in spinocerebellar degenerations	J G McLeod & J A Morgan
The use of clonazepam in the treatment of tic douloureux (a preliminary report)	B Chandra*
Serial nerve conduction studies in patients with maturity onset diabetes mellitus	G Danta
Measurement of cerebrospinal fluid IgG in the diagnosis of multiple sclerosis	E W Willoughby
Histamine-receptor blockade with cimetidine in the monkey cranial circulation	G D A Lord, E J Mylecharane, J W Duckworth & J W Lance
Performance changes during recovery from closed head injury	D Gronwall*
The continual administration of neostigmine and the neuromuscular junction	J D Gillies & J Allen

Volume 14 – 1977

CONTENTS

Transient ischaemic attacks	J P Whisnant
Post-irradiation extracranial cerebrovascular disease	P F Bladin & J Royle
Tremor in alcoholic brain disease	S Bajada & A Fisher
A case of dacrystic epilepsy	C Y Huang & G A Broe
An investigation into reading epilepsy	G Danta, P J Dowling & S R Hammond
The late form of pure familial spastic paraplegia	J Vernea & G R Symington
Motor neuron disease in Australia (State of New South Wales)	J W Lance, J Enis & J W Duckworth
The carpal tunnel syndrome: a clinical and electrophysiological study in 250 patients	S C Loong
Ocular motor involvement in post-infective polyneuropathy	W M Carroll & F L Mastaglia
Syndrome of ophthalmoplegia, ataxia and areflexia	C E Storey, G Selby & P M Williamson
The H reflex in the forearm muscles in normal subjects and patients with mild pyramidal syndrome	J Vernea

THE FLOWERING OF A WARATAH

Intestinal giardiarsis, steatorrhoea and peripheral nerve dysfunction	M L Bassett, T A Cook & G Danta
Intermittent hydrocephalus due to cysts of the septum pellucidum: a study of three cases	S S Gubbay, R Vaughan & J S Lekias
Brachiocephaliac afteritis in a young female (Takayasu's disease)	B S Gilligan
A case of Creutzfeldt-Jakob disease	R A Rodda
Saccadic velocities in multiple sclerosis and myasthenia gravis	F L Mastaglia, J L Black & D W K Collins
Diagnostic significance of autoantibodies and HLA in myasthenia gravis and multiple sclerosis	R L Dawkins, F L Mastaglia & P Kay
Electrophysiological and immunological studies in optic neuritis	R Garrick, J C Walsh & J G McLeod
Relapsing allergic neuritis	J D Pollard & G Selby
Clinical electrophysiological and pathological features of three cases of cerebromacular degeneration in childhood	J I Manson, R F Carter, M E Haynes & C G Keith
Peroneal muscular atrophy with autosomal dominant inheritance	J G McLeod & P A Low
Acupuncture for chronic back pain: patients and methods	G Mendelson, H Kranz, M A Kidson, S T Loh, D F Scott & T S Sehvood
Observations on vascular neuropathies	H Urich
Pharmacokinetics of drugs used for petit mal 'absence' epilepsy	M J Eadie, J H Tyrer, G A Smith & L McKauge
Factors influencing plasma carbamazepine concentrations	C M Lander, M J Eadie & J H Tyrer
Phenobarbitone dosage in the neonate – preliminary communication	R A Ouvrier & R Goldsmith
Therapeutic problems related to tonic status epilepticus	P F Bladin, F J Vajda & G R Symington
Plasma sodium valproate levels and clinical response in epilepsy	M Anthony, H Hinterberger & J W Lance
Spinal and cortical evoked potentials in multiple sclerosis	R Garrick & J G McLeod
Electrophysiological and computerised tomography findings in multiple sclerosis: a comparative study	F L Mastaglia, J L Black, L A Cala & D W K Collins
Computerised tomography findings in multiple sclerosis and Schilder's disease	L A Cala & F L Mastaglia
Computerised tomography of the cranium in patients with epilepsy: a preliminary report	L A Cala, F L Mastaglia & T L Woodings
Parietal lobe atrophy: a report on two patients	J C Walsh & J L Allsop
Distal chronic spinal muscular atrophy involving the hands	D J O'Sullivan & J G McLeod
Myosins in murine muscular dystrophy	R B Fitzsimons, J F Y Hob & J G McLeod
A syndrome of myopathy and polycythaemia in a young man	B A Kakulas
Effects of neostigmine and pyridostigmine at the neuromuscular junction	J D Gillies & J Allen

Appendix VII Contents of the Journals

Volume 15 – 1978

CONTENTS

The E Graeme Robertson Memorial Lecture 1978:	
Graeme Robertson and the golden age of neurology	R Hooper
Central pain mechanisms	A W Duggan
A review of some aspects of the pharmacology of levodopa	J G L Morris
The pharmacology of anticonvulsant drugs	M J Eadie
A case of spinal cysticercosis	I T Lorentz
Parasitic diseases of the nervous system in Thailand	A Vejjajiva
Vertebral metastases and spinal cord compression	B A Kakulas, C G Harper, K Shibasaki & G M Bedbrook
Wernicke-Korsakov syndrome lesions in coronial necropsies	R Rodda, R Cummings & K S Millingen
Association of central nervous system sarcoma with familial polyposis coli	P M Williamson & K V Smith
Preliminary observations on the pharmacokinetics of methylphenobarbitone	M J Eadie, F Bochner, W D Hooper & J H Tyrer
Sodium valproate: dose-plasma level relationships and interdose fluctuations	F J E Vajda, G W Mihaly, J L Miles, P M Morris & P F Bladin
A comparison of the absorption of phenobarbitone given via the oral and the intramuscular route	J K Graham
Posterior fossa arachnoid cysts: two case reports	G H Purdie & R H C Rischbieth
The causalgia syndrome treated with regional intravenous guanethidine	J T Holland
Detection of experimental carotid ulceration by radionucleotide labelled particles	G A Donnan, W J McKay, D P Thomas & P F Bladin
Acupuncture analgesia for chronic low back pain	G Mendelson, M A Kidson, S T Loh, D F Scott, T S Selwood & H Kranz
Visuo-motor skill and visual perception in left and right handed children of superior intelligence	R Mellick, I Klajic, H Grahame & B Higgins
Individual free fatty acids and migraine	M Anthony
Autonomic dysfunction in the Landry-Guillain-Barre syndrome	R R Tuck & J G McLeod
Electromyographic study of polysynaptic responses from muscles not supplied by the stimulated nerve: preliminary report	J Vernea
Memory disorder in vertebrobasilar disease	G A Donnan, K W Walsh & P F Bladin
Delayed radiation-induced damage to the brachial plexus	R Burns
An evaluation of bromocriptine in the treatment of Parkinson's disease	R A MacKenzie & J W Lance
Neurological features of polyarteritis nodosa	G L Walker
Primary empty sella syndrome and benign intracranial hypertension	S Davis, B Tress & J King
Occipital neuralgia	S R Hammond & G Danta
Some specific neurological complications of acute lymphocytic leukaemia of childhood	D B Appleton, A F Isles & J R Tieman

THE FLOWERING OF A WARATAH

The contribution of evoked potentials in the functional assessment
of the somatosensory pathway   F L Mastaglia, J L Black, R Edis & D W K Collins

Patterns of response to levodopa in Parkinson's disease   F J E Vajda, G A Donnan & P F Bladin

Volume 16 – 1979

CONTENTS

The E Graeme Robertson Memorial Lecture 1979:
    I. Aspects of cuprogenic disorder in Wilson's Disease in India   D K Dastur & D K Manghani

    II. Pathology and pathogenesis of chronic myelopathy in atlanto-axial dislocation, with operative or postoperative haematomyelia or other cord complications   D K Dastur

Thoracic outlet syndrome secondary to childhood poliomyelitis   N W Knuckey & S S Gubbay

A retrospective study of carotid endarterectomy   G D Ohlrich & J R Kukums

The stroke syndrome of long intraluminal clots with incomplete vessel obstruction   G A Donnan & P F Bladin

Neuromyotonia in the spinal form of Charcot-Marie-Tooth Disease   J W Lance, D Burke & J Pollard

Contribution of single motor units to the surface electromyogram   J L Veale & W J Russell

Brain infarction in young men   R J Burns, P C Blumbergs & M A Sage

The application of prolonged EEG telemetry and videotape recording to the study of seizures and related disorders   V Vignaendra, J Walsh & S Burrows

The epoxide of carbamazepine   L McKauge, J H Tyrer & M J Eadie

The neurological aspects of atrial myxoma   R Beran & E P Hicks

Cerebellar malformations: some pathogenetic considerations   H Urich

Adrenoleucodystrophy: a study of four patients   P G Procopis & R A Ouvrier

Primary lymphoma of the central nervous system – a case report   R A Mackenzie & S C Braye

Hypoglycaemia secondary to pancreatic islet cell adenoma   G L Coffey, D J O'Sullivan & W J Burke

Idiopathic communicating hydrocephalus: the prognostic significance of ventricular size after shunting   K S Millingen

Factors likely to affect the development of multiple sclerosis in patients presenting with optic neuritis in a tropical and subtropical area   P J Landy, M Innis & R Boyle

Antipyrine half-life as a measure of hepatic enzyme induction: clinical applications in a chronic epileptic population   E Byrne, A W Harman, D B Frewin & J F Hallpike

Urticaria pigmentosa – change in conscious state associated with rise in plasma histamine levels   G A Donnan & B J Jarrott

Oscillations in performance in levodopa-treated Parkinsonians: treatment with bromocriptine and 'Deprenyl'   C M Lander, A Lees & G Stern

Ischaemic optic neuropathy   J King

Clinical application of the patterned light visual evoked response (a two-year experience at the Adelaide Children's Hospital)   J I Manson, P F Weston & R G Beran

Observations on voluntary nystagmus	A Fisher, H Davies & S Wallis
Motor fibre refractory period and motor conduction velocity range	J Vernea
Trimethadione embryopathy: case report with review of the literature	R H Rischbieth
Two-dimensional echo encephalography in paediatric neurology	J I Manson, P F Weston & R Gent
Carbamazepine in two pregnancies	E P Hicks
Lepromatous leprosy as a model of schwann cell pathology and lysosomal activity	D K Daslur & G L Porwal*
The neuropathology of a case of Pick's disease	R A Rodda
Idiopathic scoliosis, Scheurmann's disease and myopathy: two case reports	R B Fitzsimons
Computerised tomography in the leucodystrophies	P G Procopis
Familial trigeminal and glossopharyngeal neuralgia	N W Knuckey & S S Gubbay
Lipoma of the cauda equina: case report and review of the literature	R H C Rischbieth
Some aspects of the clinical use of clonazepam in refractory epilepsy	C M Lander, G A Donnan, P F Bladin & F J E Vajda

Volume 17 – 1980

CONTENTS

The E Graeme Robertson Memorial Lecture 1980:

Myasthenia gravis: a clinical review	W J Burke
Music and neurology	J B Morley
A W Campbell: Australia's first neurologist	M J Eadie
Innovation in electroencephalography	F Ying-K'un, H Ching-Chin & K Tan-Hua*
Clinico-electroencephalographic studies in multiple sclerosis	F Ying-K'un
Patient perspectives of epilepsy	R G Beran & T Read
The clearance of anticonvulsant drugs in pregnancy	C M Lander, I Livingstone, J H Tyrer & M J Eadie
The effects of anticonvulsants on memory function in epileptic patients: preliminary findings	A T Butlin, L Wolfendale & G Danta
Method of source derivation for the EEG	L S Basser
Spontaneous dissecting aneurysms of the cervical internal carotid artery	J P Rice
Barlow's syndrome and cerebral emboli: a common cause of stroke in young patients?	K M R Grainger
Carotidynia: aetiology, diagnosis and treatment	B R Chambers, G A Donnan, R J Riddell & P F Bladin
Progressive multifocal leukoencephalopathy	J O King, D H L Hart, J R Sullivan, V M Surtees & R McD Anderson
Muscle disease and viruses	L Herzberg, G B Hamell, J Papadimitriou & N Tan
Transcutaneous sympathetic stimulation: effects on autonomic nervous function	S Bajada & A Touraine
Subacute cholinergic dysautonomia in childhood	I J Hopkins, L K Shield & M Harris
A clinical and electrophysiological study of neurologically induced winging of the scapula	S R Hammond & G Danta
The anatomy of occipital neuralgia	N Bogduk

The mitochondrial myopathies: 9 case reports and a literature review	R B Fitzsimons
Immunological studies of brain-specific antigens	R D Helme & J L Stow
Experimental neurogenic pulmonary oedema after discrete lesions in the ventrolateral medulla oblongata	W W Blessing
Neuropathology of the cortical lesions of the Parkinsonian-dementia (PD) complex of Guam	N T Tan, B A Kakulas, C L Masters, J C Gibbs & D C Gajdusek

Volume 18 – 1981

CONTENTS

The E Graeme Robertson Memorial Lecture 1981: Stretch-compression neuropathy	Sir Sydney Sunderland
Myasthenia gravis: immune mechanisms and implications	J Newsom-Davis
Disordered muscle tone and movement	J W Lance
Hypotensive central spinal cord infarction: A clinicopathological study of 3 cases of aortic disease	P C Blumbergs, D Chin & J P Rice
A comparison of Australian caucasian and aboriginal brain weights	C Harper & L Mina
Bilateral optic nerve hypoplasia	R A Ouvrier, D Lewis, G Procopis, F A Billson, M Silink & M de Silva
Acetylcholine receptor antibodies in the diagnosis and management of myasthenia gravis	G A Nicholson & L R Griffiths
Serum induced demyelination: an electrophysiological and histological study	J D Pollard, B Harrison & P Gatenby
Compression of the tibial nerve by the tendinous arch of origin of the soleus muscle	F L Mastaglia, J Venerys, B A Stokes & R Vaughan
Hypokalaemic periodic paralysis unresponsive to acetazolamide	R H Rischbieth
A case of cortical deafness	C S Kneebone & R J Burns
Metachromatic leucodystrophy in children	P G Procopis
Preservation of acquired music performance functions with a dominant hemisphere lesion: a case report	D Erdonmez & J B Morley
Changes in peripheral and central nerve conduction with aging	A Mackenzie & H Phillips II
Evaluation of therapists by patients with epilepsy	C Sutton & R G Beran
How worthwile is plasma primidone level measurement?	M J Eadie, R Heazlewood & J H Tyrer
Stroke syndromes in young people	B R Chambers, P F Bladin, K McGrath & A J Goble
Carotid endarterectomy at Royal Brisbane Hospital and Princess Alexandra Hospital, Brisbane	G D Ohlrich & J R Kukums
Retention of urine and sacral paraesthesia in anogenital herpes simplex infection	R H Edis
Substance P in the central nervous system	R D Helme & D W White
Optic nerve decompression in benign intracranial hypertension	C J Kilpatrick, D V Kaufman, J E K Galbraith & J O King
Familial occurrence of meningioma: a case report	R Pamphlett & R A Mackenzie
Senile Parkinsonism and DOPA pharmacokinetics	G A Broe, M A Evans & E J Triggs

Assessment of disability in multiple sclerosis: a new approach
to epidemiological study   R G Beran, V R Jennings & T Read

Volume 19 – 1982

CONTENTS

The E Graeme Robertson Memorial Lecture 1982:
    Multiple sclerosis: 50 years on   J Sutherland
Measles encephalitis   R T Johnson, D E Griffin, R Hirsh & A Vaisberg*
Experimental demyelinating optic neuropathy   W M Carroll, A Jennings & F L Mastaglia
Immunological studies in myotonic dystrophy   G L Walker, F L Mastagia, R J M Lane & U Karagol

Substance P in the trigeminal system at postmortem: evidence
for a role in pain pathways in man   R D Helme & J L Fletcher
Comparison of diagnostic tests in myasthenia gravis   G A Nicholson, J G McLeod & L R Griffiths

Hormonal influence on water permeability across the
blood-brain barrier   A C Reid, G M Teasdale & J McCulloch*
Myelopathy associated with decompression sickness:
a report of six cases   F L Mastaglia, R I McCallurn & D N Walder
The hypereosinophilic syndrome   G H Putdie, D Kotasek & R H C Rischbieth
Concentric sclerosis   G Yu-Pu & G Shu-Fang*
Amoebic meningitis also occurs in NSW   P G Procopis, Z Stuart & A Kan
Encephalitis in infectious mononucleosis   D H Todman
Hypopituitarism with arachnoid cyst   R H C Rischbieth
Diffuse infiltrating astrocytoma (gliomatosis cerebri) with 22-year history
       P C Blumbergs, D K F Chin & J F Hallpike
Oculopharyngeal dystrophy: clinicopathological study
of an Australian family   P C Blumbergs, D Chin, D Burrow, R J Burns & J P Rice
Hemimasticatory and hemifacial spasm: a common pathophysiology?   P D Thompson & W M Carroll
A case of Lhermitte-Duclos disease   P McCombe & B A Warren
Developmental anomalies affecting the fourth ventricular
outflow region: a report of four cases   G L Coffey, D J O'Sullivan & T J Connelley
Neurophysiological evidence of aging in Down's syndrome   R A Mackenzie, H Creasey & C Y Huang

Parenchymal brain lesions in spontaneously hypertensive
stroke-prone rats   R A Rodda, T Brain & S Jones
Embolisation of cerebral arteriovenous malformations   P G McManis, G M Selby & W A Sorby
Senile dementia and hydrocephalus due to carotid dolichoectasia   C Huang, Y W Chan & R Wang
Carotid plaques and retinal emboli: a clinical, angiographic
and morphological study   S F Berkovic, P F Bladin, L R Ferguson, J P Royle & D P Thomas
Steady-state valproate pharmacokinetics
during long-term therapy   M J Eadie, V Heazlewood, L McKauge & J H Tyrer

Hepatotoxicity of sodium valproate	S F Berkovic, P F Bladin, D B Jones, R A Smallwood & F J E Vajda
Absence status in adults	S F Berkovic & P F Bladin
Demographics of an epileptic population	R G Beran, C Sutton & T Read

Volume 20 – 1984

CONTENTS

The E Graeme Robertson Memorial Lecture 1983:

The long-term prognosis of Parkinson's disease	G Selby
Anticonvulsant effects on the memory performance of epileptics	A T Butlin, G Danta & M L Cook
Experience with continuous ambulatory EEG monitoring	S F Berkovic, P F Bladin, M D Connelly, L A Gossat, G R Symington & F J E Vajda
Convulsive status epilepsy: is there a role for thiopentone-induced narcosis?	K Burton & J T Holland
Anticonvulsants, folic acid and memory dysfunction in epileptics	A T Butlin, G Danta & M L Cook
Dilatation in the carotid vascular territory of the cat in response to activation of cell bodies in the locus coeruleus	P J Goadsby, G A Lambert & J W Lance
An analysis of the decision-making process in the management of malignant gliomas	R Iansek & J I Balla
Latency of late responses in lesions of lumbosacral nerve roots	P T Yeo
Fatal migraine	G Selby & J A Fryer
Neurovascular disturbances in headache patients	P D Drummond & J W Lance
Symptomatic hydrocephalus due to an elongated and ectatic basilar artery	R H Edis & T M H Chakera
Dexamethasone: pharmacokinetics in neurological patients	M J Eadie, T R O'R Brophy, G Ohlrich & J H Tyrer
Rubral tremor: clinical features and treatment of three cases	S F Berkovic & P F Bladin
Segmental motor paralysis in herpes zoster	J P Rice
Progressive myoclonic epilepsy, nerve deafness and spinal muscular atrophy	J W Lance & W A Evans
Neurological complications of mycoplasma pneumoniae infection	M A Hely, P M Williamson & T R Terenty
Psychometric and cranial CT study in myotonic dystrophy	G L Walker, R Rosser, F L Mastaglia & J N Walton
Scapuloperoneal myopathy	D H Todman & R A Cooke
Brainstem auditory evoked responses and quantitative saccade studies in multiple sclerosis: a comparative evaluation	W Knezevic, F L Mastaglia, J L Black & D W K Collins
Neuropathological findings in a case of coexistent progressive supranuclear palsy and Alzheimer's disease	D G Milder, C F Elliott & W A Evans
Central pontine myelinolysis with widespread extrapontine lesions: a report of two cases	R M Kalnins, S F Berkovic & P F Bladin
The plasticity of the Purkinje cell	H Urich

F-response studies. Computer analysis and recovery cycle	F L Mastaglia, W M Carroll & G W Thickbroom
Vasoactivity of cerebrospinal fluid from patients with brain swelling	A C Reid, M Stewar & G M Teasdale

Volume 21 – 1985

CONTENTS

The E Graeme Robertson Memorial Lecture 1984:

Some disorders of the central grey matter in children: clinical and radiological diagnosis	J Aicardi
Adult-onset rod disease: a clinicopathological reappraisal	E Byrne
Peripheral neuropathy in IgM kappa paraproteinaemia: clinical and ultrastructural studies in two patients	J D Pollard, J G McLeod & D Feeney
Duchenne de Boulogne and human facial expression	R A Cuthbertson
Use of total and free anticonvulsant serum levels in clinical practice	R G Beran, J H Lewis, J L Nolte & A P Westwood
Valproate hepatotoxicity: a review and report of two instances in adults	R G Dickinson, M L Basset, J Searle, J H Tyrer & M J Eadie
Adult Lennox Gastaut syndrome: features and diagnostic problems	P F Bladin
Adult Lennox Gastaut syndrome: patients with large focal structural lesions	P F Bladin
The effect of infusion of various peptide antisera on vasodilatation in the cat common carotid vascular territory	P J Goadsby & G J Macdonald
The prognostic significance of intraventricular haemorrhage	P Kerr, R Iansek, R D Helme, A Rosengarten
Ocular and ocular motor aspects of primary thalamic haemorrhage	A Fisher & W Knezevic
Familial myasthenia gravis: a study of three families	D Chin & S S Gubbay
Brainstem auditory evoked responses in hereditary spinocerebellar ataxias	W Knezevic & E G Stewart-Wynne
Triplicate post-traumatic sciatic nerve palsy: evoked potentials in the diagnosis	V M Synek & A E Hardy
Neuropathological findings in a case of chronic inflammatory polyneuropathy	D C Milder, D H L Rail & G A Broe
Availability of drug assay results and dosage advice improves antiepileptic care in a specialist neurology outpatient clinic	L L Ioannides-Demos, A J McLean, J Wodak, N Tong, U Heinzow, M Horne, P M Harrison & B S Gilligan
Clinical experience with clobazam: a new 1,5 benzodiazepine in the treatment of refractory epilepsy	F J E Vajda, P F Bladin & B J Parsons
Examination of the problems confronting those with epilepsy	R G Beran & P L Flanagan
A simple and validated tool for the clinician to assess psychosocial status when conducting anticonvulsant drug trials	P J Flanagan & R G Beran
Peripheral neuropathy with gammopathy responding to plasmapheresis	J Frayne & R J Stark
Peripheral autonomic surface potential: a quantitative technique for recording autonomic neural function in man	W Knezevic & S Bajada
Vulnerability of the dorsal root ganglion in experimental allergic encephalomyelitis	M P Pender & TA Sears

Experimental allergic encephalomyelitis: effect of neonatal exposure to neuroantigen or neuroantigen immune cells on subsequent reactivity as adults — D O Willenborg & G Danta

Spatial contrast sensitivity in patients with multiple sclerosis — R Carter & G Danta

A decision analytic approach to the role of visual evoked response and cerebrospinal fluid abnormalities in the management of singular spinal sclerosis — R Iansek & J I Balla

Cerebral abscess in leukaemia: an unusual presentation of a rare complication — M C Patterson, I H Bunce & M J Eadie

Ophthalmological complications of cryptococcal meningitis — J D Blackie, G Danta, T Sorrell & P Collignon

Cryptococcal infection of the central nervous system — P A Sandstrom

Infantile Refsum's disease: a peroxisomal storage disorder? — J I Manson, A C Pollard, A Poulos & R F Carter

Phytanic acid oxidase deficiency in childhood — G A Wise, B J Duffy, J D Mitchell, A C Pollard, A Poulos & J Pollard

Volume 22 – 1986

CONTENTS

Edrophonium test in myasthenia: quantitative oculography — I M Willlams, P Dickinson & A C Sum

A case of invasive thymoma associated with myasthenia gravis, myositis and demyelinating neuropathy — H Miller, B D Shenstone, R Joffe & S Kannangara

Chronic subdural haematomas presenting with Parkinsonian signs — R F Peppard, E Byrne & D Nye

Global stereopsis in stroke patients — B Fenelon, K Grant, A Delahunty, R Neill, D Dunlop, P Dunlop, B Frost & A Quayle

Extradural malignancy simulating brachial neuritis — P C Gates, P A Kempster, D Risebin & J I Balla

Peripheral sympathetic conduction velocity calculated from surface potentials — T J Day, D Offerman & S Bajada

Myopathy with fatiguability — myositis or myasthenia? — R Peppard, E Byrne & X Dennet

A clinical study of convulsive syncope — P A Kempster & J I Balla

Effects of age on the axon reflex response to noxious chemical stimulation — R D Helme & S McKernan

The use of lisuride in severe Parkinson's disease — D Chin, Y L Yu & C Y Huang

The natural history of syringomyelia — N E Anderson, E W Willoughby & P Wrightson

Thoracic intervertebral disc protrusion with spinal cord compression — B Gilligan & J Frayne

Substance P in human hypothalamus — R D Helme & K Thomas

The neuropathology of progressive autonomic failure of central origin (the Shy-Drager syndrome) — B A Kakulas, N Tan & V J Ojeda

Cryoglobulinaemic neuropathy – a clinical spectrum — R F Peppard, E Byrne, R McD Anderson & B J Clarke

Non-bacterial thrombotic endocarditis and stroke	R A L Macdonell, R M Kalnins & G A Donnan
Evaluation of an introductory course in neurology	J I Balla & H Edwards
Lumbosacral nerve plexus compression by ovarian-fallopian cysts	P T Yeo & A C Grice
Genito-femoral neuropathy	R H Rischbieth
Transfer factor as a therapy for multiple sclerosis: a follow-up study	J A Frith, J G McLeod, A Basten, J D Pollard, S R Hammond, D B Williams & P A Crossie
The neurochemical and clinical effects of 1-methyl-4-phenyl-1,2,3,6-tetra-hydropyridine in small animals	G A Donnan, S J Kaczmarczyk, T Solopotias, P Rowe, R M Kalnins, F J E Vajda & F A O Mendelsohn
Normative data for somatosensory evoked potentials from upper limb nerves in middle-aged subjects	V M Synek

Volume 23 – 1987

CONTENTS

The E Graeme Robertson Memorial Lecture, 1985:

Neurology of the sphincters	M Swash
Crossed facilitation and post-contraction depression of abductor pollicis brevis motor neurones	W Knezevic, F L Mastaglia, G W Thickbroom & W M Carroll
Unusual paraspinal muscle lesions in ankylosing spondylitis	B A Kakulas, I Morrison, E T Owen & R Kitridou
The pyriformis syndrome: review and case presentation	V M Synek
Clonic perseveration	G L Morris & J Leicester
The basis for aspirin dosage in stroke prevention	R A Brandon & M J Eadie
Cerebral infarction due to presumed haemodynamic factors in ambulant hypertensive patients	G D McLaren & G Danta
Subcortical arteriosclerotic encephalopathy: Binswanger's disease	S E Mathers, B R Chambers, J R Merory & I Alexander
Cranial CT scan appearances that correlate with patient outcome in acute stroke	G J Hankey, S J Davis, E G Stewart-Wynne & T M H Chakera
Clinically unsuspected cardiac disease in patients with cerebral ischaemia	P Gates, R Peppard, P Kempster, A Harris & M Pierce
Electrically evoked skin vasodilatation: a quantitative test of nociceptor function in man	R A Westerman, A Low, A Pratt, J S Hutchinson, J Szolcsanyi, W Magerl, H O Handwerker & W M Kozak
Neurogenic flare responses in chronic rheumatic pain syndromes	R D Helme, G O Littlejohn & C Weinstein

Neurogenic plasma extravasation in response to mechanical, chemical and thermal stimuli	P V Andrews & R D Helme
Magnetoencephalography: locating the source of P_{300} via magnetic field recording	E Gordon, G Sloggett, I Harvey, C Kraiuhin, C Rennie, C Yiannikas & R Meares
Gliomas presenting outside the central nervous system	B J Brew & R Garrick
Neoplastic angioendotheliosis	B J Brew, D J O'Sullivan, P Darveniza, G Selby, J Fryer & W Evans
Cryptococcal infections of the central nervous system: a ten year experience	J A Waterson & B S Gilligan
Clobazam in the treatment of epilepsy	C Kilpatrick, R Bury, R Fullinfaw & R Moulds
The management of epilepsy in women of child-bearing age and the Australian experience of valproate in pregnancy	M A W Curran*
Intensive neuromonitoring for complex partial seizures: focal seizure pattern variability in surgical patients	P F Bladin
Tolerance to the anticonvulsant effects of clonazepam and clobazam in the amygdaloid kindled rat	F J E Vajda, S J Lewis, Q L G Harris, B Jarrott & N A Young
Evaluation of the first 18 months of a specific rehabilitation programme for those with epilepsy	R G Beran, M Major & L Veldze
Impairment of consciousness in migraine	P A Kempster, R Iansek & J. Balla
Cervical spondylosis and headaches	R Iansek, J Heywood, J Karnaghan & J I Balla
Whiplash headache	J Balla & J Karnaghan
Diagnostic strategies of fifth year medical student in a neurological case. The importance of the first hypothesis	M Gibson, J Kaaden & J I Balla
An analysis of cranial computerized tomography scanning in private neurological practice	G J Hankey & E G Stewart-Wynne
Acute encephalopathy following petrol sniffing in two aboriginal patients	R H Rischbieth, G N Thompson, A Hamilton-Bruce, G H Purdie & J N Peters
Bilateral intracerebral haemorrhage presenting with supranuclear ophthalmoplegia, bradykinesia and rigidity	G J Hankey & E G Stewart-Wynne
Amnesia following right thalamic haemorrhage	M M Tsoi, C Y Huang, A O M Lee & Y L Yu
Ventriculo-peritoneal shunting of acute hydrocephalus in vein of Galen malformation	K K Pun, Y L Yu, C Y Huang & E Woo
Isolated unilateral hypoglossal nerve palsy due to a chondroid chordoma	K Millingen & M Prentice
Herpes zoster arteritis: pathological findings	R A Mackenzie, P Ryan, W E Karnes & H Okazaki
Otocerebral mucormycosis – a case report	R A L Macdonell, G A Donnan, R M Kalnins, M J Richards & P F Baldin
Lumboperitoneal shunting as a cause of visual loss in benign intracranial hypertension	B J Brew, R Garrick & T J Connelley

Volume 24 – 1987

CONTENTS

Pregnancy and multiple sclerosis. An Australian perspective	J A Frith & J G McLeod
Diagnostic value of cerebrospinal fluid myelin basic protein in patients with neurological illness	L Davies, J G McLeod, A Muir & W J Hensley
Pseudo-multiple sclerosis: a clinico-epidemiological study	G J Hankey & E G Stewart-Wynne
Unreported symptomatic and asymptomatic ischaemic heart disease in patients presenting with TIA or minor stroke detected by the London School of Hygiene cardiovascular questionnaire and Minnesota coding of a routine ECG	P Gates, S Marwood, M Jelinek & M Scott
Lacunar infarction: a 12 month study	J Reimers, C de Wytt & B Seneviratne
A case-control study of cerebrovascular disease in Western Australia	K Jamrozik, E Stewart-Wynne, G Ward, P Giele, J Perica & C Phatouros
The Perth community stroke study: attack rates for stroke and TIA in Western Australia	E Stewart-Wynne, K Jamrozik & G Ward
Paramedian thalamic and midbrain infarction: the 'mesencephalothalamic syndrome'	J A Waterston, R J Stark & B S Gilligan
Spinal arteriovenous malformations: some diagnostic difficulties with illustrative cases	E Byrne, R McD Anderson, K Henderson, J Cummins, P McNeill & E Gilford
Lipids in cerebrovascular disease: is there an association?	L Herzberg, J R L Maserei & A Taylor
Selection criteria for surgery in patients with refractory epilepsy	R Mackenzie, J S Smith, J Matheson, C Bucovaz, M Dwyer & C Morris
Post-temporal lobectomy seizures	P F Bladin
Scalp and intracerebral P_{300} in surgery for temporal lobe epilepsy	A Puce & P F Bladin
Clinical relevance of therapeutic drug level estimation with respect to clonazepam and carbamazepine: preliminary report	R G Beran, J Lewis, J Nolte & E Yip
Changes in clearance of sodium valproate with changes in dose	C J Kilpatrick, R W Bury, R O Fullinfaw & R F W Moulds
Oxcarbazepine: preliminary clinical and pharmacokinetic studies on a new anticonvulsant	W D Hooper, R G Dickinson, P R Dunstan, S C Pendlebury & M J Eadie
Glossopharyngeal neuralgia	J King
Pathological changes in the vagus nerve in diabetes and chronic alcoholism	Y-P Gui, J G McLeod & J Baverstock
Non-invasive tests of neurovascular function	R A Westerman, R E Widdop, J Hannaford, C Hogan, R Roberts & P Zimmet
Diabetic focal myelopathy	T J Anderson, I MacG Donaldson & R S Scott
Hereditary motor neuron disease	G Selby

THE FLOWERING OF A WARATAH

Visual evoked responses in diabetes   K S Millingen, P T Yeo & S Kamaldeen

Electroencephalographic abnormalities in patients with normal contrast computerised axial tomography brain scans   V M Synek, E B Walker, N A Shaw & N E Anderson

Herpes zoster arteritis: clinical and angiographic features   G K Herkes, C E Storey, R Joffe & R A Mackenzie

Listeria rhombo-encephalitis   J Frayne & P Gates

Listeria brain abscess associated with steroid therapy: successful non-surgical treatment   R Leung, E Woo, Y L Yu & C Y Huang

Acquired aphasia of childhood with epilepsy: the Landau-Kleffner syndrome   G J Hankey & S S Gubbay

Neurological sequelae of lightning stroke   J H Frayne & B S Gilligan

Measurement of flare responses in patients with pain   R D Helme

The effects of capsaicin denervation on leucocyte and complement components of the inflammatory response   R D Helme, A Eglezos & P V Andrews

Protein metabolism in Duchenne muscular dystrophy, monoclonal and mixed skeletal muscle cultures   A J Corbett

Dr James Parkinson   L Herzberg

Volume 25 – 1988

CONTENTS

Preparing neurologists for the 21st century   R Porter

History of multiple sclerosis. An Australian perspective   J A Frith

Is there still a place for carotid endarterectomy   G Matalanis & R J Lusby*

The eye in stroke: amaurosis fugax, ischaemic optic neuropathy and chronic ocular ischaemia   J King

Transient ischaemic attacks: controversies in treatment. A review   B Gilligan

Dementia, gait disturbance, incontinence and hydrocephalus   B R Chambers & A J Hughes

Absence of anti-myelin antibodies and serum demyelinating factors in most patients with chronic inflammatory demyelinating polyradiculoneuropathy   P A McCombe, J D Pollard & J G McLeod

A family with late onset autosomal dominant cerebellar degeneration   S Collins, L Sedal, J King & I Donaldson

Spinal subdural abscess   E G Butler, P J Dohrmann & R J Stark

Effects of topical capsaicin on normal skin and affected dermatomes in herpes zoster   R A Westerman, R G D Roberts, R R Kotzmann, D A Westerman, C Delaney, R E Widdop & B E Carter

Abnormalities of visual evoked responses in hyperprolactinaemia   P T Yeo, S Kamaldeen & D Walker

Somatosensory evoked potentials, electroencephalography and CT scans in the assessment of the neurological sequelae of decompression sickness   C Yiannikas & R Beran

The flight of colours test. Its value as an indicator of dysfunction of the visual pathways   M A Hamilton-Bruce & A B Black

A prospective study of the predictire value of electroencephalographic
abnormalities for epileptic loss of consciousness   S Collins & R Iansek

Transition from alpha to theta pattern coma in fatal cerebral anoxia   V M Synek & B J L Synek

Choreoathetosis and thalamic haemorrhage   R J Freilich & B R Chambers

Neurologists' use and interpretation of antiepileptic drug monitoring
in the treatment of epilepsy   R G Beran, E Y S Yip & J J Ashley

Further clinical and pharmacokinetic observations on the new
anticonvulsant, oxcarbazepine   R G Dickinson, W D Hooper, S C Pendlebury, D Moses & M J Eadie

Necropsy study of GABA/benzodiazepine receptor binding sites in
brain tissue from chronic alcoholic patients   J J Kril, P R Dodd, A L Gundlach, N Davies, W E J Watson, G A R Johnston & C G Harper

Volume 26 – 1989

CONTENTS

Optic neuritis and its significance   W I McDonald

Epilepsy in Gowers' understanding, a century ago   M J Eadie

Effect of haemodilution on experimental cerebral ischaemia   K Yamashita, S Kobayashi, S Yamaguchi & T Tsunematsu*

Spinal cord lesions induced by antigalactocerebroside serum   F L Mastaglia, W M Carroll & A R Jennings

Sympathetic neurons modulate plasma extravasation in the rat
through a non-adrenergic mechanism   Z Khalil & R D Helme

Concordance between different measures of small sensory and
autonomic fibre neuropathy in diabetes mellitus   R A Westerman, C Delaney, A Ivamy-Phillips, M Horowitz & A Roberts

Hereditary motor and sensory neuropathy type ii followed in the
next two generations by a clinically distal motor neuropathy   G Selby

The P300 event-related potential and regional cerebral blood flow
in patients with Alzheimer's disease   E Gordon, C Kraiuhin, Y Zurynski, C Rennie, P Landau, A Singer, A Howson & R Meares

The relationship between reaction time and latency of the P300
event-related potential in normal subjects and Alzheimer's disease   C Kraiuhin, C Yiannikis, S Coyle, E Gordon, C Rennie, A Howson & R Meares

Evaluation of evoked potentials and cerebrospinal fluid analysis in
the differential diagnosis of multiple sclerosis   M A Hamilton-Bruce, A B Black, D J Chappell & P R Pannail

Neurological complications of sarcoidosis   R C Y Chen & J G McLeod

Can psychometric tools be used to analyse pain in a geriatric
population?   R D Helme, B Katz, S Gibson & T Corran

Validity of a revised EEG coma scale for predicting survival in
anoxic encephalopathy   V M Synek

The addition of bromocriptine to long-term dopa therapy in Parkinson's disease   G Selby

Daily salivary anticonvulsant monitoring in patients with
intractable epilepsy   G K Herkes & M J Eadie

Possible extension of SPECT cerebral imaging in the investigation of
epilepsy using radioiodinated benzodiazepines   D J Maddalena, R G Beran, A Jenkinson & G M Snowdon

Minocyline-induced benign intracranial hypertension   C M Lander

Factors influencing the yield of cranial CT scanning in a private neurological practice   D C Reutens & E G Stewart-Wynne

A review of 20 cases of spastic dysphonia   S Whyte & P Darveniza

CNS cryptococcosis: unusual aspects   J I Cochius, R J Burns & J O Willoughby

Cerebral infarction in cryptococcal meningitis   Y L Yu, E Woo, F L Chan, T Y K. Chan & G C Y Chan*

Iophendylate-induced basal arachnoiditis   C K Wong, E Woo & W L Yu*

Infarction of the conus medullaris – clinical and radiographic features   G K Herkes, G Selby & W A Sorby

Cerebral deposits of carcinoid tumour   E G Butler, R J Stark, K Siu & R A Sinclair

Obstructive hydrocephalus caused by multiple sclerosis   E G Butler & B S Gilligan

Posterior cortical atrophy   R S Delamont, J Harrison, M Field & R S Boyle

Focal cerebral ischaemia induced by postural change   L Sedal & J Heywood

Orthostatic tremor—a case report   D Thyagarajan & P Gates

Traumatic hypoglossal nerve palsy   R S Delamont & R S Boyle

Volume 27 – 1990

CONTENTS

The value to the clinical neurologist of electromyography in the 1990s   E Stolberg

The evolution of J. Hughlings Jackson's thought on epilepsy   M J Eadie

Thirteen years longitudinal study of computed tomography, visual electrophysiology and neuropsychological changes in Huntington's chorea patients and 50% at-risk asymptomatic subjects   L A Cala, J L Black, D W K Collins, R M Ellison & S A Zubrick

Mitomycin C induces a delayed and prolonged demyelination and conduction block due to Schwann cell destruction   K Westland, J D Pollard & A J Sumner

Pleuropulmonary fibrosis due to bromocriptine treatment for Parkinson's disease   D H Todman, W A Oliver & R L Edwards

Commencement of a paediatric EEG-video telemetry service   A Bye, P Lamont & L Healy

P300 event-related potentials in de novo Parkinson's disease   J S Graham, C Yiannikas, E Gordon, S Coyle & J G L Morris

Revised LEG coma scale in diffuse acute head injuries in adults   V M Synek

Magnetoencephalography and late component ERPs   E Gordon, C Rennie & L Collins

Physical disability after stroke in the Perth community stroke study   C Anderson, K Jamrozik & E Stewart-Wynne

Perth community stroke study: design and preliminary results   C Anderson, E Stewart-Wynne, K Jamrozik, P Buryill & T Chakera

Volume 28 – 1991

CONTENTS

The E Graeme Robertson Memorial Lecture – 1991:

Vertebrobasilar embolism   L R Caplan

Superior sagittal sinus thrombosis   A Mohammed, J G McLeod & J Hallinan

The influence of age on atrial fibrillation as a risk factor for stroke   R X You, J J McNeil, S J Farish, H M O'Malley & G A Donnan

Preliminary experience with 99mTc-HMPAO SPECT in cerebral ischaemia   A E Baird, G A Donnan, M Austin, M R Newton & W J McKay

Mechanisms and clinical features of internal watershed infarction   A E Baird, G A Donnan & M Saling

Regional cerebral blood flow and recognition memory in elderly normals: potential application to Alzheimer's disease   R S Schwartz, C Burke, J Sears, E Gordon, J Batchelor, G Kostalas, R Meares & C Yiannikas

Colour duplex flow imaging in carotid arterial disease: correlation with intra-arterial digital angiography   D H Todman, D J Hewson, B Seneviratne & P Walsh

Pattern of memory deficits in a controlled psychometric study of thalamic haemorrhage   A Au, Y L Yu, M Tsoi & C M Chang*

A clinical and pathological study of progressive supranuclear palsy   J Frasca, P C Blumbergs, P Henschke & R J Burns

Ataxia telangiectasia presenting as an extrapyramidal movement disorder and ocular motor apraxia without overt telangiectasia   A Churchyard, R Stell & F L Mastaglia

Familial spastic paraplegia: an electrophysiological study of central sensory conduction pathways   P K Panegyres, G H Purdie, M A Hamilton-Bruce & R H C Rischbieth

Lithium neurotoxicity   G L Sheean

The chronic fatigue syndrome: a reappraisal and unifying hypothesis   E Byrne

Lack of neurological abnormalities in Lewis rats with experimental chronic serum sickness   P A McCombe & M P Pender

Sensorimotor peripheral neuropathy in rheumatoid arthritis   P A McCombe, A C Klestov, A E Tannenberg, J B Chalk & M P Pender

Palmar cold threshold test and median nerve electrophysiology in carpal tunnel compression neuropathy   R A Westerman & C A Delaney

Intravenous immunoglobulin therapy in the inflammatory neuropathies   A Churchyard, T Day, K Grainger & F L Mastaglia

A prospective study of acute radioculopathy after scoliosis surgery   J W Dunne, P L Silbert & M Wren

Bicycling induced pudendal nerve pressure neuropathy   P L Silbert, J W Dunne, R H Edis & E G Stewart-Wynne

Botulinum toxin treatment of spasmodic torticollis   L Davies & I T Lorentz

The value of non-invasive spinal cord monitoring during spinal surgery and interventional angiography   J W Dunne & C M Field

Late-onset acid maltase deficiency in a Chinese girl   K S Wong, C Lai & H K Ng*

Interoperator variability in quantitative electroencephalography	M A Hamilton-Bruce, K L Boundy & G H Purdie
The use of magnetic resonance imaging in neurological practice – a local experience	D Chin & P Lo*
Neuropsychological assessment in lamotrigine treated epileptic patients	G K Banks & R G Beran
Zeta waves: a distinctive type of intermittent delta wave studied prospectively	J W Dunne & P L Silbert
Intrathecal baclofen for severe spasticity: five years experience	E G Stewart-Wynne, P L Silbert, S Buffery, D Periman & E Tan
Noxious heat hyperalgesia test instrument	R A Westerman, R W Carr, W Brenton, J C Kiln, I Pano, A Rabavilas, C A Delahunty & R D G Roberts

Volume 29 – 1992

CONTENTS

The E Graeme Robertson Memorial Lecture 1992:

Interesting Neurological Syndromes	J W Lance
History of neurology in Australia	G Selby
XIXth century pre-Jacksonian concepts of epileptogenesis	M J Eadie
Update on surgical treatment of epilepsies	J Engel Jr
Psychosocial aspects of epilepsy and of epilepsy surgery	P F Bladin
The influence of other anticonvulsants on the plasma concentration of E-2-en-valproate	D B McLaughlin, G E McKinnon & M J Eadie
Video-audio/EEG monitoring in epilepsy – the Queen Elizabeth Hospital experience	S A Koblar, A B Black & G J Schapel
Salivary concentrations of antiepileptic drugs, oestradiol and progesterone throughout pregnancy in epileptic women	G K Herkes & M J Eadie
Automatisms – the current legal position related to clinical practice and medicolegal interpretation	R G Beran
Video EEG analysis of non-ictal events in children	A S Bye & J Nunan
P300 event-related potentials correlated with cerebral blood flow in nondemented patients with lacunar infarction	K Yamashita, S Kobayashi, H Koide, K Okada & T Tsunematsu*
Vigabatrin – plasma enantiomer concentration and clinical effects	G Sheean, T Schramm, D S Anderson & M J Eadie
Predicting survival after stroke: experience from the Perth community stroke study	C S Anderson, K D Jamrozik & E G Stewart-Wynne
Thrombolytic therapy in vertebrobasilar occlusion	D Thyagarajan, R J Stark, J Frayne, B S Gilligan & N Sacharias
Comparison of tramcranial doppler with DSA in vertebrobasilar ischaemia	L M Cher, B R Chambers & V Smidt
Confounding factors in non-invasive tests of neurovascular function in diabetes mellitus	R A Westerman, L E Lindblad, D Wajnblum, R G D Roberts & C A Delaney
Frontal signs following subcortical infarction	A J Corbett, H Bennett & S Kos

The molecular genetics of mitochondrial cytopathies: the
Melbourne experience   D Thyagarajan, E Byrne, X Dennet & S Marzuki

Anti-ganglioside antibodies in peripheral neuropathy   P A McCombe, R Wilson & R L Prentice

Hereditary sensory radicular neuropathy: defective neurogenic
inflammation   R A Westerman, A Block, A Nunn, C A Delaney, A Hahn, X Dennett & R W Carr

Reflex sympathetic dystrophy: altered axon reflex and autonomic
responses   R A Westerman, I Parto, A Rabavilas, A Hahn, A Nunn, R G D Roberts & H Burry

Enigmatic trigeminal sensory neuropathy diagnosed
by facial skin biopsy   P L Silbert, G R Kelsall, J M Shepherd & S S Gubbay

Late radiation associated neurological injury   A G Kerrnode, T J Day & W M Carroll

Postinfectious myelitis, encephalitis and encephalomyelitis   C M Chang, H K Ng, Y W Chan, S Y Leung, K Y Fong & Y L Yu

The cervical spine in fatal motor vehicle accidents   J Leditschke, R M D Anderson & W S C Hare*

Low osmolar and non-ionic x-my contrast media and cortical
blindness   A G Kermode, T Chakera & F L Mastaglia*

Effect of ritanserin, a highly selective 5-HT2 receptor antagonist,
on Parkinson's disease   J Henderson, C Yiannikas & J S Graham*

Volume 30 – 1993

CONTENTS

The E Graeme Robertson Memorial Lecture 1993:

     Mitochondrial genes and neurological disease   A E Harding

The explosive copula of Thomas Willis   M J Eadie

Motor neuropathies and antiglycolipid antibodies   G Serratrice

Motor nerve biopsy: feasibility and safety   P Gates, E Byme, P McKelvie, L Robert, B Tomlinson, X Dennett, W Morrison & P McNeill

The role of skin nociceptive afferent nerves in blister healing   R A Westerman, R W Carr, C A Delaney, M J Morris & R G D Roberts

Kennedy's disease: clinical presentation and laboratory diagnosis   M W Faragher, W-T Choi, H E MacLean, G L Warne & J D Zajac

Orthostatic tremor (shaky legs syndrome)   P C Gates

Acute myopathy in status asthmaticus   J D Blackie, P Gibson, K Murree-Allen & W P Saul

Watershed cerebral infarction associated with perioperative
hypotension   R P Gerraty, E J Gilford & P C Gates

Regional cerebral blood flow during memory recognition and
neuropsychological performance in patients referred for
investigation of dementia   C Burke, J Batchelor, R S Schwartz, J Snars, E Gordon & C Yiannikas

EEG monitoring during angiographic balloon test carotid occlusion:
experience in sixteen cases G K Herkes, M Morgan, V Grinnell, W Sorby, J Wong, D Rowe & J Stroud

Basilar artery occlusion following yoga exercise: a case report K Y Fong, R T F Cheung, Y L Yu, C W Lai & C M Chang*

Pentoxifylline in the treatment of acute ischaemic stroke – a reappraisal in Chinese stroke patients Y W Chan & C S Kay*

Single photon emission computed tomography in intractable infantile seizures A M Bye, J Parle & W Haindl

Plasma vigabatrin enantiomer ratios in adults and children L Nagarajan, T Schramm, D B Appleton, C J Burke & M J Eadie

Apparent hydrocephalus and chronic multiple sclerosis: a report of two cases T O'Brien, M Paine, K Matotek & E Byrne

Volume 31 – 1994

CONTENTS

The understanding of epilepsy across three millennia M J Eadie

The mystery of one red ear J W Lance

Insulin sensivity and sensory nerve function C A Delaney, J V Mouser & R A Westerman

Response to l-dopa and evolution of motor fluctuations in the early phase of treatment of Parkinson's disease M Shif & P A Kempster

Huntington's disease in Hong Kong Chinese: epidemiology and clinical picture C M Chang, E L Yu, K Y Fong, M T H Wong, Y W Chan, T H K Ng, C M Leung & V Chan*

Isaac's syndrome: report of a case responding to valproic acid T J O'Brien & P Gates

Routine use of lamotrigine, a new anti-epileptic medication, and the value of measuring its blood levels R G Beran, K Sheehan & M I Tilley

Rhinocerebral mucormycosis presenting as periorbital cellulitis with blindness: report of 2 cases T J O'Brien & P McKelvie

Primary cerebral abscess due to nocardia asteroides presenting as stroke R T F Cheung, Y L Yu & C M Chang

Alzheimer's disease and Alzheimer-type of cerebral degenerations in Chinese H K Ng

Appendix VIII

E Graeme Robertson Memorial Lecturers and Lecture Titles

Year	Lecturer	Title
1978	R Hooper	Graeme Robertson and the golden age of neurology
1979	D Dastur	Aspects of cuprogenic disorder in Wilson's disease in India: Pathology and pathogenesis of chronic myelopathy in atlanto-axial dislocation, with operative or peri-operative haematomyelia or other cord complications
1980	W G Burke	Myasthenia gravis: a clinical review
1981	S Sunderland	Stretch-compression neuropathy
1982	J M Sutherland	Multiple sclerosis fifty years on
1983	G Selby	The long-term prognosis of Parkinson's disease
1984	J Aicardi	Some disorders of the central grey matter in children: clinical and radiological diagnosis
1985	H J Barnett	Vascular disease
1986	M Swash	Neurology of the sphincters
1987	R Baloh	Neuro-otology
1988	W I McDonald	Optic neuritis and its significance
1989	J Morgan Hughes	The molecular biology of mitochondrial disease
1990	E Stalberg	The value to the clinical neurologist of electromyography in the 1990s
1991	L R Caplan	Vertebro-basilar embolism
1992	J W Lance	Interesting neurological syndromes
1993	A Harding	Mitochondrial genes and neurological disease
1994	W Landau	
1995	J B Posner	Neurological paraneoplastic syndromes: a review of diagnosis and prospects for therapy
1996	M J Eadie	Concerning a very noble lady of a most curious shape
1997	J G McLeod	Multiple sclerosis in Australia
1998	–	
1999	B A Kakulas	Molecular genetics in the diagnosis of neuro-muscular disease

Index

A

Abbie, A	1, 34, 49, 118
Abbott, K	96
Abercrombie, J	3
Academic neurology	98, 101, 120, 127, 160
Adams, D	93, 128
Adams, R	95
Adelaide Children's Hospital	95, 96, 109
Adis Press	146, 148
Adrian, E D (Lord)	19
Affiliate-in-Training	133, 138
Ainslie, J	69, 122
Alcoholic insanity	45, 46
Alfred Hospital	15, 28, 36, 55-57, 59, 66, 72, 73, 79, 89-92, 101, 114, 116, 118, 119, 123, 125
Allen, I	78, 128
Allsop, J	89, 91, 116
Alzheimer's disease	41
Amyotrophic lateral sclerosis	14, 47, 48
Anderson, R	83, 119
Andrews, C	98
Aneurysm	8, 63, 112
Angiography	8, 73
Annual General Meetings	80, 83, 100
Annual Scientific Meeting	143, 147, 149
Annual subscription	79, 85, 132, 138, 139, 146, 148
Anthony, M	90, 106
Anticonvulsant drug monitoring	88
Appleton, D B	94
Arachnoiditis	63
Argyll-Robertson pupil	33
Arnhem Land	112
Arteriography	15
Aspirin	107, 115
Austin Hospital	92, 93, 101, 108, 109, 113, 153
Australasian Annals of Medicine	84, 144
Australasian Medical Gazette	4, 13, 14, 23, 36, 50
Australian and New Zealand Society of Neuropathologists	155
Australian Association of Neurologists	42, 57, 60, 62, 66, 68, 69, 71-73, 75, 77-81, 83-85, 88, 89, 92, 99, 121, 122, 124, 127, 128, 131-135, 138, 139, 141-143, 147-155
Australian Brain Foundation	152
Australian Capital Territory	98
Australian Centre for Clinical Neuropharmacology	92
Australian Commonwealth Government	154
Australian Council for Rehabilitation of the Disabled	155
Australian Headache Society	153
Australian Institute of Tropical Medicine	29, 30
Australian Medical Association	153, 154
Australian Medical Journal	4, 11, 14
Australian Neurological Foundation	74, 132, 151, 152
Australian 'X' disease	27-31, 41
Autonomic neuropathies	114

B

Bajada, S	97

Balla, J	92	**C**	
Bancroft	10, 13, 27, 34	Cade, J	107
Banney, D	94	Calcium	33, 115
Beaney Scholar in Pathology	57	Cameron, J	94, 116
Beech, E	96, 122	Campbell, A W	6, 14, 19, 27, 29, 30, 35, 38, 39, 43-53, 55, 59, 68, 90, 112, 118, 125, 159
Bentley	7		
Beran, R	109		
Bergin, J	128, 129	Carnegie, P	111
Beri beri	13	Carotid artery disease	68
Berkovic, S	92, 101, 108	Carotido-cavernous fistula	14
Bernard, C	111	Carroll, W	97, 135
Billings, J	56, 57, 75-77, 84, 91, 92	Cerebellar degeneration	41, 112, 119
Birkett, N	16, 83	Cerebellar laminar degeneration	41
Bismuth subgallate encephalopathy	116	Cerebello-olivary atrophy	41, 68, 112
Black, A	96	Cerebellum	37, 41, 46, 49, 53, 117
Black, B	6	Cerebral cortex	7, 46-51
Bladin, P	92, 101, 108, 113	Cerebral palsy	50
Blessing, W	96, 110	Cerebral sclerosis	48
Boeke	16, 21	Cerebral tumour	10, 41, 72, 73
Bogduk, N	107, 118	Cerebral vascular disease	6, 8, 34, 68, 112, 113, 119
Bolk	49		
Bostock, J	14, 35	Cerebro-spinal fluid	14, 15, 29
Botulism	14	Chair of Medicine	98, 100, 101
Boyce, G	95	Challis Chair of Anatomy	16, 20
Boyle, R	94	Chambers, B	93
Bradfield, J	94	Charcot-Marie-Tooth disease	114
Bradley, K	57, 80, 118	Cheek, D	26
Brain	3, 7, 8, 14-16, 30, 33, 34, 40, 46-48, 50, 60, 63, 83, 93, 100, 104-106, 110, 118, 151, 152	Child Neurologists	153
		Chorea	11
		Chronic inflammatory demyelinating poly-neuropathy	114
Bramwell, B	158		
Breinl, A	24, 27, 29, 30, 50	Churchill-Livingstone	147
Brew, B	90	Ciguatera poisoning	116
Brisbane	2, 13, 23, 24, 27-29, 31, 32, 35, 72, 88, 93-95, 100, 101, 104, 107, 109-112, 115, 116, 120, 128, 145, 146	Cleland, J B	8, 9, 12, 27-30, 50, 116
		Clements, F	26, 27
		Clinical and Experimental Neurology	139, 143, 146-150, 155
Brodman, K	51	Clioquinol	116
Broe, A	101	Cluines Ross	34
Broken Hill	24, 28, 29	Coast Hospital	13, 45, 90
Bromide	7, 35, 37	Coffey, G	90
Brothers, C	11, 109	College of Neurologists	151
Burke, C	94	College of Radiologists of Australasia	63
Burke, D	90, 101, 117	Collins, A	28
Burke, W	83, 89, 117, 123	Collins, K	93
Burnell, G	28, 29, 110	Computed tomography	63, 88, 108
Burnet, Sir M	31, 63	Concord Hospital	91
Burns, R	95, 96, 101, 116, 124, 135	Constitution	73, 79-81, 83, 131-134, 156
Burrow, D	95	Cook, R	111
Byrne, E	92, 101, 114	Corbett, J	94, 95

Index

Corresponding Affiliate Member	133
Corresponding Member	133
Council	24, 57, 66, 68, 69, 76, 78-81, 83-85, 123, 124, 127, 131-134, 138, 139, 141 143, 144, 146, 147, 151, 155
Cox, L B	9, 10, 12, 14, 15, 55-60, 64, 72, 73, 77-80, 84, 91, 92, 114, 118, 119, 132, 135, 159
Critchley, M	60, 83, 85
Cullen, W	2, 3
Curthoys, I	118
Curtis, D	59, 114, 115, 132
Cytoarchitectonics	49-51

D

Danta, G	98, 111
Darveniza, P	90
Davis, E	92
Davis, S	91, 101, 113
Dawson, L A	91, 123
Dawson, W	9, 41, 43
De Crespigny, C	9, 12, 33
Dementia	41
Dementia praecox	41
Demyelination	12, 33, 111, 114
Denny-Brown, D	61
Dew, H	10
DeWytt, C	94
Dexamethasone	115
Diabetic pseudo-tabes	14
Dinner, annual	155
Diptheritic paralysis	14
Directory of Neurology in Australia	148
Disseminated sclerosis	11, 19, 47
Donnan, G	92, 101, 113
Drug Advice Committee	154
Dunne, J	97

E

E Graeme Robertson Book Collection	141
E Graeme Robertson Memorial Lecture	143
Eadie, M J	28, 53, 94, 101, 107, 109, 110, 112, 115, 116, 128, 132, 145-147
Ebeling, P	92, 113
Eccles, Sir J	115, 117
Eclampsia	7, 24
Edis, R	97
Education and Research Foundation	152

Edwards, V	94, 95
Electroencephalography	95, 96, 119, 153
Electromyography	113
Ellery, R	9, 35
Elliott Smith, Sir G	16, 51
Encephalitides	33, 41
Encephalitis	9, 11, 19, 27-31, 33, 39, 50, 63, 70, 104, 110, 111, 119
Encephalitis lethargica	11, 19, 27, 28, 33, 39, 110
Encephalography	63
Encephalomyelitis	29, 41, 63, 70
Ephedrine	14, 19
Epidemiology of multiple sclerosis	111
Epilepsy	2, 7, 8, 31-33, 35, 37, 41, 50, 63, 68, 78, 92, 107-109, 125, 153, 154
Epilepsy Society of Australia	108, 153
Epileptogenesis	7, 32, 108
Epiloia	14
Ergotamine	6, 115
Ewan, G	35

F

Fagan, E	90
Financial Matters	85, 138
Fine, R	51, 73, 90, 127
Finger-cherry blindness	35
Fisher, A	83, 96, 97, 122
Fitzsimons, R	114
Flashman, J F	11, 35, 39-41, 53, 118
Flinders University	95, 101, 109, 110
Fore people	103
Fremantle Hospital	69, 97, 122
Friedreich's ataxia	41, 50
Frith, J	11, 12, 111
Frontal lobe lesions	61
Fry, H V	35, 95
Fulton, J F	43, 49, 51

G

Gadjusek, C	103
Galvanised iron tanks	24, 25
Game, J A	56, 59, 60, 73, 74, 77, 79, 80, 84, 91, 92, 99, 101, 102, 132, 135, 138, 151, 152
Gandevia, S	117
General Advisory Committee	154
General Business Meeting	81
General paresis of the insane	9, 46, 47

Gibson, J L	14, 23-25	Hopkins, W	14
Gillies, D	90	Hornabrook, R	105
Gilligan, B S	73, 92, 135	Horne, M	93, 101
Glial biology	41	Hornsby Hospital	90, 126
Glioma	59, 118	Hunter, J I	16-21, 36, 41, 90, 102, 118
Goadsby, P	106, 107	Hurst, E W	12, 33
Goondiwindi	29	Hydatid cyst	10
Gordon, J V	83, 95, 124, 132	5-Hydroxyindoleacetic acid	106, 107
Goulston, D	34	Hyponatraemia	26
Gowers, Sir W	3, 32	Hysterical fever	50
Grainger, K	97		
Grant, J	110		

I

Infantile paralysis	29
Influenza pandemic	28
insanity	40, 45, 46
Insigne	141, 144, 155
Insular sclerosis	11
Intercolonial Medical Congress	23
Intercolonial Medical Journal of Australasia	4
Intercolonial Quarterly Journal of Medicine and Surgery	4
International EEG Society	154
Intracranial tumours	59

Grattan-Smith, P	90
Gubbay, S	97
Guillain-Barré syndrome	14, 66, 114

H

Haematomyelia	41
Haemorrhagic encephalomyelitis	41
Hallpike, J	95
Halmagyi, M	91, 118
Hamilton, D	9, 34, 90
Hammond, S	111
Hammond, W	3
Hankey, G	97, 113
Harboard, M	96
Hare, F	31, 32
Harper, C	119
Head, Sir H	47
Head injury	36, 60, 68
Headache	6, 24, 31, 32, 104-107, 117, 118, 153
Heidelberg Repatriation Hospital	73
Helme, R	101
Hemiplegia	2
Hereditary neuropathies	114
Herkes, G	91
Herpes zoster	47
Herzberg, L	97
Hicks, E P	96
Hinterberger, H	106
Holland, J T	91
Honorary Assistant Secretary	132, 138
Honorary Member Emeritus	58, 68, 69, 124, 127, 132, 134
Honorary Membership	72, 83
Honorary Secretary	73, 79, 132, 133, 135, 138
Hooper, R	60
Hopkins, I	93

J

J B Murphy Lecture	18
Jackson, J H	7, 32, 44, 50, 141, 158
Jamieson, K	93
Jayasinghe, G	95
John Hunter Hospital	91
Journal of Clinical Neuroscience	138, 139, 147, 148, 155

K

Kakulas, B	114, 119
Kaye, A	147
Kenny, G	20-22
Kilpatrick, C	92, 115
King, J	92, 135
Kneebone, C	95
Knezevic, W	97
Kuru	103-105, 119

L

Labyrinth	49
Lance, JW	60, 90, 100, 105-107, 117, 118, 132, 135
Lander, C M	94, 146

Landy, P J	93, 94, 111	Merory, J	92, 93
Latham, O	11, 12, 16-18, 28, 29, 33, 35, 40-42, 53, 68, 83, 112, 118, 119	Migraine	2, 6, 31, 32, 50, 90, 106, 107, 115, 127
Launceston	97	Miller, Sir D	10, 89, 123
Layton, W	111	Miller, H	152
Lead poisoning	23-26	Millingen, K	97, 124, 125
Leber's optic atrophy	114	Monash Medical Centre	93, 101
Leicester, J	91	Monash University	93
Leprosy	12, 13	Morgan, F	76
Lethlean, K	90	Morley, J B	92, 95
Lewisham Hospital	36, 90	Morris, J	88, 91, 101, 110, 135, 148
Localisation of cerebral function	48	Moss, G	55, 69, 77, 79, 81, 96, 122, 132
Localisation of function	7, 38, 48, 49	Movement disorder group	153
Lorente de Nó	51	Multiple sclerosis	11, 12, 33, 40, 41, 110, 111, 124, 125, 128
Lorenz, I	91	Murphy, Sir E	93
Luke, H	80	Murray Valley encephalitis	31, 63, 119
Lumbar puncture	8, 14, 24, 119	Myasthenia gravis	14, 34, 36, 114, 123
		Myelography	15
M		Myopathy	14
Macewen, Sir W	10, 17	Myotonia	14, 34, 50, 117
Machado-Joseph disease	112	Myotonia congenita	14, 50
Mackiewicz, J	118		
Maclaughlin, D	94	**N**	
MacLennan and Petty	146	National Gallery of Victoria	58, 59
Mann, P	94	National Health and Medical Research Council	76, 146, 147
Manson, J	96		
Marie's cerebellar ataxia	14	National Hospital for Nervous Diseases	3, 38, 44, 73, 76, 107, 141, 158, 160
Mastaglia, F	97, 101, 114		
Masters, C	119	Necktie	155
Maudsley, H	12, 35, 39, 62	Neostigmine	14, 34, 35
Maxwell, I	95	Nephritis	24
McCombe, P	94, 114	Neuralgia	6, 14, 49, 60
McLeod, J G	91, 100, 101, 111, 113, 117, 135	Neuroanatomy	51, 118
		Neurological rehabilitation	153
Measles	33	Neurological training	52, 55, 56, 77, 78, 81, 83, 92, 93, 95, 100, 119-121, 124, 133, 151, 154
Medical Journal of Australia	4, 5, 13, 17-19, 24-28, 34, 36, 39, 42, 43, 45, 48, 50, 60, 66, 78		
		Neurology in Australia	4, 35, 52, 56, 118, 127, 143, 148, 150, 152, 158-160
Melbourne Children's Hospital	24		
Melbourne Hospital	8, 38, 39, 55, 60, 62-64, 91-93, 101, 113	Neuropathology	41, 42, 50, 53, 55, 57, 60, 63, 118, 119
Mellick, R	90	Neuropharmacology	92, 101, 109, 114, 115
Membership growth	134	Neurophysiology	18, 117, 125
Meningioma	10	Neurosis	50
Meningitis	6, 9, 78	Neurosurgical Society of Australasia	78, 142, 147, 155
Meningococcal infection	70		
Meralgia paraesthetica	14, 37	Neurosyphilis	6, 9, 15, 66
Mercury	9, 27, 37		

Neurotoxicology	115	Pneumoencephalography	15, 52, 60, 63
Neuro-ophthalmology group	153	Pockley, F A	23
New South Wales	10, 13, 17, 18, 22, 27-31, 36, 40, 43, 67, 84, 89-91, 93, 94, 98, 100, 101, 106, 107, 153	Poliomyelitis	6, 9, 19, 21, 22, 29, 30, 50, 63, 111
		Pollard, J	91, 101, 114
New Zealand	39, 78, 105, 128, 134, 155	Polyarteritis nodosa	73
Nicholson, G	114	Polyneuritis	14, 116
Noad, Sir K	41, 52, 55, 66-68, 77-79, 84, 89, 132	Positron emission tomography	108
		Post-encephalitic Parkinsonism	19, 28
Northcott Neurological Centre	66, 91, 99, 106	President	22, 39, 48, 57, 59, 62, 68, 73, 74, 79, 84, 85, 122, 127, 132, 133, 135, 138, 141, 143, 146, 148, 151

O

Ohlrich, G	94	President-elect	133
Oligodendrogliomas	61	Preswick, G	90
Olivo-ponto-cerebellar atrophy	14, 41, 112	Prince Henry Hospital	90, 92
Optic neuritis	23, 111	Prince of Wales Children's Hospital	90
Ordinary Members	80, 81, 83-85, 133, 134, 139, 148	Princess Alexandra Hospital	94
		Princess Margaret Hospital	97
Originating Members	66, 68, 69, 71, 75, 77-79, 81, 134	Proceedings of the Australian Association of Neurologists	62, 139, 143, 148, 149
Ouvrier, R	90, 114	Procopis, P	90
Overseas Membership	133	Provisional Membership	80-83, 88, 127, 134
O'Neill, J	90	Psychosis	50
O'Sullivan, D	90	Purdie, G	96

Q

		Queen Elizabeth Hospital	95

P

Papal Knighthood	76, 129	Queen Square	3, 38, 44, 61, 62, 64, 66, 73, 76, 78, 85, 92, 95, 97, 99, 105, 107, 118-120, 123-125, 128, 141, 151
Papilloedema	23, 24		
Paralysis	2, 12, 14, 17, 23, 29, 30, 34		
Paramyoclonus multiplex	14		
Parkinsonism	10, 11, 19, 28, 104, 110, 125	Queen Victoria Hospital	92, 95
		Queensland Branch of the British Medical Association	24, 25
Parkinson's disease	10, 11, 110		
Paroxysmal neuroses	31		
Pelekanos, J	94		
Pender, M P	94, 111, 146	**R**	
Penfold, W	26	Rabies	10
Penicillin	9	Radiology	14, 56, 122
Peripheral nerve diseases	37	Rail, L R	83, 84, 90, 105
Peripheral nerve disorder	56, 114	Rainhill Asylum	45
Pernicious anaemia	38, 47	Reid, W L	11, 32
Personal chair	97, 100-102	Reimers, J	95
Phenobarbitone	8	Rennie, G	9, 14, 32, 33, 35-39, 107, 159
Phenytoin	8, 109, 115	Repatriation Hospital, Greenslopes	94
Phillips, G	10, 15, 19	Retinitis pigmentosa	19
Photogenic epilepsy	63	Retired Member	133
Pineal	47	Reye, D	105
Pink disease	25-27	Reye's syndrome	105

Index

Rice, J P 95, 135
Rischbeith, R 95, 96, 124
Robertson, E G 8, 10, 31, 33, 55, 56, 60-64, 76-80, 84, 91, 92, 97, 104, 123, 132, 135, 141, 143-145, 159
Romberg, M 158
Royal Alexandra Hospital for Children 24, 45, 66, 105
Royal Australasian College of Physicians 33, 36, 38, 39, 57, 62, 66-69, 72, 73, 76, 78, 84, 85, 90, 119, 120, 122-125, 128, 138, 142, 150-152, 154
Royal Australasian College of Surgeons 72
Royal Australian and New Zealand College of Psychiatrists 39
Royal Brisbane Hospital 93-95, 128
Royal Canberra Hospital 98
Royal Children's Hospital, Brisbane 94
Royal Children's Hospital, Melbourne 93
Royal College of Physician of London 36, 39, 40, 57, 61, 62, 66-69, 76, 120, 122-124, 126, 128
Royal College of Physicians of Edinburgh 57, 128
Royal Commission 22
Royal Hobart Hospital 97, 125
Royal Melbourne Hospital 55, 64, 91-93, 101, 113
Royal Newcastle Hospital 91, 123
Royal North Shore Hospital 89-91, 110, 126, 127
Royal Perth Hospital 55, 69, 96, 97, 122
Royal Prince Alfred Hospital 28, 36, 55, 66, 89-91, 101, 116, 118, 123, 125
Royal Society 48, 50, 85, 115
Royle, N D 5, 16-20, 102

S

Sadka, M 69, 96, 97, 122
Saines, N 94
Salpêtrière 3, 158
Sandstrom, P 94
Sarnat, H 97
Schapel, G 95
Schüller, A 56
Schwieger, A 57, 58, 83, 91, 92

Scientific and educational activities 77, 142
Scopa, J 97
Second Asian and Oceanian Congress of Neurology 62, 142
Secretariat 138
Selby, G 65, 66, 83, 84, 89-91, 106, 110, 116, 119, 124-127, 132, 135, 146
Sewell, Sir S 12, 35, 38, 39, 60, 62
Sherrington, Sir C 47, 48, 50, 53
Shield, L 93
Siejka, S 97
Silberstein, P 97
Silburn, P 94
Sippe, C 32, 35
Sir Charles Gairdner Hospital 96, 97
Sister Kenny 21, 22
Smith, G E, see Elliott Smith
Smith, S A 25
Somerville, B 107
South Australia 13, 33, 95, 96, 124
Southby, R 26
Spasticity 15-20, 22, 102, 117
Spheno-palatine neuralgia 60
Spinal cord transection 37
Spinal heterotopias 47
Spino-cerebellar degenerations 111, 112
Springthorpe, J W 7
St Vincent's Hospital 38, 56
St. George's Hospital 107
Staples, C 94
Stark, R 92
Stawell, Sir R 11, 14, 28
Stell, R 97
Stewart Lectureship 57, 99
Stewart-Wynne, E 97, 113
Stroke 2, 6, 8, 92, 112, 113, 115, 153
Stroke Society 153
Subacute combined degeneration 14
Subacute myelo-optic neuropathy 116, 127
Sulphonamides 9
Sunderland, Sir S 56, 57, 59, 71-73, 77, 79-81, 98, 100, 118
Susman, E L 9, 55, 65, 66, 68, 77-80, 84, 89, 90, 125
Sutherland, J M 93-95, 100, 101, 109-112, 120, 128, 132
Sydney Hospital 28, 55, 59, 67, 68, 81, 83, 84, 89-92, 100, 101, 124

Symington, G	92	**V**	
Symonds, Sir C	83	Vacuolation of the nerve cell	46
Sympathectomy	17, 18, 21	Vajda, F	92, 101, 109, 115
Syphilis	9, 40, 47, 50	Van Cleef Foundation	148
Syringomyelia	50	Varicella	33
		Ventriculography	15, 52
T		Victoria	9, 11, 13, 14, 28, 31, 39, 45, 53, 58, 59, 91-97, 109
Tabes dorsalis	9, 48	Video-EEG monitoring,	108
Tait, W H	109	Voluntary movement	37
Tasmania	11, 13, 28, 62, 97, 109, 125		
Teething powders	27	**W**	
Terenty, T	91	Waddy, H	96
Thallium	116	Walsh, J	91, 114
Thompson, P	12, 96	Walsh,	97
Tick-bite paralysis	12, 34	Waratah	141, 144
Tissot, S	158	Wasserman reaction	40, 41
Tolhurst, J	9, 60	Western Australia	96, 97, 122
Townsville	24, 27, 29, 30, 95	Westmead Hospital	91, 101, 110
Toxoplasma encephalomyelitis	63	White, J	63, 141
Trahair, G	15, 90	Widal test	41
Training of Australian neurologists	150	Wilkinson, H J	20, 21, 28, 33, 118
Transfer factor	111	Williams and Wilkins-Adis	146
Trepanning	8	Williamson, P	91, 127
Trigeminal neuralgia	6, 49	Willis, T	3, 9, 31, 49, 141, 158
Trumble, H	55, 57, 60, 72	Willoughby, J	96, 101, 109
Tsutsugamushi fever	68	Wise, G	90
Tuck, R	98, 114	Woden Valley Hospital	98
Turner, A J	24, 25	Wolfenden, W	91
Turner, B	119	Wolff, H G	32
Tyrer. J H	2, 83, 93, 100, 101, 107, 112, 115, 120, 128, 141, 145, 146	Wood Jones, F	72
		Word blindness	14
		World Federation for Neurology	154
U		**X**	
Uncinate epilepsy	68	X disease	33, 50, 110
University of Adelaide	30, 34, 35, 50, 73, 84, 99, 101, 122, 124	**Y**	
University of Melbourne	38, 39, 43, 56, 57, 60, 72, 73, 76, 80, 83, 84, 92, 99	Yeo, P T	97
		Youngman, N V	7, 8, 15, 93, 107
University of New South Wales	90, 98, 100, 101, 106, 107, 153	**Z**	
University of Tasmania	125	Zagami, A	107
University of Western Australia	97	Zigas, V	103, 104